AMERICAN

PSYCHIATRIC

ASSOCIATION

PRACTICE

GUIDELINES

AMERICAN
PSYCHIATRIC
ASSOCIATION

PRACTICE
GUIDELINES

American Psychiatric Association

Published by the
American Psychiatric Association
Washington, DC

Note: The authors have worked to ensure that all information in this book concerning drug dosages, schedules, and routes of administration is accurate as of the time of publication and consistent with standards set by the U.S. Food and Drug Administration and the general medical community. As medical research and practice advance, however, therapeutic standards may change. For this reason and because human and mechanical errors sometimes occur, we recommend that readers follow the advice of a physician who is directly involved in their care or the care of a member of their family.

Copyright © 1996 American Psychiatric Association
ALL RIGHTS RESERVED
Manufactured in the United States of America on acid-free paper
First Edition
99 98 97 96   4 3 2 1

American Psychiatric Association
1400 K Street, N.W., Washington, DC   20005

ISSN 1067-8743
Hardback ISBN 0-89042-305-9
Paperback ISBN 0-89042-306-7

AMERICAN PSYCHIATRIC ASSOCIATION

STEERING COMMITTEE ON PRACTICE GUIDELINES

JOHN S. McINTYRE, M.D.
Chair

SARA C. CHARLES, M.D.
Vice-Chair

DEBORAH A. ZARIN, M.D.
Director, Practice Guideline Program

HAROLD ALAN PINCUS, M.D.
Director, Office of Research

Kenneth Z. Altshuler, M.D.
William H. Ayres, M.D.
Paula J. Clayton, M.D.
Ian Cook, M.D.
Leah Dickstein, M.D.
Gerald H. Flamm, M.D.

Steven L. Jaffe, M.D.
Justine M. Kent, M.D.
Sheldon Miller, M.D.
Louis Alan Moench, M.D.
Roger Peele, M.D.
Joel Yager, M.D.

Consultants and Liaisons

Richard Kent Harding, M.D.
  (Consultant)
Grayson Norquist, M.D.
  (Consultant)
Thomas Bittker, M.D. *(Liaison)*

Marcia Goin, M.D. *(Liaison)*
Maria Lymberis, M.D.
  (Liaison)
John Oldham, M.D. *(Liaison)*
Bruce Phariss, M.D. *(Liaison)*

Leslie Seigle
Project Manager

Contents

Statement of Intent

These guidelines are not intended to be construed or to serve as standards of care. Standards of care are determined on the basis of all clinical data available for an individual case and are subject to change as scientific knowledge and technology advance and patterns evolve. These parameters of practice should be considered guidelines only. Adherence to them will not ensure a successful outcome in every case, nor should they be construed as including all proper methods of care or excluding other acceptable methods of care aimed at the same results. The ultimate judgment regarding a particular clinical procedure or treatment course must be made by the psychiatrist in light of the clinical data presented by the patient and the diagnostic and treatment options available.

These practice guidelines have been developed by psychiatrists who are in active clinical practice. In addition, some contributors are primarily involved in research or other academic endeavors. It is possible that through such activities many contributors have received income related to treatments discussed in this guideline. A number of mechanisms are in place to minimize the potential for producing biased recommendations due to conflicts of interest. The guidelines have been extensively reviewed by members of APA as well as by representatives from related fields. Contributors and reviewers have all been asked to base their recommendations on an objective evaluation of the available evidence. Any contributor or reviewer who believes that he or she has a conflict of interest that may bias (or appear to bias) his or her work has been asked to notify the APA Office of Research. This potential bias is then discussed with the work group chair and the chair of the Steering Committee on Practice Guidelines. Further action depends on the assessment of the potential bias.

Introduction

Deborah A. Zarin, M.D.
John S. McIntyre, M.D.
Harold Alan Pincus, M.D.

This volume contains the first five practice guidelines to be developed by the American Psychiatric Association (APA). Each of these Guidelines has been published in the *American Journal of Psychiatry* and also as an individual monograph through American Psychiatric Press, Inc.

The term *practice guideline* refers to a set of patient care strategies developed to assist physicians in clinical decision making. The APA is continually developing new and revised guidelines, which will be published as they are completed.

Readers should note that guidelines are not intended to be "standards of care." The Statement of Intent (p. ix) clarifies the intended role of guidelines.

Although the APA has published specific recommendations about the practice of psychiatry since 1851, the current commitment of resources to the practice guideline development process represents a qualitative change in the APA's role in establishing guidelines. Such a change raises many questions.

Why Is the APA Developing Practice Guidelines?

For nearly 150 years, the APA's fundamental aim in developing practice guidelines has been to assist psychiatrists in their clinical decision making, with the ultimate goal of improving the care of patients. The explosion of knowledge in our field over the last several decades amplifies the value of these guidelines. Furthermore, the current health care climate is characterized by rising concerns about quality of care, access to care, and cost. Efforts to respond to these problems by exerting external control over the types and amount of care that can be provided have led to new concerns about the quality of the data on which such efforts are based and the process by which the data are used to determine "appropriate" or "reimbursable" care. The realization that both treatment and reimbursement decisions are occurring, without systematic scientific and clinical input, has led the APA, along with many other medical specialty societies, to accelerate the process of documenting clearly and concisely what is known and what is not known about the treatment of patients. Although there are a number of other groups, including the federal government (through the Agency for Health Care Policy and Research), that are also developing practice guidelines, the APA has decided that the psychiatric profession should take the lead in describing the best treatments and the range of appropriate treatments available to patients with mental illnesses.

How Are Practice Guidelines Developed?

The APA guidelines are developed under the direction of the Steering Committee on Practice Guidelines. The process is designed to ensure the development of reliable and valid guidelines and is consistent with the recommendations of the American Medical Association and the Institute of Medicine. It is characterized by rigorous scientific review of the available literature, widespread review of iterative drafts, and ultimate approval by the APA Assembly and Board of Trustees. Each guideline undergoes minor revisions and updates every 3–5 years, with major revisions approximately every 10 years. The development process is fully described in the Appendix (p. 321).

What Are the Potential Benefits of This Project?

Ultimately, the aim of practice guidelines is to improve patient care. Although some have argued that no guidelines should be promulgated until "all the data are in," this is not possible given the pressure of clinical and administrative decisions. Guidelines should help practicing psychiatrists determine what is known today about how best to help their patients. In addition, psychiatrists and those charged with the allocation of health care resources must try to make the best possible decisions on the basis of currently available data. Well-developed guidelines can help in these efforts.

Toward the end of helping patients, guidelines can have other beneficial effects. They are a vehicle for educating psychiatrists, other medical and mental health professionals, and the general public about appropriate and inappropriate treatments. By demonstrating that the quality of evidence for psychiatric treatments is on par with (and in many cases exceeds) that for other medical care, guidelines contribute to the credibility of the field. Guidelines identify those areas in which critical information is lacking and in which research could be expected to improve clinical decisions. Finally, guidelines can help those charged with overseeing the utilization and reimbursement of psychiatric services to develop more scientifically based and clinically sensitive criteria.

What Are the Possible Risks?

The APA reasons that the risks of this project are small and are considerably outweighed by the benefits. One risk is that the guidelines can be misinterpreted and misused by third parties in a way that will ultimately harm patients. Although this risk rightfully concerns many psychiatrists, it is the judgment of the steering committee, the Assembly, and the Board of Trustees that the existence of guidelines helps to clarify the sources of disagreement between treating psychiatrists and reviewers and their use can be a great improvement over the use of "secret" criteria or criteria developed through less objective procedures. In addition, many have expressed the concern that guidelines can "homogenize" the care of patients and detract from psychiatrists' freedom to shape treatment in ways that they feel best suit their individual patients. Inevitably, there is a tension in writing guidelines between the desire for specificity and the desire to allow for the consideration of individual clinical circumstances. These concerns must be balanced in such a way that allows psychiatrists to make appropriate clinical decisions. This very important issue is addressed in the Statement of Intent that begins each guideline. Finally, there are concerns that the APA-approved guidelines may lead to an increase in malpractice claims. At this time, legal experts have mixed opinions about the impact of guidelines on the volume and severity of malpractice suits. However, in fact, some medical specialties that have been developing guidelines over the past decade report that guidelines seem to have had the positive effect of fewer claims and, for at least one specialty, lower malpractice insurance premiums.

How Can We Improve the Current Process?

Since the inception of the APA project in 1989, the guideline development process has evolved significantly. Specifically, the activities of the work groups developing the guidelines have been made more explicit, and the nature of the reviewers' input has been standardized. However, certain principles remain crucial to further improvement. Clearly, guidelines should be based on objective data whenever possible. Systematic reviews of the literature are an essential part of this work. However, efforts to synthesize studies in any given area are hampered by the uneven quantity and quality of research, by problems in generalizing from a literature largely derived from tertiary care research settings to more typical clinical practice, by the inherent difficulty in conducting controlled studies of some treatments for some populations, and by the difficulty in characterizing "clinical consensus." These issues will be partially addressed through the use of the APA's newly formed Practice Research Network (PRN). The PRN will ultimately involve a panel of 1,000 psychiatrists in the full range of practice settings, who will cooperate to gather data and conduct clinical research. Practice research networks have been used in other areas of medicine (e.g., family practice and pediatrics) to gather data from practice settings of relevance to the development of guidelines. For example, data about prevailing practice patterns and patient outcomes could be systematically gathered and incorporated into the guidelines. In addition, the impact of guidelines on psychiatric practice and patient outcomes could be assessed (e.g., by testing different education or dissemination strategies); ultimately, it should be possible to determine whether guidelines improve patient care.

Guidelines Being Developed

Guidelines on the following topics are currently in development:

- ❖ Schizophrenia
- ❖ Nicotine dependence
- ❖ Panic disorder and related anxiety disorders
- ❖ Alzheimer's and related dementias
- ❖ Delirium
- ❖ Geriatrics
- ❖ Mental retardation

Completed guidelines are revised at 3- to 5-year intervals.

Conclusions

The Practice Guidelines in this volume represent an important step toward the development of an "evidence-based psychiatry." The development of better research tools, the accumulation of new research data, and the iterative improvement of the process for developing guidelines will contribute to the continual development of better guidelines to aid psychiatrists in their clinical decision making.

PRACTICE GUIDELINE
FOR
PSYCHIATRIC
EVALUATION OF
ADULTS

WORK GROUP ON
PSYCHIATRIC EVALUATION OF ADULTS

Barry S. Fogel, M.D., Co-Chair
Ronald Shellow, M.D., Co-Chair

Renee Binder, M.D.
Jack Bonner III, M.D.
Leah Dickstein, M.D.
Gerald H. Flamm, M.D.
Marc Galanter, M.D.
Anthony Lehman, M.D.
Francis Lu, M.D.
Michael Popkin, M.D.
George Wilson, M.D.

Contents

Psychiatric Evaluation of Adults

Summary

The following summary is intended to provide an overview of the organization and scope of recommendations in this practice guideline. The psychiatric evaluation of patients requires the consideration of many factors and cannot adequately be reviewed in a brief summary. The reader is encouraged to consult the relevant portions of the guideline when specific recommendations are sought. This summary is not intended to stand by itself.

This guideline focuses on the purpose, site, domains, and process of clinical psychiatric evaluations. General psychiatric evaluations, emergency evaluations, and clinical consultations, conducted in inpatient, outpatient, and other settings, are discussed. The domains of these evaluations include the reason for the evaluation, history of the present illness, past psychiatric history, general medical history, psychosocial/developmental history (personal history), social history, occupational history, family history, review of systems, physical examination, mental status examination, functional assessment, diagnostic tests, and information derived from the interview process.

Processes by which information is obtained and integrated to address the aims of the evaluation are described. Methods of obtaining information discussed include the patient interview; use of collateral sources; use of structured interviews, questionnaires, and rating scales; use of diagnostic, including psychological and neuropsychological, tests; use of the multidisciplinary team; examination under medication and/or restraint; and the physical examination. The process of assessment includes diagnosis and case formulation, formulation of the initial treatment plan, decisions regarding treatment-related legal and administrative issues, addressing of systems issues, and consideration for sociocultural diversity.

Other special considerations discussed include interactions with third-party payers, privacy and confidentiality, legal and administrative issues in institutions, and evaluation of elderly persons.

Introduction

Psychiatric evaluations vary according to their purpose. This guideline is intended primarily for general, emergency, and consultation evaluations for clinical purposes. It is applicable to evaluations conducted by a psychiatrist with adult patients, age 18 or older, although sections may be applicable to younger patients. Other psychiatric evaluations (including forensic, child custody, and disability evaluations) are not the focus of this guideline.

The guideline presumes familiarity with basic principles of psychiatric diagnosis and treatment planning as outlined in standard, contemporary psychiatric textbooks and taught in psychiatry residency training programs. It was developed following a review of contemporary references and emphasizes areas of consensus in the field.

While there is broad agreement that each element of the extensive general evaluation described in the guideline may be relevant or even crucial in a particular case, the specific emphasis of a given evaluation will vary according to its purpose and the problem presented by the patient. Consideration of the domains outlined in this guideline is part of a general psychiatric evaluation, but the content, process, and documentation must be determined by applying the professional skill and judgment of the psychiatrist. The performance of a particular set of clinical procedures does not assure the adequacy of a psychiatric evaluation, nor does their omission imply that the evaluation is deficient. The particular emphasis or modifications applied by the psychiatrist to the generic evaluation offered in this guideline should be consonant with the aims of the evaluation, the setting of practice, the patient's presenting problem, and the ever-evolving knowledge base concerning clinical assessment and clinical inference. It is important to emphasize that the scope and detail of clinically appropriate documentation also will vary with the patient, setting, clinical situation, and confidentiality issues. Because of the great variation in these factors, this guideline does not include recommendations regarding the content or frequency of documentation. These determinations must be based on the specific circumstances of the evaluation.

I. Purpose of Evaluation

The purpose and conduct of a psychiatric evaluation depend on who requests the evaluation, why it is requested, and the expected future role of the psychiatrist in the patient's care. Three types of clinical psychiatric evaluations are discussed: 1) general psychiatric evaluation, 2) emergency evaluation, and 3) clinical consultation. In addition, general principles to guide the conduct of evaluations for administrative or legal purposes are reviewed. At times there may be a conflict between the need to establish an effective working relationship with the patient and the need to efficiently obtain comprehensive information. To the extent that the psychiatrist expects to directly provide care to the patient, the establishment of an effective working relationship with the patient may take precedence over the comprehensiveness of the initial interview or interviews. In these instances, emphasis is placed on obtaining information needed for immediate clinical recommendations and decisions (1).

A. General Psychiatric Evaluation

A general psychiatric evaluation has as its central component a face-to-face interview with the patient. The interview-based data are integrated with data that may be obtained through other components of the evaluation, such as a review of medical records, a physical examination, diagnostic tests, and history from collateral sources. A general evaluation usually takes more than 1 hour to complete, depending on the complexity of the problem and the patient's ability and willingness to work cooperatively with the psychiatrist. Several meetings with the patient may be necessary. Evaluations of lesser scope may be appropriate when the psychiatrist is called on to address a specific, limited diagnostic or therapeutic issue.

The aims of a general psychiatric evaluation are 1) to establish a psychiatric diagnosis, 2) to collect data sufficient to permit a case formulation, and 3) to develop an initial treatment plan, with particular consideration of any immediate interventions that may be needed to ensure the patient's safety, or, if the evaluation is a reassessment of a patient in long-term treatment, to revise the plan of treatment in accord with new perspectives gained from the evaluation.

B. Emergency Evaluation

The emergency psychiatric evaluation occurs in response to the occurrence of thoughts or feelings that are intolerable to the patient, or behavior that prompts urgent action by others, such as violent or self-injurious behavior, threats of harm to self or others, failure to care for oneself, deterioration of mental status, bizarre or confused behavior, or intense expressions of distress (2). The aims of the emergency evaluation include the following:

1. To establish a provisional diagnosis of the mental disorder most likely to be responsible for the current emergency, and to identify other diagnostic possibilities requiring further evaluation in the near term, including general medical conditions to be further assessed as potential causes of or contributors to the patient's mental condition.
2. To identify social, environmental, and cultural factors relevant to immediate treatment decisions.
3. To determine the patient's ability and willingness to cooperate with further assessment and treatment, what precautions are needed if there is a substantial risk of harm to self or others, and whether involuntary treatment is necessary.
4. To develop a plan for immediate treatment and disposition, with determination of whether the patient requires treatment in a hospital or other supervised setting and what follow-up will be required if the patient is not hospitalized.

The emergency evaluation varies greatly in length and may on occasion exceed several hours. Patients who will be discharged to the community after emergency evaluation may require more extensive evaluation in the emergency setting than those who will be hospitalized.

Patients presenting for emergency psychiatric evaluation have a high prevalence of combined general medical and psychiatric illness, recent trauma, substance use and substance-related conditions, and cognitive impairment disorders. These diagnostic possibilities deserve careful consideration. General medical and psychiatric evaluations should be coordinated so that additional medical evaluation can be requested or initiated by the psychiatrist on the basis of diagnostic or therapeutic considerations arising from the psychiatric history and interview. In many emergency settings, patients initially are examined by a nonpsychiatric physician to exclude acute general medical problems. Such examinations usually are limited in scope and rarely are definitive. Therefore, the psychiatrist may need to request or initiate further general medical evaluation to address diagnostic concerns that emerge from the psychiatric evaluation (3, 4).

C. Clinical Consultation

Clinical consultations are evaluations requested by other physicians or health care professionals, patients, families, or others for the purpose of assisting in the diagnosis, treatment, or management of a patient with a suspected mental disorder or behavioral problem. These evaluations may be comprehensive or may be focused on a relatively narrow question, such as the preferred medication for treatment of a known mental disorder in a patient with a particular general medical condition. Psychiatric evaluations for consultative purposes use the same data sources as general evaluations. Consideration is given to information from the referring source on the specific problem leading to the consultation, the referring source's aims for the consultation, information that the psychiatrist may be able to obtain regarding the patient's relationship with the primary clinician, and the resources and constraints of those currently treating the patient. Also, in the case of a consultation regarding a mental or behavioral problem in a patient with a general medical illness, information about that illness, its treatment, and its prognosis is relevant. The patient should be informed that the purpose of the consultation is to advise the party who requested it.

The aim of the consultative psychiatric evaluation is to provide clear and specific answers to the questions posed by the party requesting the consultation (5, 6). These include 1) a psychiatric diagnosis when relevant to the question posed to the consultant; 2) treatment advice, when requested, at a level of specificity appropriate to the needs of the treating clinician; and 3) recommendation for a change in treatment (e.g., in site of treatment) when the consultant finds a major diagnostic or therapeutic issue not raised by the requester but of concern to the patient or of likely relevance to treatment outcome.

The evaluation should respect the patient's relationship with the primary clinician and should encourage positive resolution of conflicts between the patient and the primary clinician if these emerge as an issue.

D. Other Consultations

Other psychiatric consultations are directed toward the resolution of specific legal, administrative, or other nonclinical questions. While the details of these evaluations, such as forensic evaluations, child custody evaluations, and disability evaluations, are beyond the scope of this guideline, several general principles apply. First, the evaluee usually is not the psychiatrist's patient and there are limits to confidentiality implicit in the aims of the evaluation; accordingly, the aims of the evaluation and the scope of disclosure should be addressed with the evaluee at the start of the interview (7, 8). Second, questions about the evaluee's legal status and legal representation should be resolved before the assessment begins, if possible. Third, many such consultations rely heavily, or even entirely, on documentary evidence or data from collateral sources. The quality and potential biases of such data should be taken into account.

The aims of these psychiatric consultations are 1) to answer the requester's question to the extent possible with the data obtainable and 2) to make a psychiatric diagnosis if it is relevant to the question.

II.   Site of the Clinical Evaluation

A.   Inpatient Settings

The scope, pace, and depth of inpatient evaluation depend on the patient population served by the inpatient service, the goals of the hospitalization, and the role of the inpatient unit within the overall system of mental health services available to the patient (9). For example, a general hospital psychiatric unit specializing in patients with combined medical and psychiatric illness will necessarily do a relatively rapid general medical evaluation of all admitted patients (10). The evaluation of stable chronic general medical conditions in a long-stay setting for the chronically mentally ill might proceed at a slower pace than in a psychiatric-medical specialty unit in a general hospital.

When a patient is admitted by someone other than the treating psychiatrist, the reason for continued hospitalization should be promptly reviewed. The necessity for hospitalization should be carefully assessed, and alternative treatment settings should be considered.

From the outset, inpatient evaluations should include consideration of discharge planning (9). If the posthospitalization disposition is not apparent, the evaluation should identify both patient factors and community resources that would be relevant to a viable dispositional plan and should identify the problems that could impede a suitable disposition. If the patient was referred to the hospital by another clinician, the inpatient evaluation should be viewed in part as a consultation to the referring source (9). Special attention is given to unresolved diagnostic issues requiring data collection in an inpatient setting.

B.   Outpatient Settings

Evaluation in the outpatient setting usually differs in intensity from inpatient evaluation, because of less frequent interviews, less involvement of other professionals, and less immediate availability of laboratory services and consultants from other medical specialties. Also, the psychiatrist in the outpatient setting has substantially less opportunity to directly observe the patient's behavior and to implement protective interventions when necessary. For this reason, during the period of evaluation the outpatient evaluator should continually reassess whether the patient requires hospitalization and whether unresolved questions about the patient's general medical status require more rapid assessment. A decision to change the setting for continued evaluation should be based on the patient's current mental status and behavior.

Advantages of the outpatient setting include economy, greater patient autonomy, and the potential for a longer longitudinal perspective on the patient's symptoms. However, the lack of continuous direct observation of behavior limits the obtainable data on how the patient's behavior appears to others. The involvement of family or significant others as collateral sources in the evaluation process deserves consideration. When substance use is suspected, data from collateral observers, drug screens, and/or determination of blood alcohol levels may be especially important.

C.   General Medical Settings

Evaluations on general medical (i.e., nonpsychiatric) inpatient units allow for some direct behavioral observation by staff and for some safeguards against self-injurious or other violent behavior by patients. However, the level of behavioral observation and potential intervention against risky behavior tends to be less than on psychiatric inpatient units.

Psychiatric interviews on general medical-surgical units often are compromised by interruptions and lack of privacy. These problems sometimes can be mitigated by careful scheduling of interviews and using a space on the unit where the patient and the psychiatrist can meet privately.

Documentation of psychiatric evaluations in general medical charts should be sensitive to the standards of confidentiality of the nonpsychiatric medical sector and the possibility that charts may be read by persons who are not well informed about psychiatric issues. Information written in general medical charts should be confined to that necessary for the general medical team and should be expressed with a minimum of technical terms.

D.   Other Settings

Evaluations conducted in other settings, such as partial hospital settings, residential treatment facilities, home care services, nursing homes, long-term care facilities, schools, and prisons, are affected by a number of factors: 1) the level of behavioral observations available and the quality of those observations, 2) the availability of privacy for conducting interviews, 3) the availability of general medical evaluations and diagnostic tests, 4) the capacity to conduct the evaluation safely, and 5) the likelihood that information written in facility records will be understood and kept confidential.

In light of these factors, it is necessary to consider whether a particular setting permits an evaluation of adequate speed, safety, accuracy, and confidentiality to meet the needs of the patient.

III. Domains of the Clinical Evaluation

General psychiatric evaluations involve a systematic consideration of the broad domains described in this guideline, and they vary in scope and intensity. The intensity with which each domain is assessed depends on the purpose of the evaluation and the clinical situation. An evaluation of lesser scope may be appropriate when its purpose is to answer a circumscribed question. Such an evaluation may involve a particularly intense assessment of one or more domains especially relevant to the reason for the evaluation.

A. Reason for the Evaluation

The purpose of the evaluation influences the focus of the examination and the form of documentation. The reason for the evaluation usually includes (but may not be limited to) the chief complaint of the patient, elicited in sufficient detail to permit an understanding of the patient's specific goals for the evaluation. If the symptoms are of long standing, the reason for seeking treatment at this specific time is relevant; if the evaluation was occasioned by a hospitalization, the reason for the hospitalization is also relevant.

B. History of the Present Illness

The history of the present illness is a chronologically organized history of current symptoms or syndromes, recent exacerbations or remissions, available details of previous treatments, and the patient's response to those treatments. In consideration of the information obtained, the patient's current mental state may be relevant. If the patient was or is in treatment with another clinician, the effects of that relationship on the current illness, including transference and countertransference issues, are considered. Factors that the patient believes to be precipitating, aggravating, or otherwise modifying the illness are also pertinent.

C. Past Psychiatric History

The past psychiatric history includes a chronological summary of all past episodes of mental illness and treatment, including psychiatric syndromes not formally diagnosed at the time, previously established diagnoses, treatments offered, and responses to treatment. The dose, duration of treatment, efficacy, side effects, and patient's adherence to previously prescribed medications are part of the past psychiatric history. Past medical records frequently contain relevant data.

The chronological summary also includes episodes when the patient was functionally impaired or seriously distressed by mental or behavioral symptoms, even if no formal treatment occurred. Such episodes frequently can be identified by asking the patient about the past use of psychotropic drugs prescribed by a nonpsychiatric physician, prior suicide attempts or other self-destructive behavior, and otherwise unexplained episodes of social or occupational disability.

D.   General Medical History

The general medical history includes available information on known general medical illnesses (e.g., hospitalizations, procedures, treatments, and medications) and undiagnosed health problems that have caused the patient major distress or functional impairment. This includes history of any episodes of important physical injury or trauma; sexual and reproductive history; and any history of neurologic disorders, allergies, drug sensitivities, and conditions causing pain and discomfort. Of particular importance is a specific history regarding diseases, and symptoms of diseases, that have a high prevalence among individuals with the patient's demographic characteristics and background, e.g., infectious diseases in users of intravenous drugs or pulmonary and cardiovascular disease in people who smoke. Information regarding all current and recent medications is part of the general medical history.

E.   History of Substance Use

The psychoactive substance use history includes past and present use of both licit and illicit psychoactive substances, including but not limited to alcohol, caffeine, nicotine, marijuana, cocaine, opiates, sedative-hypnotic agents, stimulants, solvents, and hallucinogens. Relevant information includes the quantity and frequency of use and route of administration; the pattern of use (e.g., episodic versus continual; solitary versus social); functional, interpersonal, or legal consequences of use; tolerance and withdrawal phenomena; any temporal association between substance use and present psychiatric illness; and any self-perceived benefits of use. Obtaining an accurate substance use history often involves a gradual, nonconfrontational approach to inquiry with multiple questions seeking the same information in different ways and/or the use of slang terms for drugs, patterns of use, and drug effects.

F.   Psychosocial/Developmental History (Personal History)

The personal history reviews the stages of the patient's life, with special attention to developmental milestones and to patterns of response to normative life transitions and major life events. The patient's history of formal education and history of important cultural and religious influences on the patient's life are obtained. Any involvement with the juvenile or criminal justice system is noted. A sexual history is obtained, as well as any history of physical, emotional, sexual, or other abuse or trauma (11–13). Any experiences related to political repression, war, or a natural disaster are also relevant.

An assessment of the patient's past and present levels of functioning in family and social roles (e.g., marriage, parenting, work, school) (14–16) includes the following information: number and ages of any children; capacity to meet the needs of dependent children in general and during psychiatric crises, if these are likely to occur; and the overall health, including mental health, of the children, especially when the patient's psychiatric condition is likely to affect the children through genetic or psychosocial mechanisms or to impede the patient's ability to recognize and attend to the needs of a child.

G. Social History

The social history includes the patient's living arrangements and currently important relationships. Emphasis is given to relationships, both familial and nonfamilial, that are relevant to the present illness, act as stressors, or have the potential to serve as resources for the patient. Also included is a history of any formal involvement with social agencies or the courts, as well as details of any current litigation or criminal proceedings.

H. Occupational History

The occupational history describes the sequence of jobs held by the patient, reasons for job changes, and the patient's current or most recent employment, including whether current or recent jobs have involved unusual physical or psychological stress, toxic materials, a noxious environment, or shift work. Relevant data about military experience would include volunteer versus draftee status, whether the patient experienced combat, discharge status, awards, disciplinary actions, and whether the patient suffered injury or trauma while in service.

I. Family History

The family history includes available information about general medical and psychiatric illness in close relatives, including disorders that may be familial or may strongly affect the family environment. This information includes any history of mood disorder, psychosis, suicide, and substance use disorders, as well as any treatment received and response to treatment. Items of current family health status that are of emotional importance to the patient are identified.

J.   Review of Systems

The review of systems includes current symptoms not already identified in the history of the present illness. Also relevant are sleep, appetite, vegetative symptoms of mood disorder, pain and discomfort, systemic symptoms such as fever and fatigue, and neurologic symptoms, if any of these have not already been covered in the history of the present illness. In addition, common symptoms of diseases for which the patient is known to be at particular risk because of historical, genetic, environmental, or demographic factors are a relevant part of the review of systems.

K.   Physical Examination

A physical examination is needed to evaluate the patient's general medical (including neurological) status. The scope and intensity necessary will vary according to clinical circumstances. An understanding of the patient's general medical condition is important in order to 1) properly assess the patient's psychiatric symptoms and their potential cause, 2) determine the patient's need for general medical care, and 3) choose among psychiatric treatments that can be affected by the patient's general medical status (4, 17). The physical examination includes sections concerning the following:

1.   General appearance and nutritional status.
2.   Vital signs.
3.   Head and neck, heart, lungs, abdomen, and extremities.
4.   Neurological status, including cranial nerves, motor and sensory function, gait, coordination, muscle tone, reflexes, and involuntary movements.
5.   Skin, with special attention to any stigmata of trauma, self-injury, or drug use.
6.   Any body area or organ system that is specifically mentioned in the history of the present illness or review of systems or that is relevant to determining the current status of problems mentioned in the past medical history.

Additional items may be added to the examination to address specific diagnostic concerns or to screen a member of a clinical population at risk for a specific disease. For example, a mentally retarded adult might be assessed for recognizable patterns of malformation.

L.   Mental Status Examination

The mental status examination is a systematic collection of data based on observation of the patient's behavior during the interview and before and after the interview while the patient is in the psychiatrist's view. Responses to specific questions are an important part of the mental status examination, particularly in the assessment of cognition (18).

The purpose of the mental status examination is to obtain evidence of current symptoms and signs of mental disorders from which the patient might be suffering. Further, evidence is obtained regarding the patient's insight, judgment, and capacity for abstract reasoning, to inform decisions about treatment strategy and the choice of an appropriate treatment setting. The mental status examination contains the following core elements:

1.   The patient's appearance and general behavior.
2.   The patient's expressions of mood and affect.
3.   Characteristics of the patient's speech and language (e.g., rate, rhythm, structure, flow of ideas, and pathologic features such as tangentiality, vagueness, incoherence, or neologisms).
4.   The patient's rate of movement and the presence of any purposeless, repetitive, or unusual movements or postures.
5.   The patient's current thoughts and perceptions, including the following:

    a.   Spontaneously expressed worries, concerns, thoughts, impulses, and perceptual experiences.
    b.   Cognitive and perceptual symptoms of specific mental disorders, usually elicited by specific questioning and including hallucinations, delusions, ideas of reference, obsessions, and compulsions.
    c.   Suicidal, homicidal, violent, or self-injurious thoughts, feelings, or impulses. If present, details are elicited regarding their intensity and specificity, when they occur, and what prevents the patient from acting them out (19).

6.   Features of the patient's associations, such as loose or idiosyncratic associations and self-contradictory statements.
7.   The patient's understanding of his or her current situation.
8.   Elements of the patient's cognitive status, including the following:

    a.   Level of consciousness.
    b.   Orientation.
    c.   Attention and concentration.
    d.   Language functions (naming, fluency, comprehension, repetition, reading, writing).
    e.   Memory.
    f.   Fund of knowledge (appropriate to sociocultural and educational background).

g. Calculation (appropriate to educational attainment).

h. Drawing (e.g., copying a figure or drawing a clock face).

i. Abstract reasoning (e.g., explaining similarities or interpreting proverbs).

j. Executive (frontal system) functions (e.g., list making, inhibiting impulsive answers, resisting distraction, recognizing contradictions).

k. Quality of judgment.

While systematic assessment of cognitive functions is an essential part of the general psychiatric evaluation, the level of detail necessary and the appropriateness of particular formal tests depend on the purpose of the evaluation and the psychiatrist's clinical judgment.

M. Functional Assessment

For persons with chronic diseases, and particularly those with multiple comorbid conditions, structured assessment of physical and instrumental function may be useful in assessing disease severity and treatment outcome (20). Functional assessments include assessment of physical activities of daily living (e.g., eating, using the toilet, transferring, bathing, and dressing) and instrumental activities of daily living (e.g., driving or using public transportation, taking medication as prescribed, shopping, managing one's own money, keeping house, communicating by mail or telephone, and caring for a child or other dependent) (21, 22). Impairments in these activities can be due to physical or cognitive impairment or to the disruption of purposeful activity by the symptoms of mental illness.

Formal functional assessments facilitate the delineation of the combined effects of multiple illnesses and chronic conditions on patient's lives, and such assessments provide a severity measure that is congruent with patients' and families' experience of disability. In addition, functional assessment facilitates the monitoring of treatment by assessing important beneficial and adverse effects of treatment.

Formal functional assessment may be appropriate for patients who are evidently disabled by old age or by chronic physical or mental illness.

N. Diagnostic Tests

Laboratory tests are included in a psychiatric evaluation when they are necessary to establish or exclude a diagnosis, to aid in the choice of treatment, or to monitor treatment effects or side effects (23, 24). Relevant test results are documented in the evaluation, and their importance for diagnosis and treatment is indicated in the case formulation or treatment plan (see section IV.A.4).

O. Information Derived From the Interview Process

The face-to-face interview provides the psychiatrist with a sample of the patient's inter-personal behavior and emotional processes that can either support or qualify diagnostic inferences from the history and examination and can also aid in prognosis and treatment planning. Important information can be derived by observing the ways in which the patient minimizes or exaggerates certain aspects of his or her history, whether particular questions appear to evoke hesitation or signs of discomfort, and the patient's general style of relating. Further observations concern the patient's ability to communicate about emotional issues, the defense mechanisms the patient uses when discussing emotionally important topics, and the patient's responses to the psychiatrist's comments and to other behavior, such as the psychiatrist's handling of interruptions or time limits.

IV. Evaluation Process

A. Methods of Obtaining Information

1. Patient interview

The psychiatrist's primary assessment tool is the direct face-to-face interview of the patient: evaluations based solely on review of records and interviews of persons close to the patient are inherently limited. The interview should be done in a manner that optimizes the ability to support the patient's attempts to tell his or her story, while simultaneously obtaining the necessary information. Empirical studies of the interview process suggest that the most comprehensive and accurate information emerges from a combination of a) open-ended questioning with empathic listening and b) structured inquiry about specific events and symptoms (25–28). When the purpose is a general evaluation, beginning with open-ended, empathic inquiry about the patient's concerns usually is best. Patient satisfaction with open-ended inquiry is greatest when the psychiatrist provides feedback to the patient at one or more points during the interview. Structured, systematic questioning has been shown to be especially helpful in eliciting information about substance use and about traumatic life events and in ascertaining the presence or absence of specific symptoms and signs of particular mental disorders (29–32).

The psychiatrist should discuss with the patient the purpose of the evaluation. The psychiatrist should also consider whether the time planned for the interview is adequate for the aims of the evaluation and should prioritize the aims or extend the time accordingly. A high priority should be given to the assessment of the patient's safety and the identification of any general medical or mental disorders requiring urgent treatment; the patient's most pressing concerns should also receive a high priority whenever possible. The specific method and sequence of the interview is left to the psychiatrist's clinical judgment. Since the aim of evaluative interviews often is to develop an alliance with the patient, certain inquiries might be limited initially in the service of that alliance.

The evaluation ought to be performed in a manner that is sensitive to the patient's individuality, identifying issues of development, culture, ethnicity, gender, sexual orientation, familial/genetic patterns, religious/spiritual beliefs, social class, and physical and social environment influencing the patient's symptoms and behavior (also refer to section IV.B.5). Interpreters other than family members should be used if possible when the psychiatrist and the patient do not share a common language (including sign language in persons with impaired hearing). Interpreters with mental health experience and awareness of the patient's culture can provide the best information (33). The interpreter should be instructed to translate the patient's own words and to avoid paraphrasing except as needed to translate the correct meaning of idioms and other culture-specific expressions.

2. Use of collateral sources

The psychiatrist should always consider using collateral sources of information. Collateral information is particularly important for patients with impaired insight, including those with substance use disorders or cognitive impairment, and is essential for treatment planning for patients requiring a high level of assistance or supervision because of impaired function or unstable behavior. Nonetheless, the confidentiality of the patient should be respected, except when immediate safety concerns are paramount. Family members, other important people in the patient's life, and records of prior medical and/or psychiatric treatment are frequently useful sources of information. The extent of the collateral interviews and the extent of prior record review should be commensurate with the purpose of the evaluation, the ambitiousness of the diagnostic and therapeutic goals, and the difficulty of the case.

3. Use of structured interviews, questionnaires, and rating scales

Structured interviews, standardized data forms, questionnaires, and rating scales can be useful tools for diagnostic assessment and evaluation of treatment outcome. Structured interviews increase the reliability of determining that diagnostic criteria for a particular mental disorder are present; rating scales permit quantification of symptom severity. Potential cultural, ethnic, gender, social, and age biases are relevant to the selection of standardized interviews and rating scales and the interpretation of their results (34–37).

However, these tools are not a substitute for the clinician's narrative or judgment (38, 39). In particular, diagnostic and treatment decisions for patients whose conditions approach but do not reach diagnostic criteria for major psychiatric syndromes rely heavily on clinical judgment. Clinical impressions of treatment response should consider the relative importance of specific symptoms to the patient's function and well-being and the relative impact of specific symptoms on the patient's social environment.

4. Use of diagnostic tests, including psychological and neuropsychological tests

Diagnostic tests used during a psychiatric evaluation include those that do the following:

a. Detect or rule out the presence of a disorder or condition that has treatment consequences. Examples include urine screens for substance use disorders, neuropsychological tests to ascertain the presence of a learning disability, and brain imaging tests to ascertain the presence of a structural neurological abnormality.

b. Determine the relative safety and/or appropriate dose of potential alternative treatments. For example, tests of hematologic, thyroid, renal, and cardiac function in a patient with bipolar disorder may be needed to help the clinician choose among available mood-stabilizing medications.

c. Provide a baseline that will be useful in monitoring treatment response. For example, a baseline ECG may be required to facilitate the detection of tricyclic antidepressant effects on cardiac conduction.

In each of these cases, the potential utility of a test is determined by the following:

a. The probability that the disorder or condition under question is currently present or the probability that a condition may occur at a later date and require a baseline measure for detection. This may be thought of as the prevalence of the condition in a population of similar patients.

b. The probability that the test will correctly detect the condition if it is present.

c. The probability that the test will incorrectly identify a condition that is not present.

d. The treatment implications of the potential correct and incorrect test results. The treatment implications may be nil if the test detects a condition that is already known to be present on the basis of clinical examination or history or if it detects a condition that has no impact on treatment.

Given the wide range of clinical situations that are evaluated by psychiatrists, there are no general guidelines about which tests should be "routinely" done. Rather, the principles already discussed, as well as patient preferences, should be applied. Although each patient should be considered individually, it is sometimes possible to apply "clinical rules." For example, in some cases tests may be ordered on the basis of the setting (e.g., patients seen in emergency rooms of large city hospitals may be at high risk for certain conditions that warrant diagnostic tests), the clinical presentation (e.g., certain tests are warranted for patients with new onset of delirium), or the potential treatments (e.g., patients may need certain tests before initiation of lithium therapy).

5. Working with multidisciplinary teams

Multidisciplinary teams participate in general evaluations in most institutional settings and in many outpatient clinics. When working with a multidisciplinary team, the attending psychiatrist integrates both primary data and evaluative impressions of team members in arriving at a diagnosis and case formulation. It is crucial that the psychiatrist's diagnosis and case formulation rely on data recorded in the medical record and not rest primarily on undocumented impressions of other members of the team.

Systematic observations of patients' behavior by staff are a diagnostic asset of controlled settings, such as hospitals, partial hospital settings, residential treatment facilities, and other institutions. In these settings the psychiatrist may suggest to other team members specific observations that may be particularly relevant to the diagnosis or treatment plan. Several types of observations may be recorded, according to the patient's specific situation.

a. General observations.   These are relevant to all patients in all settings and include notes on patients' behavior, complaints and statements, cooperativeness with or resistance to staff, sleep/wake patterns, and self-care.

b. Diagnosis-specific observations.   These are observations relevant to confirming a diagnosis or assessing the severity, complications, or subtype of a disorder. Examples include recording of signs of withdrawal in an alcohol-dependent patient and observations during meals for patients with eating disorders.

c. Patient-specific observations.   These are observations aimed at assessing a clinical hypothesis. An example is observation of behavior following a family meeting, for a patient in whom family conflicts are suspected of having contributed to a psychotic relapse.

d. Observations of response to treatment interventions.   Examples include systematic recording of a target behavior in a trial of behavior therapy, observations of the effects of newly prescribed medications, and nurse-completed rating scales to measure changes after behavioral or psychotherapeutic interventions.

6.   Examination under medication and/or restraint

The initial evaluation of a severely ill patient sometimes requires the use of psychotropic medication, seclusion, and/or physical restraint in order to provide for the safety of the patient and/or others, to allow collection of diagnostic information, and to enable the conduct of a physical examination and diagnostic testing. Resort to such measures should be justified by the urgency of obtaining the information and should be in compliance with applicable laws. The psychiatrist should consider how any special circumstances of the interview or examination may influence clinical findings; parts of the examination that cannot be completed or that are grossly influenced by the use of medication, seclusion, and/or restraint should be repeated if possible when the patient is able to cooperate.

7.   Physical examination

The physical examination may be performed by the psychiatrist or another physician. Moreover, the psychiatrist may supplement an examination by another physician (e.g., perform a focused neurological examination). The psychiatrist should be informed about the scope and pertinent findings of examinations performed by other physicians. Considerations influencing the decision of whether the psychiatrist will personally perform the physical examination include potential effects on the psychiatrist-patient relationship, the purposes of the evaluation, and the psychiatrist's proficiency in performing physical examinations.

The psychiatrist's close involvement in the patient's general medical evaluation and ongoing care can improve the patient's care by promoting cooperation, facilitating follow-up, and permitting prompt reexamination of symptomatic areas when symptoms change.

In most cases, the physical examination by a psychiatrist should be chaperoned. Particular caution is warranted in the physical examination of persons with histories of physical or sexual abuse or with other features that could increase the possibility of the patient's being distressed as a result of the examination (e.g., a patient with an erotic or paranoid transference to the psychiatrist). All but limited examinations of such patients should be chaperoned.

B.   The Process of Assessment

The actual assessment process during a psychiatric evaluation usually involves the development of initial impressions and hypotheses during the interview and their continual testing and refinement on the basis of information obtained throughout the interview and from mental status examination, diagnostic testing, and other sources (40).

1.   Diagnosis and case formulation

On the basis of information obtained in the evaluation, a differential diagnosis is developed. The differential diagnosis comprises conditions (including personality disorders or personality traits) described in the current edition of the *Diagnostic and Statistical Manual of Mental Disorders* (DSM) of the American Psychiatric Association. The DSM classification and the specific diagnostic criteria are meant to serve as guidelines to be informed by clinical judgment in the categorization of the patient's condition(s) and are not meant to be applied in a cookbook fashion. (Other issues in the use of DSM and its application in developing a psychiatric diagnosis are discussed in DSM-IV, pp. xv–xxv and 1–13 [41].) General medical conditions are established through history, examination, medical records, conferences with or referrals to other physicians, diagnostic tests, and independent examinations performed by the psychiatrist. A multiaxial system of diagnosis provides a convenient format for organizing and communicating the patient's current clinical status, other factors affecting the clinical situation, the patient's highest level of past functioning, and the patient's quality of life (41, pp. 25–31).

Information is obtained and compiled to permit an assessment of the patient's adaptive strengths, stressors implicated in the present illness, and support available in the patient's environment. The method of deriving this information should be sensitive to the patient's individuality, identifying issues of development, culture, ethnicity, gender, sexual orientation, familial/genetic patterns, religious/spiritual beliefs, social class, and physical and social environment influencing the patient's symptoms and behavior.

The case formulation includes information specific to the individual patient that goes beyond what is conveyed by the diagnosis. The scope and depth of the formulation vary with the purpose of the evaluation. Elements commonly include psychosocial and developmental factors that may have contributed to the present illness; the patient's particular strengths and weaknesses; social resources and the ability to form and maintain relationships; issues related to culture, ethnicity, gender, sexual orientation, and religious/spiritual beliefs; likely precipitating or aggravating factors in the illness; and preferences, opinions, and biases of the patient relevant to the choice of a treatment (33, 42–53). Additional elements may be based on a specific model of psychopathology and treatment, e.g., psychodynamic or behavioral. The diagnosis and case formulation together facilitate the development of a treatment plan.

2. Initial treatment plan

A psychiatrist conducting an evaluation to guide treatment should include an initial treatment plan that includes answers to the questions that were posed and/or a plan for obtaining additional necessary information.

The initial treatment plan begins with an explicit statement of the diagnostic, therapeutic, and rehabilitative goals for treatment. In the case of patients who initially will be treated in an inpatient or partial hospital setting, this implies apportioning the therapeutic task between a hospital phase and a posthospital phase. On the basis of the goals, the plan specifies further diagnostic tests and procedures, further systematic observations to be made, and specific therapeutic modalities to be applied.

All potentially effective treatments should be considered. More detailed consideration of the risks and benefits of treatment options may be needed in the following circumstances: when a relatively risky, costly, or unusual treatment is under consideration; when involved parties disagree about the optimal course of treatment; when the patient's motivation or capacity to benefit from potential treatment alternatives is in question; when the treatment would be involuntary or when other legal or administrative issues are involved; or when external constraints limit available treatment options.

3. Decisions regarding treatment-related legal and administrative issues

Within the scope of general evaluation, certain areas might require special emphasis if there is an outstanding legal or administrative issue. Assessment should be undertaken with these issues in mind. Discussions of informed consent, if carried out during the evaluation for the purpose of treatment planning, require documentation. Thus, when a patient's competence to consent to treatment is in question, questioning to determine mental status should be extended to include items that test the patient's decision-making capacity.

On the basis of the history, examination, symptoms, diagnosis, and case formulation, the psychiatrist makes and justifies decisions regarding voluntary versus involuntary status; the patient's capacity to make treatment-related decisions; the appropriateness and/or necessity of the site, intensity, and duration of the treatment chosen; and the level of supervision necessary for safety.

4. Addressing systems issues

In addition to generating goals for the patient's diagnosis and individual treatment, the evaluation may lead to the development of goals for intervention with the family, other important people in the patient's life, other professionals (e.g., therapists), general medical providers, and governmental or social agencies (e.g., community mental health centers or family service agencies). Goals are developed in response to data from the initial evaluation indicating that various aspects of the care system have an important role in the patient's illness and treatment. Plans may be needed for addressing problems in the care system that are seen as important to the patient's illness, symptoms, function, or well-being and that appear amenable to modification. These plans should consider feasibility, the patient's wishes, and the willingness of other people to be involved.

5. Consideration for sociocultural diversity

The process of psychiatric evaluation must take into consideration and respect the diversity of American subcultures and must be sensitive to the patient's ethnicity and place of birth, gender, social class, sexual orientation, and religious/spiritual beliefs (54). Respectful evaluation involves an empathic, nonjudgmental attitude toward the patient's explanation of illness, concerns, and background. An awareness of one's possible biases or prejudices about patients from different subcultures and an understanding of the limitations of one's knowledge and skills in working with such patients may lead to the identification of situations calling for consultation with a clinician who has expertise concerning a particular subculture (41, pp. 843–849; 55–57). Further, the potential effect of the psychiatrist's sociocultural identity on the attitude and behavior of the patient should be taken into account in the formulation of a diagnostic opinion.

V. Special Considerations

A. Interactions With Third-Party Payers and Their Agents

Third-party payers and their agents frequently request data from psychiatric evaluations to make determinations about whether a hospital admission or a specific treatment modality will be covered by a particular insurance plan. Despite the blanket consents to release information to payers that most patients must sign to obtain insurance benefits, the psychiatrist should, whenever feasible, inform the patient what specific information has been requested and obtain specific consent to the release of that information. With valid consent, the psychiatrist may release information to a third-party reviewer, supplying the third-party reviewer with sufficient information to understand the rationale for the treatment and why it was selected over potential alternatives. The psychiatrist may withhold information about the patient not directly relevant to the utilization review or preauthorization decision.

B.   Privacy and Confidentiality

Psychiatrists should follow APA standards for confidentiality in dealing with the results of psychiatric evaluations. Evaluations should be conducted in the most private setting compatible with the safety of the patient and others. The identity and presence of persons other than the psychiatrist at a diagnostic interview should be explained to the patient, and the presence of these persons should be acceptable to the patient unless compelling clinical or safety reasons justify overriding the patient's objection. Psychiatrists should not make audiotape or videotape recordings of patient interviews without the knowledge and consent of the patient or the patient's legal guardian (58).

C.   Legal and Administrative Issues in Institutions

When a patient is admitted to a hospital or other residential setting, the patient's legal status should be promptly clarified. It should be established whether the admission is voluntary or involuntary, whether the patient gives or withholds consent to evaluation and recommended treatment, and whether the patient appears able to make treatment-related decisions. If there is a potential legal impediment to necessary treatment, action should be taken to resolve the issue.

In every institution, whether public or private, fiscal and administrative considerations limit treatment options. Usually there are constraints on length of stay and on the intensity of services available. Further constraints can arise from the absence or inadequate funding of aftercare services or of a full continuum of care. The initial assessment of treatment needs should not be confounded unduly with concerns about financing or availability of services, although the actual treatment may represent a compromise between optimal treatment and external constraints. When this results in a major negative effect on patient care, efforts should be made to find alternatives and the patient, family, and/ or third-party payer should be informed of the limitations of the current treatment setting and/or resources. A common example is the situation in which a patient's safety requires a level of supervision not available in a given facility. Another example is when a patient requires a general medical workup that cannot be carried out in a freestanding psychiatric facility and requires the patient's transfer to a general hospital.

D. Evaluation of Elderly Persons

While advanced chronological age alone does not necessitate a change in the approach to the psychiatric evaluation, the strong association of old age with chronic disease and related impairments may increase the need for emphasis on certain aspects of the evaluation. The general medical history and evaluation, cognitive mental status examination, and functional assessment may need to be especially detailed because of the high prevalence of disease-related disability, use of multiple medications, cognitive impairment, and functional impairment in older people. The psychiatrist should attempt to identify all of the general medical and personal care providers involved with the patient and to obtain relevant information from them if the patient consents. The personal and social history includes coverage of common late-life issues, including the loss of a spouse or partner, the loss of friends or close relatives, residential moves, the new onset of disabilities, financial concerns related to illness or disability, and intergenerational issues, such as informal caregiving or financial transfers between members of different generations.

The psychiatrist may need to accommodate the evaluation to patients who cannot hear adequately. Amplification, a quieter interview room, and enabling lip reading are possible means to do this. When elderly patients are brought for psychiatric evaluation by a family member, special effort may be necessary to ensure them of the opportunity to talk to the psychiatrist alone.

VI.   Development Process

The development process is detailed in a document available from the APA Office of Research, "APA Practice Guideline Development Process." Key features of the process included the following:

❖   a literature review (see the following description);
❖   initial drafting by a work group that included psychiatrists with clinical and research expertise in psychiatric evaluation;
❖   the production of multiple drafts with widespread review, in which 32 organizations and over 106 individuals submitted comments (see section VII);
❖   approval by the APA Assembly and Board of Trustees; and
❖   planned revisions at 3- to 5-year intervals.

Two types of literature were reviewed. Major texts published since 1983 on general psychiatry or psychiatric evaluation were identified by using the card catalogue at a medical school library. Primary sources and major review articles were identified by using MED-LINE (1973–1993) and PsycLIT (1987–1993) and using references given in the texts. Key words for computer searches included the following:

Diagnostic Interview Schedule
    and evaluation
Interview-Psychological (including Psychiatric)
    and family history
    and adult
    and forensic
    and methods
    and initial
Mental-Disorders-Diagnosis
    and interview
    and physical examination
    and outcome
    and tests
Mental Status Examination
Psychiatric-status-rating scales
Psychiatric
    and validity
    and admission
Psychological
    and discharge
    and evaluation
    and emergency
    and interview

The literature search was augmented by numerous references suggested by reviewers. It showed a predominance of expert opinion and psychometric studies of specific tests, with a small number of studies linking the evaluation process to clinical outcome.

VII. Individuals and Organizations That Submitted Comments

Paul Stuart Appelbaum, M.D.
Bernard S. Arons, M.D.
Boris M. Astrachan, M.D.
Joseph Autry, M.D.
F.M. Baker, M.D., M.P.H.
Richard Balon, M.D.
Ruth T. Barnhouse, M.D.

Cole Barton, Ph.D.
Jerome S. Beigler, M.D.
Jules R. Bemporad, M.D.
Charles H. Blackinton, M.D.
Mary C. Blehar, Ph.D.
Linda Bond, M.D.
Barbara A. Bonorden, M.S.

William H. Bristow, Jr., M.D.
John W. Buckley, M.D.
Robert Paul Cabaj, M.D.
Claudio Cepeda, M.D.
Daniel S. Chaffin, M.D.
Gordon H. Clark, Jr., M.D.
Norman Clemens, M.D.
Jacquelyn T. Coleman
John D. Cone, M.D.
Namir Damluji, M.D.
Carol Dashoff
Dave M. Davis, M.D.
Barbara G. Deutsch, M.D.
Park Dietz, M.D., Ph.D.
Richard S. Epstein, M.D.
Lois T. Flaherty, M.D.
Jean-Guy Fontaine, M.D.
Robert Fusco, M.D.
Glen Owens Gabbard, M.D.
Donald Gallant, M.D.
Elizabeth Galton, M.D.
Elena Garralda, Ph.D.
Jerry H. Gelbart, M.D.
Earl L. Giller, M.D., Ph.D.
Katharine Gillis, M.D.
Linda G. Gochfeld, M.D.
Stephen M. Goldfinger, M.D.
Larry S. Goldman, M.D.
Melvin G. Goldzband, M.D.
James Goodman, M.D.
Tracy R. Gordy, M.D.
Sheila Hafter Gray, M.D.
David Arlen Gross, M.D.
J.D. Hamilton, M.D.
Edward Hanin, M.D.
Steven C. Hayes, Ph.D.
Michel Hersen, M.D.
Steven K. Hoge, M.D.
Jeffrey S. Janofsky, M.D.
Mary A. Jansen, Ph.D.
Brad Johnson, M.D.
Robert A. Kimmich, M.D.

Donald F. Klein, M.D.
Thomas M. Kozak, Ph.D.
Kachigere Krishnappa, M.D.
Jeremy Lazarus, M.D.
Robert L. Leon, M.D.
William L. Licamele, M.D.
Elliot D. Luby, M.D.
Velandy Manohar, M.D.
John C. Markowitz, M.D.
Ronald L. Martin, M.D.
Jerome A. Motto, M.D.
Charles B. Mutter, M.D.
Carol Nadelson, M.D.
Henry Nasrallah, M.D.
James E. Nininger, M.D.
George W. Paulson, M.D.
Herbert S. Peyser, M.D.
Katharine Phillips, M.D.
Edward Pinney, M.D.
Ghulam Qadir, M.D.
Jonas R. Rappeport, M.D.
Victor I. Reus, M.D.
Richard E. Rhoden, M.D.
Michelle Riba, M.D.
Barbara R. Rosenfeld, M.D.
Pedro Ruiz, M.D.
James Ray Rundell, M.D.
Jo-Ellyn M. Ryall, M.D.
Joseph D. Sapira, M.D.
Jerome M. Schnitt, M.D.
Marc A. Schuckit, M.D.
Paul M. Schyve, M.D.
Stephen Shanfield, M.D.
Sheldon N. Siegel, M.D.
Edward Silberman, M.D.
Andrew Edward Skodol II, M.D.
Stanley L. Slater, M.D.
Terry Stein, M.D.
Nada L. Stotland, M.D.
Paul Summergrad, M.D.
Margery Sved, M.D.
Kenneth J. Tardiff, M.D.

William R. Tatomer, M.D., M.P.H.

Clark Terrell, M.D.

Ole Johannes Thienhaus, M.D., M.B.A.

Josef H. Weissberg, M.D.

Joseph J. Westermeyer, M.D., Ph.D.

Robert M. Wettstein, M.D.

Rhonda Whitson, R.R.A.

Howard V. Zonana, M.D.

American Academy of Child and Adolescent Psychiatry

American Academy of Neurology

American Academy of Psychiatrists in Alcoholism and Addiction

American Academy of Psychiatry and the Law

American Academy of Psychoanalysis

American Association of Community Psychiatrists

American Association of Psychiatric Administrators

American Association of Psychiatrists From India

American Association of Suicidology

American College of Emergency Physicians

American Medical Association

American Nurses Association

American Psychoanalytic Association

American Psychological Association

American Psychosomatic Society

American Sleep Disorders Association

American Society for Adolescent Psychiatry

American Society of Addiction Medicine

American Society of Clinical Hypnosis

Association for Academic Psychiatry

Association for Child Psychoanalysis

Association for the Advancement of Behavior Therapy

Association of Gay and Lesbian Psychiatrists

Center for Substance Abuse Prevention

Department of Veterans Affairs

Joint Commission on Accreditation of Healthcare Organizations

National Association of Veterans Affairs Chiefs of Psychiatry

National Institute of Mental Health

Pakistan Psychiatric Society of North America

Royal College of Psychiatrists

Society of Biological Psychiatry

Substance Abuse and Mental Health Services Administration

VIII.   References

The following coding system is used to indicate the nature of the supporting evidence in the summary recommendations and references:

[A] *Randomized clinical trial.*   A study of an intervention in which subjects are prospectively followed over time; there are treatment and control groups; subjects are randomly assigned to the two groups; both the subjects and the investigators are blind to the assignments.

[B] *Clinical trial.*   A prospective study in which an intervention is made and the results of that intervention are tracked longitudinally; study does not meet standards for a randomized clinical trial.

[C] *Cohort or longitudinal study.*   A study in which subjects are prospectively followed over time without any specific intervention.

[D] *Case-control study.*   A study in which a group of patients is identified in the present and information about them is pursued retrospectively or backward in time.

[E] *Review with secondary data analysis.*   A structured analytic review of existing data, e.g., a meta-analysis or a decision analysis.

[F] *Review.*   A qualitative review and discussion of previously published literature without a quantitative synthesis of the data.

[G] *Other.*   Textbooks, expert opinion, case reports, and other reports not included above.

1.   Margulies A, Havens LL: The initial encounter: what to do first? Am J Psychiatry 1981; 138:421–428 [F]

2.   Bassuk EL: The diagnosis and treatment of psychiatric emergencies. Compr Ther 1985; 11(7):6–12 [F]

3.   Hall RC, Gardner ER, Popkin MK, Lecann AF, Stickney SK: Unrecognized physical illness prompting psychiatric admission: a prospective study. Am J Psychiatry 1981; 138:629–635 [C]

4.   Anfinson TJ, Kathol RG: Laboratory and neuroendocrine assessment in medical-psychiatric patients, in Psychiatric Care of the Medical Patient. Edited by Stoudemire A, Fogel BS. New York, Oxford University Press, 1993 [F]

5.   Garrick TR, Stotland NL: How to write a psychiatric consultation. Am J Psychiatry 1982; 139:849–855 [G]

6.   Karasu TB, Plutchik R, Conte H, Siegel B, Steinmuller R, Rosenbaum M: What do physicians want from a psychiatric consultation service? Compr Psychiatry 1977; 18:73–81 [C]

7.   Appelbaum PS, Gutheil TG: Clinical Handbook of Psychiatry and the Law. Baltimore, Williams & Wilkins, 1991 [F]

8.   Group for the Advancement of Psychiatry: The Mental Health Professional and the Legal System: Report 131. Washington, DC, Group for the Advancement of Psychiatry, 1991 [F]

9.   Sederer LI: Brief hospitalization, in American Psychiatric Press Review of Psychiatry, vol 11. Edited by Tasman A, Riba MB. Washington, DC, American Psychiatric Press, 1992 [F]

10. Fogel BS, Summergrad P: Evolution of the medical-psychiatric unit in the general hospital, in Handbook of Studies on General Hospital Psychiatry. Edited by Judd FK, Burrows GD, Lipsitt DR. New York, Elsevier, 1991 [G]

11. Lowenstein RJ: An office mental status examination for complex chronic dissociative symptoms and multiple personality disorder. Psychiatr Clin North Am 1991; 14:567–604 [G]

12. Herman JL: Trauma and Recovery. New York, Basic Books, 1992, pp 115–129 [G]

13. March JS: What constitutes a stressor: the "Criterion A" issue, in Posttraumatic Stress Disorder: DSM-IV and Beyond. Edited by Davison JRT, Foa EB. Washington, DC, American Psychiatric Press, 1993 [F]

14. Rey JM, Stewart GW, Plapp JM, Bashir MR, Richards IN: Validity of Axis V of DSM-III and other measures of adaptive function. Acta Psychiatr Scand 1988; 77:535–542 [C]

15. Sohlberg S: There's more in a number than you think: new validity data for the Global Assessment Scale. Psychol Rep 1989; 64:455–461 [F]

16. Harder DW, Strauss JS, Greenwald DF, Kokes RF, Ritzler BA, Gift TE: Predictors of outcome among adult psychiatric first admissions. J Clin Psychol 1992; 46:119–128 [C]

17. Schiffer RB, Klein RF, Sider RC: The Medical Evaluation of Psychiatric Patients. New York, Plenum, 1988, pp 3–33 [G]

18. Trzepacz PJ, Baker RW: The Psychiatric Mental Status Examination. New York, Oxford University Press, 1993, pp 3–12 [G]

19. Tardiff K: The current state of psychiatry in the treatment of violent patients. Arch Gen Psychiatry 1992; 49:493–499 [G]

20. Applegate WB, Blass JP, Williams TF: Instruments for the functional assessment of older patients. N Engl J Med 1990; 322: 1207–1214 [F]

21. Katz S: Assessing self-maintenance: activities of daily living, mobility, and instrumental activities of daily living. J Am Geriatr Soc 1983; 31:721–727 [F]

22. American Psychiatric Association: Position statement on the role of psychiatrists in assessing driving ability (official actions). Am J Psychiatry 1995; 152:819 [G]

23. Anfinson TJ, Kathol RG: Screening laboratory evaluation in psychiatric patients: a review. Gen Hosp Psychiatry 1992; 14:248–257 [F]

24. White AJ, Barraclough B: Benefits and problems of routine laboratory investigations in adult psychiatric admissions. Br J Psychiatry 1989; 155:65–72 [F]

25. Cox A, Hopkinson K, Rutter M: Psychiatric interviewing techniques, II—naturalistic study: eliciting factual information. Br J Psychiatry 1981; 138:283–291 [C]

26. Hopkinson K, Cox A, Rutter M: Psychiatric interviewing techniques, III—naturalistic study: eliciting feelings. Br J Psychiatry 1981; 138:406–415 [C]

27. Cox A, Rutter M, Holbrook D: Psychiatric interviewing techniques, V—experimental study: eliciting factual information. Br J Psychiatry 1981; 139:29–31 [B]

28. Cox A, Holbrook D, Rutter M: Psychiatric interviewing techniques, VI—experimental study: eliciting feelings. Br J Psychiatry 1981; 139:144–152 [B]

29. Maier W, Philipp M, Buller R: The value of structured clinical interviews. Arch Gen Psychiatry 1988; 45:963–964 [C]

30. Robins L: Diagnostic grammar and assessment: translating criteria into questions. Psychol Med 1989; 19:57–68 [F]

31. Watson CG, Juba MP, Manifold V, Kucala T, Anderson PE: The PTSD interview: rationale, description, reliability, and concurrent validity of a DSM-III-based technique. J Clin Psychol 1991; 47:179–188 [C]

32. Skre I, Onstad S, Torgersen S, Kringlen E: High interrater reliability for the Structured Clinical Interview for DSM-III-R axis I (SCID I). Acta Psychiatr Scand 1991; 84:167–173 [C]

33. Westermeyer JJ: Cross-cultural psychiatric assessment, in Culture, Ethnicity, and Mental Illness. Edited by Gaw AC. Washington, DC, American Psychiatric Press, 1993 [F]

34. Escobar JI, Burnam A, Karno M, Forsythe A, Landsverk J, Golding JM: Use of the Mini-Mental State Examination (MMSE) in a community population of mixed ethnicity: cultural and linguistic artifacts. J Nerv Ment Dis 1986; 174:607–614 [C]

35. Lopez S, Nunez JA: Cultural factors considered in selected diagnostic criteria and interview schedules. J Abnorm Psychol 1987; 96:270–272 [F]

36. Flaherty JA, Gaviria FM, Pathak D, Mitchell T, Wintrob R, Richman JA, Birz S: Developing instruments for cross-cultural psychiatric research. J Nerv Ment Dis 1988; 176:257–263 [F]

37. Roberts RE, Rhoades HM, Vernon SW: Using the CES-D Scale to screen for depression and anxiety: effects of language and ethnic status. Psychiatry Res 1990; 31:69–83 [C]

38. Kovess V, Sylla O, Fournier L, Flavigny V: Why discrepancies exist between diagnostic interviews and clinicians' diagnoses. Soc Psychiatry Psychiatr Epidemiol 1992; 27:185–191 [C]

39. Harrington R, Hill J, Rutter M, John K, Fudge H, Zoccolillo M, Weissman M: The assessment of lifetime psychopathology: a comparison of two interviewing styles. Psychol Med 1988; 18: 487–493 [C]

40. Nurcombe B, Fitzhenry-Coor I: How do psychiatrists think? clinical reasoning in the psychiatric interview: a research and education project. Aust NZ J Psychiatry 1982; 16:13–24 [F]

41. American Psychiatric Association: Diagnostic and Statistical Manual of Mental Disorders, 4th ed (DSM-IV). Washington, DC, APA, 1994 [G]

42. Perry S, Cooper AM, Michels R: The psychodynamic formulation: its purpose, structure, and clinical application. Am J Psychiatry 1987; 144:543–550 [F]

43. Barrett DH, Abel GG, Rouleau JL, Coyne BJ: Behavioral therapy strategies with medical patients, in Psychiatric Care of the Medical Patient. Edited by Stoudemire A, Fogel BS. New York, Oxford University Press, 1993

44. Miller NE: Behavioral medicine: symbiosis between laboratory and clinic. Annu Rev Psychol 1983; 34:1–31

45. Powell G (ed): The Psychosocial Development of Minority Group Children. New York, Brunner-Mazel, 1983 [F]

46. Dickstein L: New perspectives on human development, in American Psychiatric Press Review of Psychiatry, vol 10. Edited by Tasman A, Goldfinger S. Washington, DC, American Psychiatric Press, 1991 [F]

47. Gaw A (ed): Culture, Ethnicity, and Mental Illness. Washington, DC, American Psychiatric Press, 1993 [G]

48. Notman M, Nadelson C: Women and Men: New Perspectives on Gender Differences. Washington, DC, American Psychiatric Press, 1991 [F]

49. Stein T: Changing perspectives on homosexuality, in American Psychiatric Press Review of Psychiatry, vol 12. Edited by Oldham J, Riba M, Tasman A. Washington, DC, American Psychiatric Press, 1993 [F]

50. McGoldrick M, Pearce J, Giordano J (eds): Ethnicity and Family Therapy. New York, Guilford Press, 1982 [G]

51. Barnhouse R: How to evaluate patients' religious ideation, in Psychiatry and Religion: Overlapping Concerns. Edited by Robinson L. Washington, DC, American Psychiatric Press, 1986 [G]

52. Kroll J, Sheehan W: Religious beliefs and practices among 52 psychiatric inpatients in Minnesota. Am J Psychiatry 1989; 146: 67–72 [C]

53. Westermeyer J: Psychiatric Care of Migrants: A Clinical Guide. Washington, DC, American Psychiatric Press, 1989 [G]

54. Gonzalez CA, Griffith EEH, Ruiz P: Cross-cultural issues in psychiatric treatment, in Treatments of Psychiatric Disorders, 2nd ed. Edited by Gabbard GO. Washington, DC, American Psychiatric Press, 1995

55. Pinderhughes E: Understanding Race, Ethnicity and Power. New York, Free Press, 1988 [F]

56. American Psychiatric Association: Guidelines regarding possible conflict between psychiatrists' religious commitments and psychiatric practice (official actions). Am J Psychiatry 1990; 147: 542 [G]

57. American Psychiatric Association: Position statement on bias-related incidents (official actions). Am J Psychiatry 1993; 150:686 [G]

58. Macbeth JE, Wheeler AM, Sither JW, Onek JN: Legal and Risk Management Issues in the Practice of Psychiatry. Washington, DC, American Psychiatric Press, 1994 [F]

PRACTICE GUIDELINE

FOR

EATING DISORDERS

WORK GROUP ON EATING DISORDERS

Joel Yager, M.D., Chair

Arnold Andersen, M.D.
Michael Devlin, M.D.
James Mitchell, M.D.
Pauline Powers, M.D.
Alayne Yates, M.D.

Contents

Eating Disorders

This practice guideline was published in February 1993 in the *American Journal of Psychiatry*.

Reference Coding System

The following coding system is used to indicate the nature of the supporting evidence in the summary recommendations and references:

[A] Randomized controlled clinical trial, crossover design with randomly assigned treatment sequence
[B] Nonrandomized case-control study, repeated measures design, follow-up study
[C] Nonrandomized cohort study
[D] Clinical report with nonrandomized historical comparison groups
[E] Case report or series
[F] Expert consensus
[G] Data consolidation and reanalysis, e.g., meta-analysis
[H] Epidemiologic report
[I] Subject review
[J] Other, e.g., published instrument, published abstract, published letter

Literature Review Process

The following sources were reviewed:

1. Eating disorders, in Treatments of Psychiatric Disorders: A Task Force Report of the American Psychiatric Association, vol 1. Washington, DC, APA, 1989
2. The following authoritative volumes published within the past decade:

Agras WS: Eating Disorders: Management of Obesity, Bulimia and Anorexia Nervosa. Oxford, Pergamon Press, 1987

Andersen AE (ed): Males With Eating Disorders. New York, Brunner/Mazel, 1990

Andersen AE: Practical Comprehensive Treatment of Anorexia Nervosa and Bulimia. Baltimore, Johns Hopkins University Press, 1985

Bell RM: Holy Anorexia. Chicago, University of Chicago Press, 1985

Bemporad JR, Herzog DB (eds): Psychoanalysis and Eating Disorders. New York, Guilford Press, 1989

Beumont PJ, Burrows GD, Casper RC (eds): Handbook of Eating Disorders Part I: Anorexia and Bulimia Nervosa. New York, Elsevier, 1987

Blinder BJ, Chaitin BF, Goldstein R (eds): The Eating Disorders: Medical and Psychological Bases of Diagnosis and Treatment. Great Neck, NY, PMA, 1988

Brownell KD, Foreyt JP (eds): Handbook of Eating Disorders: Physiology, Psychology, and Treatment of Obesity, Anorexia and Bulimia. New York, Basic Books, 1986

Brumberg JJ: Fasting Girls: The Emergence of Anorexia Nervosa as a Modern Disease. Cambridge, MA, Harvard University Press, 1988

Carruba MO, Blundell JE (eds): Pharmacology of Eating Disorders. New York, Raven Press, 1986

Crisp AH: Anorexia Nervosa: Let Me Be. London, Academic Press, 1980

Fichter MM (ed): Bulimia Nervosa: Basic Research, Diagnosis and Therapy. New York, John Wiley & Sons, 1990

Garfinkel PE, Garner DM: Anorexia Nervosa: A Multidimensional Perspective. New York, Brunner/Mazel, 1982

Garfinkel PE, Garner DM (eds): The Role of Drug Treatments for Eating Disorders. New York, Brunner/Mazel, 1987

Garner DM, Garfinkel PE (eds): Handbook of Psychotherapy for Anorexia Nervosa and Bulimia. New York, Guilford Press, 1985

Garner DM, Garfinkel PE (eds): Diagnostic Issues in Anorexia Nervosa and Bulimia Nervosa. New York, Brunner/Mazel, 1988

Gislason IL: Eating disorders in childhood (ages 4 through 11), in The Eating Disorders: Medical and Psychological Bases of Diagnosis and Treatment. Edited by Blinder BJ, Chaitin BF, Goldstein RS. Great Neck, NY, PMA, 1988

Hall RCW (ed): Eating Disorders: Diagnostic and Treatment Issues, vol 1. Psychiatr Med 1989 (Suppl); 7:3

Hall RCW (ed): Eating Disorders: Diagnostic and Treatment Issues, vol 2. Psychiatr Med 1989 (Suppl); 7:4

Hornyak LM, Baker EK (eds): Experiential Therapies for Eating Disorders. New York, Guilford Press, 1989

Hsu LKG: Eating Disorders. New York, Guilford Press, 1990

Johnson C (ed): Psychodynamic Treatment of Anorexia Nervosa and Bulimia. New York, Guilford Press, 1991

Johnson C, Connors ME: The Etiology and Treatment of Bulimia Nervosa. New York, Basic Books, 1987

Kaye WH, Gwirtsman HE (eds): A Comprehensive Approach to the Treatment of Normal Weight Bulimia. Washington, DC, American Psychiatric Press, 1985

Mitchell JE (ed): Anorexia Nervosa and Bulimia: Diagnosis and Treatment. Minneapolis, University of Minnesota Press, 1985

Orbach S: Hunger Strike: The Anorectic's Struggle as a Metaphor for Our Age. New York, WW Norton, 1986

Piran N, Kaplan AS (eds): A Day Hospital Group Treatment Program for Anorexia Nervosa and Bulimia Nervosa. New York, Brunner/Mazel, 1990

Powers PS, Fernandez RC (eds): Current Treatment of Anorexia Nervosa and Bulimia. Basel, Karger, 1984

Root MPP, Fallon P, Friedrich WN: Bulimia: A Family Systems Approach to Treatment. New York, WW Norton, 1986

Schneider LH, Cooper SJ, Halmi KA (eds): The Psychobiology of Human Eating Disorders: Preclinical and Clinical Perspectives. Annals of the New York Academy of Sciences, vol 575. New York, New York Academy of Medicine, 1989

Schwartz HJ (ed): Bulimia: Psychoanalytic Treatment and Theory, 2nd ed. Madison, CT, International Universities Press, 1990

Sours J: Starving to Death in a Sea of Objects. New York, Jason Aronson, 1980

Touyz SW, Beumont PJ: Eating Disorders: Prevalence and Treatment. Baltimore, Williams & Wilkins, 1985

Vandereycken W, Kog E, Vanderlinden J (eds): The Family Approach to Eating Disorders. Great Neck, NY, PMA, 1989

Wilson CP, Hogan CC, Mintz IL (eds): Fear of Being Fat: The Treatment of Anorexia Nervosa and Bulimia, 2nd ed. Northvale, NJ, Jason Aronson, 1985

Wilson CP, Hogan CC, Mintz IL (eds): Psychodynamic Technique in the Treatment of Eating Disorders. Northvale, NJ, Jason Aronson, 1992

Yager J, Gwirtsman HE, Edelstein CK (eds): Special Problems in Managing Eating Disorders. Washington, DC, American Psychiatric Press, 1991

3.   The following review articles and book chapters:

Blinder BJ: Eating disorders in psychiatric illness. Clin Applied Nutrition 1991; 1:73–85

Casper RC, Offer D: Weight and dieting concerns in adolescents: fashion or symptom? Pediatrics 1990; 86:384–390

Cox GL, Merkel WT: A qualitative review of psychosocial treatments for bulimia. J Nerv Ment Dis 1989; 177:77–84

DiNicola VF, Roberts N, Oke L: Eating and mood disorders in young children. Psychiatr Clin North Am 1989; 12:873–893

Hall RC, Beresford TP: Medical complications of anorexia and bulimia. Psychiatr Med 1989; 7:165–192

Hall RC, Hoffman RS, Beresford TP, Wooley B, Hall AK, Kubasak L: Physical illness encountered in patients with eating disorders. Psychosomatics 1989; 30:174–191

Herzog DB, Copeland PM: Eating disorders. N Engl J Med 1985; 313:295–303

Jacobs BW, Isaacs S: Pre-pubertal anorexia nervosa: a retrospective controlled study. J Child Psychol Psychiatry 1986; 27:237–250

Kreipe RE, Churchill BH, Strauss J: Long-term outcome of adolescents with anorexia nervosa. Am J Dis Child 1989; 143:1322–1327

Nussbaum M, Shenker IR, Baird D, Saravay S: Follow-up investigation in patients with anorexia nervosa. J Pediatr 1985; 106:835–840

Palla B, Litt IF: Medical complications of eating disorders in adolescents. Pediatrics 1988; 81:613–623

Pomeroy C, Mitchell JE: Medical complications and management of eating disorders. Psychiatr Annals 1989; 19:488–493

Steiner H, Mazar C, Litt IF: Compliance and outcome in anorexia nervosa. West J Med 1990; 153:133–139

Yager J: The treatment of eating disorders. J Clin Psychiatry (Suppl) 1988; 49:18–25

Yager J: Psychotherapeutic strategies for bulimia nervosa. J Psychotherapy Practice Research 1992; 1:91–102

Yager J: Bulimia nervosa, in Integrating Pharmacotherapy and Psychotherapy. Edited by Bietman BD, Klerman GL. Washington, DC, American Psychiatric Press, 1991

Yates A: Current perspectives on the eating disorders, II: treatment, outcome and research directions. J Am Acad Child Adolesc Psychiatry 1990; 29:1–9

4.   A MEDLINE computerized search was conducted in March 1990 using the following key words:

1.   Eating Disorders and Treatment, yielding 151 references.
2.   Anorexia Nervosa and Treatment, yielding 188 references.
3.   Bulimia Nervosa and Treatment, yielding 115 references.

Abstracts were reviewed for pertinent data-based studies.

I. Disease Definition, Epidemiology, and Natural History

These guidelines address anorexia nervosa and bulimia nervosa only; they do not address eating disorders not otherwise specified, pica, or rumination. The discussion of diagnoses in these guidelines are based on DSM-III-R criteria. Anorexia nervosa and bulimia nervosa affect large numbers of persons, with 90%–95% of cases occurring in females. With the obvious exception of concerns regarding menstrual function and female sexuality, issues of assessment and treatment for male patients (1) generally parallel those for females. DSM-III-R criteria for anorexia nervosa and bulimia nervosa are outlined below. Some aspects of diagnosis and treatment may require special consideration for the very young.

A. DSM-III-R Criteria

1. For anorexia nervosa

a. Refusal to maintain body weight over a minimal normal weight for age and height, e.g., weight loss leading to maintenance of body weight 15% below that expected; or failure to make expected weight gain during period of growth, leading to body weight 15% below that expected.
b. Intense fear of gaining weight or becoming fat, even though underweight.
c. Disturbance in the way in which one's body weight, size, or shape is experienced, e.g., the person claims to "feel fat" even when emaciated, believes that one area of the body is "too fat" even when obviously underweight.
d. In females, absence of at least three consecutive menstrual cycles when otherwise expected to occur (primary or secondary amenorrhea). (A woman is considered to have amenorrhea if her periods occur only following hormone, e.g., estrogen, administration).

2. For bulimia nervosa

a. Recurrent episodes of binge eating (rapid consumption of a large amount of food in a discrete period of time).
b. A feeling of lack of control over eating behavior during the eating binges.
c. The person regularly engages in either self-induced vomiting, use of laxatives or diuretics, strict dieting or fasting, or vigorous exercise in order to prevent weight gain.
d. A minimum average of two binge eating episodes a week for at least 3 months.
e. Persistent overconcern with body shape and weight.

B. Epidemiology and Characteristics of Eating Disorders

The prevalence of eating disorders appears to be increasing (2, 3) and may range from 1%–4% of adolescent and young adult women in predominantly white upper-middle- and middle-class student groups (3–7). Although the prevalence of these disorders elsewhere in the population is much lower (8), increasing numbers of cases are being seen in males, minorities, and women of all age groups. Some experts feel that increasing numbers of cases are being seen in prepubertal children. Homosexual men may be at greater risk than heterosexual men (9). Bulimia nervosa is more common than anorexia nervosa (10).

Weight preoccupation is a primary symptom in both anorexia nervosa and bulimia nervosa. Many patients demonstrate both anorexic and bulimic behaviors. Anorexia nervosa appears in restricting and bulimic subtypes; up to 50% of anorexia nervosa patients develop bulimic symptoms, significant numbers of patients who are initially bulimic develop anorexic symptoms, and restricting and bulimic subtypes may occasionally alternate in the same patient (11–16). For these reasons some consider the disorders to occur along a continuum. Patients with the restricting subtype ("dieters") limit energy intake to as few as several hundred kilocalories per day, limit food selection, and often demonstrate obsessive-compulsive symptoms regarding food and other matters. Patients with the bulimic subtype suffer from frequent eating binges, usually purge, and are often self-destructive (13). Patients with either subtype may exercise for hours daily (17) and may demonstrate bizarre food preferences, social isolation, diminished sexual interest, and depression. Anorexia nervosa patients who purge but who do not objectively binge eat are often encountered. Careful assessment of exactly what each patient means by a "binge" is imperative.

Physical complications of anorexia nervosa include all serious sequelae of malnutrition, including cardiovascular compromise. Prepubertal patients may have arrested sexual maturation, general physical development, and growth and may not grow to anticipated heights. Even patients who look and feel deceptively well and who have normal ECGs often have bradycardia and other manifestations of impaired cardiac function, such as drop in orthostatic blood pressure and increase in pulse rate, and may be prone to sudden death (18). Prolonged amenorrhea (more than 6 months) is associated with potentially irreversible osteopenia and a correspondingly higher rate of pathological fractures (19). Patients may suffer from dehydration, electrolyte disturbances, gastrointestinal motility disturbances, infertility (20), hypothermia and other evidence of hypometabolism, and from the psychological sequelae of starvation described later in the text.

Although laboratory findings may be normal in spite of profound malnutrition, abnormalities may include neutropenia with relative lymphocytosis, abnormal liver function, hypoglycemia, hypercortisolemia, hypercholesterolemia, hypercarotenemia, low serum zinc levels, widespread disturbances in endocrine functioning (including low T_3 levels which are reversible with weight restoration and generally should not be treated with replacement therapy), and electrolyte disturbances (21–23). Abnormal computerized tomography (CT) scans of the brain may be found in more than half of patients with anorexia nervosa (24), and patients with weight loss may exhibit decreased metabolic rate (25).

Physical complications of bulimic behaviors include electrolyte disturbances (notably, a hypokalemic, hypochloremic alkalosis in patients who vomit), mineral and fluid imbalances, hypomagnesemia, gastric and esophageal irritation and bleeding, large bowel abnormalities due to laxative abuse, erosion of dental enamel, parotid enlargement, and accompanying hyperamylasemia. Mallory-Weiss esophageal tears occur rarely. Abuse of ipecac to induce vomiting may cause cardiomyopathies (with sudden death) or peripheral muscle weakness (26). Resting bradycardia, hypotension, and decreased metabolic rate are observed in some bulimic patients and may reflect decreased activity in the sympathetic nervous system and the thyroid axis (27). In addition, although bulimic patients may appear physically within the standards of healthy weight, they may show psychological correlates of starvation, so that definitive psychological assessment may be difficult to accomplish before eating and weight are stabilized.

Symptoms of eating disorders are seen in heterogeneous psychiatric populations suffering from varied types and degrees of psychopathology, character organizations, and levels of ego functioning (15, 16, 28–32). Early histories of patients with eating disorders are often complicated by medical and surgical illnesses, separations, family deaths, and behavioral disturbances. Whether the prevalence of these problems is higher among persons with eating disorders in comparison to those with other forms of psychopathology is not known. Sexual abuse has been reported in 20%–50% of patients with bulimia nervosa (33), but this rate may be similar to that found in other psychiatric populations (34). For those who have been victimized, the abuse is a major treatment consideration and assessment for abuse is very important (35).

Patients with relatively uncomplicated eating disorders are encountered in college populations and among younger age groups, but many patients seeking treatment at tertiary psychiatric treatment centers are far more complex. Comorbid major depression and/or dysthymia have been reported in 50%–75% of anorexia nervosa patients (28). In addition, obsessive-compulsive disorder may be found in about 10%–13% of cases (28, 36), with a lifetime prevalence of obsessive-compulsive disorder in anorexia nervosa of about 25% (28). Among patients with bulimia nervosa, increased rates have been reported for anxiety (43%) and chemical dependency (49%) disorders (37), bipolar disorder (12%) (38), and personality disorders (or at least substantial personality trait disturbances) (50%–75%) (39–41). Due to disputes regarding diagnostic criteria, disagreement exists regarding comorbidity rates for borderline personality disorder and eating disorders, with reported estimates varying widely between 2% and 60% (42). Additionally, many bulimic eating-disordered patients have dissociative symptoms, sexual conflicts and disturbances, and a variety of impulsive behaviors that frequently involve overspending, shoplifting, promiscuity, and self-mutilation (15, 16, 32, 43).

First-degree female relatives of patients with anorexia nervosa have increased rates of anorexia nervosa (44). Twins of patients with bulimia nervosa also have increased rates of bulimia nervosa, with monozygotic twins having higher concordance than dizygotic twins. The evidence regarding rates of bulimia in other first-degree female relatives is controversial (3). In addition, families of patients with bulimia nervosa have increased rates of substance abuse (particularly alcoholism) (45), affective disorders (37), and obesity (46).

II. Treatment Principles and Alternatives

A. Goals of Treatment

Treatment interventions are first aimed at nutritional rehabilitation and the restoration of normal eating patterns to correct the biological and psychological sequelae of malnutrition that may perpetuate eating-disordered behavior. The concurrent longer-term goals are to diagnose and help resolve the associated psychological, family, social, and behavioral problems so that relapse does not occur.

1. Malnutrition and other biologically mediated problems

Consensus currently exists that many of the physical and psychological symptoms of eating disorders may result from malnutrition (47). Volunteers who submit to starvation and semistarved prisoners of war develop food preoccupation, food hoarding, abnormal taste preferences, binge eating and other disturbances of appetite regulation, symptoms of depression, obsessionality, apathy, irritability, and other personality changes. These disturbances reverse with refeeding, although it may take considerable time following weight restoration for them to abate completely (48). Complete psychological assessment may not be possible until some degree of weight normalization is achieved (49).

Although biological hypotheses have suggested that primary hypothalamic or suprahypothalamic abnormalities account for profound disturbances in hormones, neurotransmitters, and neuromodulators (50–53), and other hypotheses have suggested that eating disorders may be variants of affective disorders (54, 55), all of these hypotheses are rendered somewhat questionable because virtually all of the biological disturbances and many of the mood disturbances abate with nutritional rehabilitation (44, 56, 57). However, treatment studies suggest that, at least for some patients, specific relationships may exist between mood, bulimic behaviors, and responses to specific antidepressant medications (58).

2. Psychological, behavioral, and social deficits

Formulations regarding psychological abnormalities seen in patients with eating disorders are based on psychodynamic (30, 59, 60), psychoanalytic (15, 32, 61, 62), cognitive (63, 64), learning (65), family systems (66–68), sociocultural (69, 70), and feminist (71) theories. One prominently held view asserts that central psychological features of patients with eating disorders include a sense of pervasive ineffectiveness which results in an attempt to gain self-control in the sphere of weight, difficulties in interpreting inner sensations, including hunger and satiety, and difficulties in both interpreting and tolerating many affective states. Deficits in self-structure, self-esteem, self-coherence and self-regulation, and incomplete and ambivalent object relations may leave these patients ill-equipped for the developmental tasks of separation/individuation and result in a weak sense of personal and gender identity and in a pervasive sense of ineffectiveness and helplessness. The relative contributions of autonomous constitutional factors, developmental difficulties with separation/individuation, difficulties with self-esteem regulation, pathogenic family styles of interaction, and pathogenic social input are thought to be important but have not been empirically established (72). Preoccupation with appearance and weight may become the focus for attempts at mastery during developmentally stressful periods such as adolescence. Women with greater degrees of conflict regarding maturation, separation, sexuality, self-esteem, or compulsivity or greater difficulties in tension regulation may be more prone than others to develop eating disorders. For example, anorexia nervosa can provide a means for avoiding both physical and psychological aspects of sexuality (30, 59). Initially, patients may be rewarded for thinness by family and peers, and peers may even compete in this regard. However, as symptoms become habitual, many patients experience a growing sense of the eating disorder becoming their core identity. Other patients persistently deny the abnormality or the severity of their eating disorders.

3. Culturally mediated distortions

Constructs such as self-worth and attractiveness have become closely associated with dieting and weight control for women in Western culture (69, 70, 73) and among immigrant women undergoing rapid cultural change (74). Challenging distorted values related to shape without attacking individual bases for self-esteem is a delicate task requiring clinical sensitivity (64, 75).

B. Treatment of Anorexia Nervosa: Indications, Efficacy, and Safety

Anorexia nervosa is a medically, psychopathologically, and interpersonally complex, serious, and often chronic condition that requires ongoing commitment and attention to the multiple, interdigitating diagnoses and to a comprehensive treatment plan that involves medical management, individual psychotherapy, and family therapy.

At the present time the best initial results appear linked to weight restoration accompanied by individual and family psychotherapies when the patient is medically ready to participate.

1. Nutritional rehabilitation and treatment setting

There is general agreement that weight restoration should be a central, early treatment goal for the seriously underweight patient (76). Weight restoration per se in these patients may result in improvement in obsessional thinking, mood, and personality disturbance.

a. Target weights. The ultimate weight target should be a return to an individually determined healthy body weight, one at which normal reproductive function resumes (77–79) and bone demineralization is reversed (80). The relationship between an individual's healthy weight and "ideal weights" published in standard tables (e.g., Metropolitan Life Insurance Company 1983 [81], National Center for Health Statistics 1973 [82]) is quite variable; some patients have always been slim and others may require a weight of 115% or more of published ideal weight for height to achieve a healthy status. Weight at discharge in relation to the healthy target weight may vary depending on the patient's ability to feed herself, her motivation and ability to participate in aftercare programs, and the adequacy of aftercare, including partial hospitalization.

Because several different "standards" of ideal body weight exist and healthy weights may be more properly understood in terms of ranges rather than specific numbers, many eating disorders consultants are moving toward the use of the body mass index as a standard measure of nutritional status rather than percentages of ideal body weight: body mass index = weight (kg)/ height (m)^2. Healthy ranges for body mass index are related to the age of the patient, and appropriate tables should be consulted (83, 84).

b. Choice of setting. Although some underweight patients who are less than 20% below average weight for height may be successfully treated outside of the hospital, such treatment usually requires a highly motivated patient, cooperative family, and brief duration of symptoms. Such patients may be treated in outpatient programs with close monitoring for several weeks to assess their response (85–87). Most severely underweight patients and those with physiological instability require inpatient medical management and comprehensive treatment for support of weight gain. Decisions to hospitalize on a psychiatric versus general medical or adolescent/pediatric unit depend on the patient's medical status and on the skills and abilities of local psychiatric and medical staff and local programs to care for the patient's medical and psychiatric problems (88).

Increasingly, partial hospitalization day hospital programs are being utilized in attempts to decrease the length of some inpatient hospitalizations and, for milder cases, in place of hospitalization. However, such programs cannot always easily replace traditional hospital programs or shorten lengths of stay, especially for patients with lower initial weights (e.g., those who are 70% of average weight for height, or below) (89). In order to benefit from partial hospitalization, patients must be motivated to participate in an intensive treatment program with mutually agreed-upon expectations of symptomatic change, including weight gain and/or decreased binge eating or purging, and must also demonstrate ability to relate in a group setting (90).

c. Inpatient programs. Regardless of the treatment setting, the availability of staff trained in and knowledgeable about the care of persons with eating disorders is critical. Where the staff does not have the training or experience to deal with patients with eating disorders, the psychiatrist or other qualified professionals must spend time educating, consulting with, and supervising the staff and managing their reactions to the patient's condition. Such work with the staff, though time consuming, is essential to the success of the treatment (91).

Both positive (e.g., praise) and negative (e.g., restriction of exercise or bed rest) reinforcers can influence the rates at which patients eat and gain weight, and combinations of informational feedback regarding weight gain and caloric intake, large meals, and behavioral programs may produce good short-term therapeutic effects (92). Moreover, a meta-analysis of treatment programs using medications or psychotherapy suggested that medication programs alone have failed to produce consistent weight gain in anorexia nervosa. Programs utilizing behavior therapy were more efficient, resulting in shorter hospital stays (92). However, the speed of weight gain during inpatient treatment is no assurance of long-term outcome.

Some studies have shown that "lenient" behavioral programs utilizing initial bed rest and the threat of returning the patient to bed if weight gain does not continue may be as effective and perhaps in some situations more efficient than "strict" programs in which meal-by-meal caloric intake or daily weight is tied precisely to a schedule of privileges such as time out of bed, time off the unit, and permission to exercise or receive visitors (93, 94). Lenient programs are more likely to enlist the patient's cooperation and sense of participation and control; they also increase staff satisfaction by reducing the policing functions. In strict programs, staff are more likely to develop conflicted relationships with patients that interfere with supportive and empathic aspects of the treatment process. The relative merits of various degrees of strictness and leniency require further study. However, some basic milieu practices may be necessary, such as routinely restricting unaccompanied use of the bathroom for a period of time following meals to discourage purging. These practices may be individualized depending on the patient's past history and personality structure.

Most consultants believe that nasogastric tube feeding or even total parenteral nutrition may be required only rarely and in life-threatening situations. There is significant recognition of the danger of rapid refeeding (e.g., severe fluid retention and cardiac failure) and of forced nasogastric or parenteral feeding. These interventions should not be used routinely. However, some severely malnourished anorexic patients may accept nasogastric feeding more willingly than eating, especially in the early stages of renourishment. In situations where forced feeding is considered, careful thought should be given to clinical circumstances, family opinion, and relevant legal and ethical dimensions of the patient's treatment.

d. Hospital stay.   Research addressing optimal length of hospitalization is sparse. In one study, significantly fewer relapses were observed in patients able to complete an inpatient treatment program (discharged at normal weight) compared with those who left the hospital before completing treatment (95).

2.   Psychosocial treatment

The exact role of psychotherapy in the acute treatment of the hospitalized, severely malnourished patient remains unclear. Although some studies question the utility of individual or family psychotherapy during the acute refeeding stage (96), there is general consensus that the patient and her family have to be engaged from the very beginning of treatment and should be educated as to the nature of the patient's condition, the relationships among semistarvation and the symptoms of anorexia nervosa, psychodynamic, family, and sociocultural issues, and related matters (97, 98). This engagement can serve as a foundation for the later use of more insight-oriented therapies. Family or individual/ couples psychotherapy for parents is frequently useful in helping young patients achieve age-appropriate separation and symptom alleviation. One study showed that 1 year following discharge from the hospital, patients with anorexia nervosa with onset at or before age 18 and with a duration of fewer than 3 years showed greater improvement with family therapy than individual psychotherapy; in contrast, older anorexia nervosa patients did better with individual therapy than with family therapy (99). However, patients in this study were not assigned to *both* family and individual treatment, a combination frequently used in practice.

Since many patients have difficulty talking about their problems, clinicians have also tried a variety of nonverbal therapies, such as creative arts therapies, and have reported them to be useful (100).

Consultants agree that having the same psychiatrist treat the patient throughout hospitalization and aftercare, using therapeutic modalities that best fit the circumstances, constitutes a desirable approach whenever practical.

Many types of therapies have been reported to be of value in case series (49). Although intensive psychodynamic psychotherapy may sometimes be ineffective with emaciated patients during the acute weight restoration phase, many consultants see psychodynamic or interpersonal psychotherapies as very useful for subsequent psychological maturation during weight maintenance. The experience of a large number of psychoanalytically trained psychiatrists suggests that good results may be obtained by psychoanalysis or psychoanalytic psychotherapy in nondebilitated patients when underlying personality disorders are important in contributing to the illness. Psychiatrists treating patients from a strictly psychoanalytic perspective will focus on longer-term treatment-oriented goals, not focused on, but resulting in, weight restoration. The experience of these clinicians suggests that in most cases their results are as rapid as, and more durable than, most other methods of treatment (32, 101). Many clinicians favor cognitive-behavioral psychotherapies for maintaining healthy eating behavior and cognitive or interpersonal psychotherapies for inducing mature insights and promoting more effective coping (102, 103). The use of various modalities considered coercive by patients with anorexia nervosa, for whom control is of such importance, is an issue to be carefully weighed.

3. Medications

Few controlled studies of the use of medications for anorexia nervosa have been published. In one study lower-weight patients with the restricting subtype who were receiving intensive inpatient treatment seemed to benefit, albeit to a small degree, from cyproheptadine; amitriptyline had some value as well (104). Results from studies with lithium (105), clomipramine (in lower-than-usual doses) (106), and pimozide (107) have been unimpressive. Because of reported increased seizure risk associated with bupropion in patients with eating disorders, this medication cannot be recommended for such patients (108, 109). There have been no controlled pharmacologic studies conducted solely with child or early adolescent populations of patients with eating disorders.

Many different somatic treatments ranging from vitamin and hormone treatments to electroconvulsive therapy have been tried in uncontrolled studies. None has been shown to have specific value (23). Medications used most often on an empirical basis include antidepressants for patients with depressions that persist in spite of or in the absence of weight gain; low doses of neuroleptics for marked obsessionality, anxiety, and psychotic-like thinking; and antianxiety agents used selectively before meals to reduce anticipatory anxiety concerning eating (110, 111). Uncontrolled trials have suggested that fluoxetine may help some patients in weight restoration (112) and weight maintenance phases (113), but many patients do not improve with this or any other currently available medication. Although fluoxetine has been reported at higher doses (e.g., 60 mg/day or more) to impair appetite and cause weight loss in normal-weight and obese patients, this effect has not been reported in anorexia nervosa patients treated at lower doses.

Most consultants 1) find that malnourished depressed patients are more prone to the side effects of and less responsive to antidepressant medications than other patients with depression; 2) are concerned that tricyclic antidepressants may add to the risk of hypotension and arrhythmia in anorexia nervosa patients, particularly in purging anorexia nervosa patients whose hydration may be inadequate and whose cardiac status may be nutritionally compromised; and 3) find that at least some symptoms of depression remit with weight gain. However, for patients with persistent depression the use of antidepressants should always be considered; these medications may be helpful if not contraindicated by cardiovascular status. For patients in whom potential cardiovascular effects of medication are of concern, consultations to evaluate cardiovascular status and to advise on the use of medication may be helpful.

Estrogen replacement to reduce calcium loss and thereby reduce the risks of osteoporosis is sometimes used in anorexia nervosa patients with chronic amenorrhea and should be considered (114). However, for adolescent patients, authorities advocate waiting at least 1 year before offering estrogen replacement (115), during which time efforts should be made to increase weight and achieve resumption of normal menses.

4.   Application of the addiction model

Given the high prevalence of substance abuse among persons with eating disorders and the likelihood that either condition may precipitate the other, where substance abuse exists it is important that a progressive treatment plan be initiated for this disorder as well (116).

Some clinicians consider that eating disorders may be usefully treated via addiction models, but no data from short- or long-term outcome studies with these methods have been reported. These programs should be equipped to care for patients with substantial psychiatric and/or general medical problems associated with their eating disorders.

C.   Prognosis in Anorexia Nervosa

Reviews of carefully done follow-up studies conducted on hospitalized or tertiary referral populations at least 4 years after onset of illness show that about 44% of patients had an overall good outcome (weight restored to within 15% of recommended weight for height and regular menstruation established), about 24% had poor outcome (weight never approached 15% under recommended weight for height and menstruation was absent or at best sporadic), about 28% had an intermediate outcome (between that of the good and poor groups), and fewer than 5% had died (early mortality). Poorer prognosis has been associated with initial lower minimum weight, the presence of vomiting, failure to respond to previous treatment, premorbidly disturbed family relationships, and marital status (being married) (117, 118). Mortality, primarily resulting from cardiac arrest or suicide, increased with length of follow-up and reached about 20% among patients followed for more than 20 years (119). Furthermore, about two-thirds of patients continued to have persistent morbid food and weight preoccupations, up to 40% had bulimic symptoms, and many had dysthymia, social phobia, obsessive-compulsive symptoms, and/or substance abuse (28). Patients with less severe degrees of illness, whose conditions therefore permit them to be treated primarily as outpatients, tend to have better outcomes. However, the chronic nature of anorexia nervosa often requires that even patients with less severe illness participate in long-term maintenance treatment programs to prevent relapse.

D.   Treatment of Bulimia Nervosa:
Indications, Efficacy, and Safety

Strategies for the treatment of bulimia nervosa include nutritional counseling and rehabilitation; individual and/or group cognitive-behavioral, behavioral, psychoanalytic, and psychodynamic approaches; family interventions; and medications (120).

1.   Hospitalization

Most consultants currently hold that hospital treatment for uncomplicated bulimia nervosa is rarely necessary and that such patients should first be treated in outpatient or day hospital programs. Hospitalization should be considered in cases complicated by suicidality, severe concurrent alcohol or drug abuse, or life-endangering medical problems not amenable to outpatient treatment. For those whose eating behavior is entirely out of control and who do not make substantial progress during an adequate trial of outpatient treatment, hospital admission aimed at breaking the binge-purge cycle may prove helpful. These periods of stabilization often require several weeks.

2. Psychosocial treatment

Patients treated for bulimia nervosa appear to improve; however, the number of patients who achieve full abstinence from binge-purge behavior is highly variable, with the minority becoming fully abstinent, according to most published studies. Many therapeutic approaches including individual cognitive-behavioral therapy, behavior therapy, focal psychotherapy (121), psychodynamic and interpersonal psychotherapy, psychoanalysis, and addiction-oriented therapy have value (122–128). Nevertheless, current research emphasizes cognitive-behavioral therapy for symptom reduction, at least in the short run (129). One study found that although cognitive-behavioral therapy, interpersonal psychotherapy, and behavior therapy were all effective in reducing binge eating and depressive symptoms, cognitive-behavioral therapy was more effective than the other two in modifying outpatients' disturbed attitudes toward shape, weight, dieting, and the use of vomiting to control shape and weight (129). When cognitive therapy was compared to short-term focal psychotherapies both were effective, but patients treated with cognitive-behavioral therapy had greater overall improvement (121). Clinicians unfamiliar with this approach may benefit from cognitive-behavioral therapy treatment manuals for bulimia nervosa (130–134). Still, given the complexities of concurrent psychopathologies in patients with bulimia nervosa, many therapeutic strategies have a role, and individual psychodynamic and interpersonal, family-oriented, and psychoanalytic therapies, which many clinicians find useful and which have yet to be used as comparison treatments in any well-designed studies, may be particularly useful for long-term functioning. For example, as eating disorders symptoms abate, some patients with prior histories of traumatization and abuse may experience an intensification of other symptoms, including posttraumatic stress disorder symptoms (135).

Conflicting evidence exists as to whether the behavioral procedure of exposure (binge eating food) plus response prevention (inhibiting vomiting) (136, 137) is superior to, adds to, or subtracts from the efficacy of cognitive-behavioral therapy alone, and evidence is available to support each of these viewpoints (138–140).

Many controlled group psychotherapy studies of bulimia have been reported, all showing treatment superior to no treatment (141–147). A recent meta-analysis of 40 group treatment studies of bulimia suggested moderate efficacy, with improvement typically maintained in those studies reporting 1-year follow-up data (148). Larger posttreatment effect sizes are associated with more hours of therapy per week and with the addition of other treatment components such as individual therapy (149). Although some reports suggest that group treatments tend to have a higher dropout rate compared to individual treatments (150), this finding has been questioned. There is some evidence that treatments that include dietary counseling and management as part of the program perform better that those that do not (125, 151), and available evidence suggests that more frequent visits early in treatment produce better results (63, 129, 152).

Virtually every type of individual psychotherapy for the treatment of bulimia nervosa has been described in uncontrolled case series, and many seem to help (49). In practice, many consultants use psychodynamically oriented and interpersonal psychotherapies after initial symptom control and, at times, to help patients with initial symptom resolution. In properly selected cases, psychoanalytic psychotherapy and psychoanalysis have been reported to successfully address the psychological conflicts associated with patients' symptoms and to lead to symptom alleviation (32). Family therapy was reported as helpful in a large case series (153). Although no systematic studies exist, some patients have found Overeaters Anonymous and similar groups to be helpful in recovery, in part because of the networking, sense of connectedness to a group, and 24-hour-per-day support against food cravings that they offer (154, 155). At the same time, controversy exists regarding the role of 12-step programs that do not address nutritional considerations and psychological/behavioral deficits when used as the sole intervention in the treatment of eating disorders (128).

3.   Medications

Double-blind placebo-controlled studies have demonstrated the efficacy of imipramine (156, 157), desipramine (158), trazodone (159), and fluoxetine (160, 161) in reducing bulimic symptoms. In the imipramine studies, the large majority of patients reduced their eating binges by at least half, and about a third became free of binge eating and purging. In the desipramine study about two-thirds of those who achieved therapeutic blood levels experienced a remission in bulimic symptoms. This is the only study thus far to demonstrate a relationship between serum drug level and symptom response in bulimia. Furthermore, the desipramine study involved only nondepressed bulimic patients.

The monoamine oxidase inhibitors (MAOIs) phenelzine (162) and isocarboxazid (163) have been shown to effectively reduce bulimic symptoms. Recent data suggest that patients with atypical depression and bulimia may preferentially respond to phenelzine in comparison to imipramine (58). Because some patients have difficulty avoiding foods containing tyramine, a careful evaluation of the patient's reliability in maintaining a tyramine-free diet is indicated when MAOIs are being considered (111, 164). Carbamazepine (165) and lithium have been less effective in treating the symptoms of bulimia (166, 167), and their occasional adjunctive use in patients with eating disorders should rest on consideration of other comorbid conditions.

To summarize, antidepressant medications can be useful in the treatment of bulimia nervosa. Doses of tricyclic and MAOI antidepressants used to treat bulimia nervosa are generally at the same levels as those used to treat mood disorders. However, higher doses of fluoxetine (60 mg/day) seem more effective than lower doses (20 mg/day) (160). Several medication trials are sometimes required to establish the proper medication for a given patient (168, 169).

4.   Psychosocial and/or medication strategies

Few studies have compared psychosocial and medication treatments (170, 171). In one study in which patients were randomly assigned to treatment or placebo groups, intensive group outpatient treatment, imipramine, and imipramine plus intensive group outpatient treatment were all better than placebo, and intensive group outpatient treatment was superior to imipramine alone in reducing binge eating, purging, and symptoms of depression (170). The intensive group outpatient treatment included many hours per week of structured meetings and lectures, and meals were provided for several weeks. The program was based on cognitive-behavioral and educational principles. Adding imipramine to intensive group outpatient treatment did not improve outcome with respect to eating behaviors per se, but did improve outcome for symptoms of depression and anxiety. However, use of active drug was also associated with a higher dropout rate.

In a study in which patients were randomly assigned to cognitive-behavioral therapy alone, cognitive-behavioral therapy plus desipramine, or desipramine alone, both cognitive-behavioral therapy groups were superior to desipramine alone. At 24 weeks, cognitive-behavioral therapy in combination with desipramine (but not cognitive-behavioral therapy alone) was superior to 16 weeks of desipramine alone in reducing binge eating and purging, dietary preoccupation, and hunger (171).

However, the use of a single antidepressant medication in these comparisons does not reflect actual clinical practice. Typically, when one antidepressant fails, a clinician will try a second or third agent, and this full range of choices often results in better antidepressant efficacy than was found in the studies mentioned (159, 168). Other medications, including narcotic antagonists and tryptophan, have been used but have received less systematic study; these medications should rarely be necessary.

E. Prognosis in Bulimia Nervosa

Little is known about the natural history or long-term outcome of bulimia nervosa. The overall short-term success rate for patients receiving psychosocial or medication treatment varies; patients have been reported to have a 50%–90% reduction in binge eating and purging, with an average of about 70% of those who complete the treatment programs reporting substantial reduction of bulimic symptoms. Those treated as outpatients seem to maintain symptomatic improvement over follow-up periods of up to 6 years; however, some symptoms often persist (172, 173). Patients who function well and have milder symptoms at the start of treatment, and so are more likely to be treated as outpatients, often have a better prognosis than those who function poorly and have disabling symptoms. In contrast, at 3 years about 27% of patients hospitalized with bulimia have a good outcome (binge eating and purging less than once a month), 40% have an intermediate outcome, and 33% a have a poor outcome (daily binge eating and vomiting or ongoing cathartic-diuretic abuse) (174). It is also well known that anorexia nervosa patients who purge are at much greater risk for developing serious medical complications (175). Very little is known about the prognosis of untreated bulimia nervosa. Over a 1- to 2-year period, bulimic patients who were never treated have reported modest degrees of spontaneous improvement, with roughly 25%–30% reductions in their overall levels of binge eating, purging, and laxative abuse (176, 177).

III. Recommendations

The following recommendations are based upon the degree and quality of the research data and/or clinical consensus.

A. General Principles of Assessment of Eating Disorders

The following are recommended:

1. Comprehensive multidimensional assessment. At the very outset, clinicians should attempt to build trust, establish mutual respect, and develop a therapeutic relationship with the patient that will serve as the basis for ongoing exploration and treatment of the problems associated with eating disorders. During data gathering, clinicians and patients may initially be helped by semistructured interview instruments, such as the Eating Disorders Examination (178), or by the many well-regarded self-report questionnaires, such as the Eating Disorders Questionnaire (179), the Diagnostic Survey for Eating Disorders (180), the Stanford Eating Disorders Questionnaire (181), or the Eating Disorders Inventory (182), although their specific validity for populations of children and young adolescents has not been reported [E,F]. The complete assessment usually requires at least several hours, and often patients and their families may not initially reveal pertinent information about sensitive issues even when directly questioned. Some important information may be uncovered only during ongoing treatment, after a trusting relationship has been established and the patient is better able to accurately identify inner emotional states.

a. Eating disorder signs and symptoms.   Initial assessment generally includes a longitudinal history regarding lifetime actual and desired weights in relation to height; onset and patterns of menstruation; food restriction and avoidances; frequency and extent of binge eating, self-induced vomiting, and spontaneous vomiting; use of laxatives, diuretics, diet pills, and ipecac; and body-image and self-image disturbances. Food intake, food preferences and peculiarities, attitudes toward food, cognitive distortions regarding food and appearance, ritualistic and compulsive behaviors regarding food and exercise, and details of other associated behavioral, psychological, and social impairments should generally also be assessed. It is often helpful in understanding the patient's problems to explore the patient's understanding of how the illness developed and the effect of any interpersonal relationships on the onset of the eating disorder. For patients whose recollections are vague, taking the detailed history of a single day or using a calendar as a timeline prompt may help elicit specific information. Much useful information is often obtainable by a less structured, open-ended approach. Family history should be obtained regarding eating disorders and other psychiatric disorders, obesity, family interactions in relation to the patient's disorder, and attitudes toward eating, exercise, and appearance [E,F]. It may be helpful to involve health professionals who routinely work with children, parents, and school personnel in the assessment of young patients.

b. Psychiatric history. Attention should be paid to concurrent psychiatric disturbances, especially affective and anxiety disorders, suicidality, substance abuse, obsessive and compulsive symptoms, and personality disturbances. Shoplifting, stealing food, and self-mutilatory behaviors should be noted. A developmental history should attend to temperament, sexual and physical abuse, and sexual history. Psychological testing may clarify personality/neuropsychological disturbances. In addition to assessing behavioral and formal psychopathological aspects of the case, it is generally useful to investigate psychodynamic and interpersonal conflicts that may be relevant to understanding and treating the patient's eating disorder and to assess the patient's potential (e.g., motivation, self-awareness, availability of affects) for psychodynamic and interpersonal psychotherapies [E,F].

c. Physical health status. A full physical examination should be performed with particular attention to vital signs, weight for height, skin, the cardiovascular system, and evidence of laxative or diuretic abuse and vomiting. A dental examination should be performed. It is generally useful to assess growth, sexual development, and general physical development in younger patients. Laboratory studies should be determined on an individual basis depending on the patient's condition and as necessary for making treatment decisions. For ambulatory patients who are not obviously underweight, tests may include a complete blood count, urinalysis, BUN/creatinine levels, and electrolyte balance. For malnourished and severely symptomatic patients, laboratory studies often also include measures of calcium, magnesium, phosphorus, amylase, and liver function and an ECG. In all cases, if the patient is more than 15% below healthy body weight or if weight loss has been rapid, significant physical compromise may be present even if the ECG, laboratory studies, and physical examination appear normal [E,F].

d. Family assessment. Assessment of the family is important whenever possible for patients of any age living at home and for others who are so enmeshed with their families as to preclude all efforts to function independently. Family assessment may be extremely useful for some patients in order to understand interactions that may contribute to ongoing illness or that may potentially facilitate recovery [E,F].

2. Coordinated care plan. The coordinated care plan requires the collaboration of a variety of professionals to provide nutritional counseling and dental assessment, work with the family, and set up behavioral programs. Other physician specialists and dentists should be consulted when necessary for management of medical (e.g., cardiac dysfunction) and dental complications [E,F].

Other options which may be recommended in individual circumstances:

1. Imaging techniques and evaluation of brain function. Although abnormalities are frequently found on magnetic resonance imaging (MRI) and CT scans of the head and EEG, the therapeutic implications of these findings are unclear. Consequently, these tests are not routinely indicated. Consultants are of mixed opinions as to whether abnormalities on such tests are likely to increase patient compliance with treatment; the large majority believe that they have little value in this regard, but others believe that presenting patients with objective evidence of brain abnormalities may increase compliance with treatment [F].

2. Other laboratory tests. Depending on potential treatment decisions that may be heavily influenced by laboratory findings, the following tests may sometimes be of value: serum amylase levels as a possible indicator of persistent or recurrent vomiting behavior; estradiol levels in amenorrheic patients (low values are suggestive of bone loss); bone mineral densitometry to assess risk for pathological fractures secondary to osteoporosis in chronic anorexia nervosa; and levels of luteinizing hormone (LH) and follicle-stimulating hormone (FSH) when amenorrhea persists at normal weight [E,F].

3. Modification of approaches. Circumstances that may require modification of the assessment and treatment approaches described in these guidelines include problems in the availability of resources, treatment-reluctant or treatment-resistant patients, substantial problems of comorbidity, and particularly difficult family/social problems [F].

B.   Treatment of Anorexia Nervosa

The following are recommended:

1. Initial treatment setting. A trial of outpatient treatment or partial hospitalization is warranted for highly motivated patients who have good social supports, are not losing weight rapidly, are metabolically stable, whose weight is not below 70% of average weight for height, and when close monitoring of physical state can be guaranteed [E,F]. However, many patients require hospital treatment. Patients with rapidly falling weight or metabolic instability need to be hospitalized earlier in the course of care than others, as may children and young adolescents [E,F]. Legal interventions may be necessary to ensure the safety of treatment-reluctant patients whose medical conditions are life-threatening.

2. Aims of treatment. The aims of treatment should be to 1) restore patients to a healthy weight (at which menses will generally resume); 2) restore healthy eating patterns; 3) treat/remediate physical complications; 4) address dysfunctional thoughts, feelings, and beliefs; 5) correct defects in affect and behavioral regulation; 6) improve associated psychological difficulties; 7) enlist family support of treatment where appropriate; and 8) prevent relapse. Many consultants believe that patients are less likely to relapse if they are hospitalized until they achieve healthy weight [E,F]. Those patients who are fully cooperative with their treatment, are achieving treatment goals, and for whom good aftercare is available may be discharged before full healthy weight is restored, with the plan that additional weight will be gained during aftercare [E].

Hospital programs should establish healthy target weights and expected rates of controlled weight gain to reassure patients that they can develop control over their own eating patterns. A supportive, encouraging staff with whom patients and families may develop realistic, trusting relationships is essential. Expectations for a reasonable rate of weight gain (e.g., 1–3 lb/week on inpatient units) and some positive and negative reinforcements (e.g., required bed rest, restriction of off-unit privileges, exercise contingent upon weight gain) should be built into the program [C,D,E,F,G]. Medical monitoring during refeeding should include vital signs, food and fluid intake and output, and observation for edema, rapid weight gain associated primarily with fluid overload, congestive heart failure, and gastrointestinal symptoms [E,F]. Outpatient programs often establish expectations of weight gain in the range of $\frac{1}{2}$–2 lb/week [F]. A patient suspected of artificially increasing her weight should be weighed in the morning after voiding, wearing only a gown; her fluid intake should be carefully monitored. Physical activity should be adapted to the food intake and energy expenditure of the patient, taking into account bone mineral density and cardiac function. The focus of an exercise program should be on physical fitness as opposed to expending calories. Staff should help patients deal with their concerns about weight gain and body image changes, as these are particularly difficult adjustments for patients to make [F].

3. Meal selection and caloric intake. Although it is most desirable to help patients to eventually choose their own meals and to not avoid any of the major food groups, initially meal selection may be best recommended by a dietitian. Usual starting intakes of 30–40 kcal/kg per day (approximately 1000–1600 kcal/day) may ultimately have to be increased to as high as 70–100 kcal/kg per day for some patients during the weight gain phase, with 40–60 kcal/kg per day during weight maintenance [C,E]. Some patients who require higher caloric intakes are exercising frequently, vomiting, or discarding food, while others may have a truly elevated metabolic rate. Nutritional assessment, education, and ongoing support are essential [A,B].

4. Medications. Medications should not be used routinely [A,C,D,E,F]. The role for antidepressants is usually best assessed following weight gain, when the psychological effects of malnutrition are resolving; however, these medications should be considered when depression persists [F].

Patients who are persistent purgers should have ongoing monitoring of serum potassium levels. Chronic hypokalemia should be treated with oral potassium supplementation [F].

5. Discharge criteria for hospitalized patients. Patients may be discharged from the hospital when they are medically stable and weight has been restored to a suitable level, behavioral symptoms have been substantially controlled, sufficient work with psychological and family factors has been undertaken assuring that aftercare treatment will be focused on relevant areas, and a targeted aftercare plan has been formulated and can be implemented.

6. Longer-term goals. Longer-term goals include improving enduring moods, personality disturbances, interpersonal relationships, and social functioning. Supportive and educative therapies should begin on initial contact. For patients accessible to insight therapy, a relationship with a therapist should be established as soon as possible [F].

7. Family involvement. Families should usually be engaged from the beginning of treatment and included in family meetings and treatment planning sessions [E,F]. Psychotherapy with the family (if possible with at least both parents, if not all family members) should be instituted when family members are able to participate without being persistently, destructively critical toward the patient and when no family member is so disruptive as to preclude productive work [F]. Hypercritical parents may first be seen without the patient present to help prepare them to participate in constructive family therapy that includes the patient. Family therapy is most useful for younger patients [A], and many experts consider family therapy to be mandatory for children and younger adolescents [F]. Marital therapy may be useful for married patients [F].

8. Psychotherapy. Psychotherapy should be tailored to the level of cognitive development, style, and complexity of the individual patient and family. Empathic support, education, insight, and problem solving should be used as soon as the patient is accessible to them. Because of the enduring and tenacious quality of many of the psychopathological and personality disturbance features and the need for considerable change and support during recovery, ongoing treatment in individual and/or group settings, at varying intervals depending on the patient's psychopathology and medical status, is frequently required for at least a year and often for several years [E,F].

9. Considerations regarding chronicity. Since many patients have a chronic course of illness, are unable to maintain a healthy weight, and often suffer from chronic depression, obsessionality, and social withdrawal, individualized treatment planning and careful case management are necessary. Treatment may require consultation with other specialists, subsequent rehospitalization, partial hospitalization, residential care, individual and/or group therapy, medications as indicated, and other social therapies [E,F]. Communication among professionals is important throughout outpatient care. With chronic patients, small progressive gains and fewer relapses may be the goals of psychological interventions. More frequent outpatient contact and other supports may sometimes help to prevent further hospitalization [E,F]. Expectations for weight gain with hospitalization may be more modest for chronic patients; achieving a safe weight rather than a healthy weight may be all that is possible.

Other options which may be recommended in individual circumstances:

1. Dietary supplements. Treatment options for nutritional rehabilitation include supplementation—and for treatment-resistant hospitalized patients, replacement—of regular food with liquid food supplements until the patient can return to normal table food [E]. Normal foods are best introduced as soon as possible to help the patient overcome "food phobias."

2. Enteral tube feedings and parenteral alimentation. Rarely used options, in most instances requiring life-threatening or very unusual circumstances, may include nasogastric tube or in extreme cases parenteral feedings. These potentially life-saving interventions should be used for as brief a period of time as is necessary while normal eating is developed [E,F]. When the patient strongly objects to nasogastric or parenteral feeding in a life-threatening situation, an ethics consultation may be useful. Most consultants agree that these interventions should be used only when indicated by the patient's medical condition and not as a means of behavioral manipulation, although some believe that in early renourishment some severely malnourished patients accept passive feeding via nasogastric tube more easily than the active choice of eating [F].

3. Medications. At some points during treatment, tricyclic antidepressants [A,E], cyproheptadine [A], fluoxetine [E], antipsychotics [A,E], and antianxiety agents [E] may be useful for some patients. Medications should not be used as the sole or primary treatment for anorexia nervosa.

4. Management models. Some programs routinely arrange for "split management" models of treatment, wherein a therapist primarily conducts the psychodynamic therapy and another psychiatrist writes orders, handles administrative and medical requirements, and works on changing the disturbed eating and weight patterns directly. For this split management model to work effectively, all personnel must work closely together, maintaining open communication and mutual respect to avoid reinforcing some patients' tendencies to play staff off against one another, i.e., to "split" the staff [F].

An alternative split management approach is to have medical care providers (e.g., specialists in internal medicine, pediatrics, adolescent medicine) manage general medical issues, such as nutrition, weight gain, exercise, and eating patterns, while the psychiatric providers address psychiatric issues.

5. Support groups. Support groups led by professionals or advocacy organizations led by lay personnel that provide patients and their families with mutual support, advice, and education about eating disorders and their treatment may be of adjunctive benefit.

Treatment approaches not recommended:

Twelve-step-based programs or other approaches that focus exclusively on the need for abstinence without attending to nutritional considerations or behavioral deficits are not recommended as the sole initial treatment approach for anorexia nervosa [F]. The potential utility of these approaches in the *adjunctive* treatment of anorexia nervosa is an unsettled issue.

C.   Treatment of Bulimia Nervosa

The following are recommended:

1. Initial treatment approach.   Patients with bulimia nervosa uncomplicated by the abuse of laxatives, alcohol or drug abuse, psychosis, suicidality, or major personality disturbances rarely require hospitalization and may achieve substantial symptom reduction with brief individual [A] or group psychotherapies [A,G]. Nutritional counseling [A], cognitive-behavioral therapy [A], and simple behavioral techniques such as planned meals and diary keeping [A] appear particularly helpful for initial symptom management, interrupting the binge-purge behaviors. With such approaches, some degree of clinical improvement is often evident within 2 to 4 months of treatment. Psychodynamically and interpersonally oriented psychotherapies [E,F] and psychoanalysis [E,F] often help such patients recognize and alleviate conflicts that contribute to their symptoms.

2. Indications for hospitalization.   Indications for hospitalization include serious concurrent medical problems, psychiatric disturbances that would warrant the patient's hospitalization independent of the eating disorder diagnosis, or severe and disabling symptoms (e.g., multiple daily binges and purges that significantly disrupt vocational performance or activities of daily living, unremitting laxative abuse) which have not responded to adequate trials of competent outpatient treatment [E,F]. In cases where other treatment options such as suitable partial hospitalization or residential programs are not available locally, hospital-based treatment may occasionally be provided initially for severely symptomatic patients [F].

3. Discharge criteria for hospitalized patients.   Patients may be discharged from the hospital following substantial control of binge-purge cycles, laxative abuse, and other disabling symptoms, and when a targeted aftercare plan has been formulated and can be implemented.

4. Antidepressant medications.   Antidepressant medications may reduce symptoms of binge eating and purging independent of the presence of depression [A]. Antidepressants may be used as one component of an initial treatment program for most patients, but should not constitute the entire treatment [A,C,E]. They may be especially helpful for patients with significant symptoms of depression, anxiety, obsessions, or certain impulse disorder symptoms, or for patients who have failed previous attempts at appropriate psychosocial therapy [F]. Often, several different antidepressant medications may have to be tried sequentially to achieve the optimum effect. Doses of tricyclic and MAOI antidepressants for treating bulimia nervosa parallel those used to treat depression, although doses of fluoxetine higher than those used for depression may be more effective for bulimic symptoms [B,C,E,F]. In cases where symptoms do not respond to medication, it is important to assure that the patient has not taken the medication shortly before vomiting. Serum levels of medication may be obtained to determine whether presumably effective levels have actually been achieved [F].

5. Psychotherapy. Because of high rates of comorbid mood, anxiety, and personality disturbances and persistent, unresolved conflicts, recovering patients may achieve more lasting changes by continuing in extended psychotherapy or psychoanalysis that addresses relapse prevention and intrapsychic and interpersonal issues that come into focus as the initial symptoms of bulimia abate [C,E,F]. Psychodynamic, interpersonal, cognitive, or psychoanalytic approaches are most useful during this period. Therapeutic work may focus on common themes of development, identity formation, sexual and aggressive difficulties, affect regulation, gender role expectations, family dysfunction, coping styles, and problem solving. Patients with concurrent anorexia nervosa and/or concurrent borderline personality disorder usually require extended treatment [E,F].

6. Family therapy. Family therapy should be considered whenever possible and especially for adolescents still living with their parents, older patients with ongoing conflicted interactions with parents, or patients with marital discord [E,F].

7. Concurrent substance abuse disorders. Unless malnutrition is severe, concurrent substance abuse disorders should usually be attended to first, since successful treatment for bulimia nervosa in the presence of an active substance abuse disorder is unlikely. Where treatment staff are competent to treat both disorders, concurrent treatment may be attempted [E,F].

Other options which may be recommended in individual circumstances:

Twelve-step programs such as Overeaters Anonymous may be helpful as an adjunct to initial treatment of bulimia nervosa and for subsequent relapse prevention [C,E]. Because of the great variability of knowledge, attitudes, beliefs, and practices from chapter to chapter and from sponsor to sponsor regarding eating disorders and their medical and psychotherapeutic treatment, and because of the great variability of patients' personality structures, clinical conditions, and susceptibility to potentially countertherapeutic practices, clinicians should carefully monitor patients' experiences with 12-step programs [F].

Treatment approaches not recommended:

Twelve-step-based programs or other approaches that exclusively focus on the need for abstinence without attending to nutritional considerations or behavioral deficits are not recommended as the sole initial treatment approach for bulimia nervosa [F].

IV. Areas for Future Research

The many gaps in our knowledge are evident, but several areas requiring considerable research stand out.

A. Biological, psychological, and social predictors of recovery and nonrecovery for treated and untreated anorexia nervosa and bulimia nervosa patients:

1. The impact of various comorbid conditions including mood, anxiety, substance abuse, personality, and other commonly encountered concurrent disorders on course and treatment response.
2. Modifications of treatment necessary in the presence of comorbid conditions.

B. Treatment evaluation and outcome studies that attend to patient preferences, long-term outcomes, and costs in relation to:

1. Incrementally intensive care programs ("stepped-care") and treatment package approaches.
2. Inpatient versus partial hospitalization programs for anorexia nervosa (to establish better criteria for defining appropriate durations for hospital and partial hospital care).
3. Newer biological agents affecting mood, anxiety, hunger, and satiety.
4. Psychodynamic, interpersonal, psychotherapeutic, and psychoanalytically based treatments.
5. Treatments based on and/or including 12-step and other recovery models.
6. Addressing the unique developmental (biological, psychological, and social) needs of children and adolescents with eating disorders.
7. Nutritional counseling strategies to successfully facilitate maintenance of healthy eating habits and weight in recovering patients.
8. Alternative treatment approaches.
9. Methods to facilitate early recognition and referral.

V. Eating Disorders Guideline Reviewers and Consultants

David W. Abbott, M.D.
Sigurd H. Ackerman, M.D.
W. Stewart Agras, M.D.
Donald Banzhaf, M.D.
Joan K. Barber, M.D.
John C. Bartlett, M.D.
Lee H. Beecher, M.D.
Jerome S. Beigler, M.D.
Peter Beumont, M.D.
Charles Bowden, M.D.
Andrew W. Brotman, M.D.
Kelly D. Brownell, Ph.D.
Ewald W. Busse, M.D.
Regina C. Casper, M.D.
Martin Ceaser, M.D.
Drew Clemens, M.D.
Kenneth D. Cohen, M.D.
James L. Curtis, M.D.
Barbara G. Deutsch, M.D.
Elke D. Eckert, M.D.
Carole K. Edelstein, M.D.
Judith L. Feldman, M.D.
James M. Ferguson, M.D.
Manfred M. Fichter, M.D.
Stanley E. Fischman, M.D.
David L. Fogelson, M.D.
Saul Z. Forman, M.D.
Max L. Gardner, M.D.
David Garner, Ph.D.
Thomas D. Geracioti, M.D.
Seymour Gers, M.D.
Marla Gokee, M.D.
Carolyn N. Gracie, M.D.
Harry E. Gwirtsman, M.D.
Anne Hall, M.D.
Richard C.W. Hall, M.D.
Katherine A. Halmi, M.D.

Robert L. Hendren, D.O.
Alfred Herzog, M.D.
David B. Herzog, M.D.
Jules Hirsch, M.D.
Charles C. Hogan, M.D.
Andrew Hornstein, M.D.
Lee-Keung George Hsu, M.D.
James I. Hudson, M.D.
Laura Humphrey, Ph.D.
David C. Jimerson, M.D.
Bernard B. Kahan, M.D.
Jack Katz, M.D.
Walter H. Kaye, M.D.
Steven G. Kessler, M.D.
Howard Kibel, M.D.
Robert Klesges, Ph.D.
Dean D. Krahn, M.D.
Felix E.F. Larocca, M.D.
Gloria Leon, Ph.D.
Stewart Levine, M.D.
Lawrence B. Lurie, M.D.
R. Bruce Lydiard, Ph.D., M.D.
Mannuccio Mannucci, M.D.
Eric R. Marcus, M.D.
Margaret S. McKenna, M.D.
Diane W. Mickley, M.D.
Charles A. Murkofsky, M.D.
James E. Nininger, M.D.
Ralph A. O'Connell, M.D.
Inge S. Ortmeyer, CISW
Herbert S. Peyser, M.D.
Janet Polivy, Ph.D.
Harrison G. Pope, M.D.
Charles W. Portney, M.D.
David B. Pruitt, M.D.
Richard Pyle, M.D.
Lynn W. Reiser, M.D.

Ana-Maria Rizzuto, M.D.
Maria P.P. Root, Ph.D.
Barbara Rosenfeld, M.D.
Bruce S. Rothschild, M.D.
F. David Russek, M.D.
Eslee Samberg, M.D.
Patricia A. Santucci, M.D.
Harvey J. Schwartz, M.D.
Keith Sedlacek, M.D.
Catherine M. Shisslak, Ph.D.
Harvey R. St. Clair, M.D.
Ruth Striegel-Moore, Ph.D.

Michael Strober, Ph.D.
Albert J. Stunkard, M.D.
George Szmukler, M.D.
J. Kevin Thompson, Ph.D.
Stephen Touyz, Ph.D.
John C. Urbaitis, M.D.
R. Dale Walker, M.D.
B. Timothy Walsh, M.D.
Nicholas G. Ward, M.D.
Theodore E. Weltzin, M.D.
C. Philip Wilson, M.D.

VI. Organizations That Submitted Comments

Academy of Psychosomatic Medicine
Alcohol, Drug Abuse and Mental Health Administration
American Academy of Child and Adolescent Psychiatry
American Academy of Clinical Psychiatrists
American Academy of Family Physicians
American Academy of Pediatrics
American Academy of Psychiatrists in Alcoholism and Addiction
American Academy of Psychiatry and the Law
American Association of Chairmen of Departments of Psychiatry
American Association of Community Psychiatrists
American Association of Psychiatric Administrators
American Association of Psychiatric Services for Children
American Association of Psychiatrists from India
American Board of Forensic Psychiatry, Inc.
American College of Neuropsychopharmacology
American College of Physicians
American College of Psychoanalysts
American Hospital Association
American Nurses Association
American Psychoanalytic Association
American Psychological Association
American Society of Addiction Medicine
Anorexia Nervosa and Related Eating Disorders
Group for the Advancement of Psychiatry

Joint Commission on Accreditation of Healthcare Organizations
National Association of Private Psychiatric Hospitals
National Association of Social Workers
National Institute of Mental Health
National Institute on Alcohol Abuse and Alcoholism
National Institute on Drug Abuse
National Mental Health Association
Research Society on Alcoholism
Society for Adolescent Medicine
U.S. Veterans Administration, Mental Health Section

VII.   References

1. Andersen AE (ed): Males with Eating Disorders. New York, Brunner/Mazel, 1990 [I]
2. Lucas AR, Beard CM, O'Fallon WM, Kurlan LT: 50-year trends in the incidence of anorexia nervosa in Rochester, Minn.: a population-based study. Am J Psychiatry 1991; 148:917–922 [H]
3. Kendler KS, MacLean C, Neale M, Kessler R, Heath A, Eaves L: The genetic epidemiology of bulimia nervosa. Am J Psychiatry 1991; 148:1627–1637 [H]
4. Schotte DE, Stunkard AJ: Bulimia vs bulimic behaviors on a college campus. JAMA 1987; 258:1213–1215 [H]
5. Drewnowski A, Hopkins SA, Kessler RC: The prevalence of bulimia nervosa in the US college student population. Am J Public Health 1988; 78:1322–1325 [H]
6. Striegel-Moore RH, Silberstein LR, Frensch P, Rodin J: A prospective study of disordered eating among college students. Int J Eating Disorders 1989; 8:499–509 [C]
7. Kurtzman FD, Yager J, Landsverk J, Wiesmeier E, Bodurka DC: Eating disorders among select female student populations at UCLA. J Am Diet Assoc 1989; 89:45–53 [H]
8. Szmukler GI: The epidemiology of anorexia nervosa and bulimia. J Psychiatr Res 1985; 19:143–153 [H]
9. Herzog DB, Newman KL, Warshaw M: Body image dissatisfaction in homosexual and heterosexual males. J Nerv Ment Dis 1991; 179:356–359 [C]
10. Whitaker A, Johnson J, Shaffer D, Rapoport JL, Kalikow K, Walsh BT, Davies M, Braiman S, Dolinsky A: Uncommon troubles in young people: prevalence estimates of selected psychiatric disorders in a nonreferred adolescent population. Arch Gen Psychiatry 1990; 47:487–496 [H]
11. Beumont PJ, George GC, Smart DE: "Dieters" and "vomiters and purgers" in anorexia nervosa. Psychol Med 1976; 36:617–622 [C]
12. Casper RC, Eckert ED, Halmi KA, Goldberg SC, Davis JM: Bulimia: its incidence and clinical importance in patients with anorexia nervosa. Arch Gen Psychiatry 1980; 37:1030–1035 [C]
13. Garfinkel PE, Moldofsky H, Garner DM: The heterogeneity of anorexia nervosa: bulimia as a distinct subgroup. Arch Gen Psychiatry 1980; 37:1036–1040 [C]
14. Kassett JA, Gwirtsman HE, Kaye WH, Brandt HA, Jimerson DC: Pattern of onset of bulimic symptoms in anorexia nervosa. Am J Psychiatry 1988; 145:1287–1288 [C]

15. Wilson CP, Hogan CC, Mintz IL (eds): Fear of Being Fat: The Treatment of Anorexia Nervosa and Bulimia, 2nd ed. Northvale, NJ, Jason Aronson, 1985 [I]

16. Wilson CP, Hogan CC, Mintz IL (eds): Psychodynamic Technique in the Treatment of Eating Disorders. Northvale, NJ, Jason Aronson, 1992 [I]

17. Yates A: Compulsive Exercise and the Eating Disorders: Toward an Integrated Theory of Activity. New York, Brunner/Mazel, 1991 [I]

18. Schocken DD, Holloway JD, Powers PS: Weight loss and the heart: effects of anorexia nervosa and starvation. Arch Intern Med 1989; 149:877–881 [I]

19. Rigotti NA, Neer RM, Skates SJ, Herzog DB, Nussbaum SR: The clinical course of osteoporosis in anorexia nervosa: a longitudinal study of cortical bone mass. JAMA 1991; 265:1133–1138 [B]

20. Stewart DE, Robinson E, Goldbloom DS, Wright C: Infertility and eating disorders. Am J Obstet Gynecol 1990; 163:1196–1199 [C]

21. Halmi KA: Anorexia nervosa and bulimia. Annu Rev Med 1987; 38:373–380 [I]

22. Herzog DB, Copeland PM: Eating disorders. N Engl J Med 1985; 313:295–303 [I]

23. Garfinkel PE, Garner DM: Anorexia Nervosa: A Multidimensional Perspective. New York, Brunner/Mazel, 1982 [I]

24. Krieg JC, Pirke KM, Lauer C, Backmund H: Endocrine, metabolic, and cranial computed tomographic findings in anorexia nervosa. Biol Psychiatry 1988; 23:377–387 [E]

25. Dempsey DT, Crosby LO, Pertschuk MJ, Feurer ID, Buzby GP, Mullen JL: Weight gain and nutritional efficacy in anorexia nervosa. Am J Clin Nutr 1984; 39:236–242 [B]

26. Mitchell JE, Seim HC, Colon E, Pomeroy C: Medical complications and medical management of bulimia. Ann Intern Med 1987; 107:71–77 [I]

27. Obarzanek E, Lesem MD, Goldstein DS, Jimerson DC: Reduced resting metabolic rate in patients with bulimia nervosa. Arch Gen Psychiatry 1991; 48:456–462 [D]

28. Halmi KA, Eckert E, Marchi P, Sampugnaro V, Apple R, Cohen J: Comorbidity of psychiatric diagnoses in anorexia nervosa. Arch Gen Psychiatry 1991; 48:712–718 [H]

29. Sours J: Starving to Death in a Sea of Objects. New York, Jason Aronson, 1980 [I]

30. Crisp AH: Anorexia Nervosa: Let Me Be. London, Academic Press, 1980 [I]

31. Rothschild B: Sexual functioning of female eating disordered patients. Int J Eating Disorders 1991; 10:389–394 [C]

32. Schwartz HJ: Bulimia: Psychoanalytic Treatment and Theory, 2nd ed. Madison, CT, International Universities Press, 1990 [I]

33. Bulik CM, Sullivan PF, Rorty M: Childhood sexual abuse in women with bulimia. J Clin Psychiatry 1989; 50:460–464 [C]

34. Pope HG Jr, Hudson JI: Is childhood sexual abuse a risk factor for bulimia nervosa? Am J Psychiatry 1992; 149:455–463 [G]

35. Root MPP, Fallon P: Treating the victimized bulimic: the functions of binge-purge behavior. J Interpersonal Violence 1989; 4:90–100 [E]

36. Kasvikis YG, Tsakiris F, Marks IM, Basogul M, Noshirvani HF: Past history of anorexia nervosa in women with obsessive compulsive disorder. Int J Eating Disorders 1986; 5:1069–1076 [C]

37. Hudson JI, Pope HG Jr, Yurgelun-Todd D, Jonas JM, Frankenburg FR: A controlled study of lifetime prevalence of affective and other psychiatric disorders in bulimic outpatients. Am J Psychiatry 1987; 144:1283–1287 [C]

38. Shisslak CM, Perse T, Crago M: Coexistence of bulimia nervosa and mania: a literature review and case report. Compr Psychiatry 1991; 32:181–184 [E]

39. Gartner AF, Marcus RN, Halmi K, Loranger AW: DSM-III-R personality disorders in patients with eating disorders. Am J Psychiatry 1989; 146:1585–1591 [C]

40. Yager J, Landsverk J, Edelstein CK, Hyler SE: Screening for Axis II personality disorders in women with bulimic eating disorders. Psychosomatics 1989; 30:255–262 [C]

41. Zanarini MC, Frankenburg FR, Pope HG Jr, Hudson JI, Yurgelun-Todd D, Cicchetti CJ: Axis II comorbidity of normal weight bulimia. Compr Psychiatry 1990; 31:20–24 [H]

42. Wonderlich SA, Mitchell JE: Eating disorders and personality disorder, in Special Problems in Managing Eating Disorders. Edited by Yager J, Gwirtsman HE, Edelstein CK. Washington, DC, American Psychiatric Press, 1991 [I]

43. Favazza AR, DeRosear L, Conterio K: Self-mutilation and eating disorders. Suicide Life Threat Behav 1989; 19:352–361 [E]

44. Strober M, Lampert C, Morrell W, Burroughs J, Jacobs C: A controlled family study of anorexia nervosa: evidence of familial aggregation and lack of shared transmission with affective disorders. Int J Eating Disorders 1990; 9:239–253 [B]

45. Mitchell JE, Hatsukami D, Pyle R, Eckert E: Bulimia with and without a family history of drug abuse. Addict Behav 1988; 13:245–251 [C]

46. Pyle RL, Mitchell JE, Eckert ED: Bulimia: a report of 34 cases. J Clin Psychiatry 1981; 42:60–64 [E]

47. Casper RC, Davis JM: On the course of anorexia nervosa. Am J Psychiatry 1977; 134:974–978 [C]

48. Keys A, Brozek J, Henschel A, Mickelsen O, Taylor HL: The Biology of Human Starvation. Minneapolis, University of Minnesota Press, 1950 [B]

49. Garner DM, Garfinkel PE (eds): Handbook of Psychotherapy for Anorexia Nervosa and Bulimia. New York, Guilford Press, 1985 [I]

50. Kaye WH, Ebert MH, Raleigh M, Lake R: Abnormalities in CNS monoamine metabolism in anorexia nervosa. Arch Gen Psychiatry 1984; 41:350–355 [E]

51. Kaye WH, Gwirtsman HE, George DT, Ebert MH: Altered serotonin activity in anorexia nervosa after long-term weight restoration: does elevated cerebrospinal fluid 5-hydroxyindoleacetic acid level correlate with rigid and obsessive behavior? Arch Gen Psychiatry 1991; 48:556–562 [C]

52. Kaye WH, Berrettini WH, Gwirtsman HE, Gold PW, George DT, Jimerson DC, Ebert MH: Contribution of CNS neuropeptide (NPY, CRH, and beta-endorphin) alterations to psychophysiological abnormalities in anorexia nervosa. Psycho pharmacol Bull 1989; 25:433–438 [E]

53. Fava M, Copeland PM, Schweiger U, Herzog DB: Neurochemical abnormalities of anorexia nervosa and bulimia nervosa. Am J Psychiatry 1989; 146:963–971 [I]

54. Cantwell DP, Sturzenberger S, Burroughs J, Salkin B, Green JK: Anorexia nervosa: an affective disorder? Arch Gen Psychiatry 1977; 34:1087–1093 [B]

55. Hudson JI, Pope HG Jr: Affective spectrum disorder: does antidepressant response identify a family of disorders with a common pathophysiology? Am J Psychiatry 1990; 147:552–564 [I]

56. Ploog DW, Pirke KM: Psychobiology of anorexia nervosa. Psychol Med 1987; 17:843–859

57. Strober M, Katz J: Do eating disorders and affective disorders share a common etiology? Int J Eating Disorders 1987; 6:171–180 [I]

58. Rothschild R, Quitkin HM, Quitkin FM, Stewart JW, Ocepek-Welikson K, McGrath PJ, Tricamo E: A double-blind placebo controlled comparison of phenelzine and imipramine in the treatment of bulimia in atypical depression. Arch Gen Psychiatry (in press) [A]

59. Bruch H: Eating Disorders: Obesity, Anorexia Nervosa and the Person Within. New York, Basic Books, 1973 [I]

60. Johnson C (ed): Psychodynamic Treatment of Anorexia Nervosa and Bulimia. New York, Guilford Press, 1991 [I]

61. Levinson NA, Hessling T, Morris M: Eating disorders, in Female Psychology: An Annotated Psychoanalytic Bibliography. Edited by Shuker E, Levinson NA. Hillsdale, NJ, Analytic Press, 1991 [I]

62. Thoma H: Anorexia Nervosa. Madison, CT, International Universities Press, 1967 [E]

63. Fairburn C: A cognitive behavioral approach to the treatment of bulimia. Psychol Med 1981; 11:707–711 [E]

64. Garner DM, Bemis K: Cognitive therapy for anorexia nervosa, in Handbook of Psychotherapy for Anorexia Nervosa and Bulimia. Edited by Garner DM, Garfinkel PE. New York, Guilford Press, 1985 [I]

65. Andersen AE: A proposed mechanism underlying eating disorders and other disorders of motivated behavior, in Males With Eating Disorders. Edited by Andersen AE. New York, Brunner/Mazel, 1990 [I]

66. Minuchin S, Rosman BL, Baker L: Psychosomatic Families: Anorexia Nervosa in Context. Cambridge, MA, Harvard University Press, 1978 [I]

67. Palazzoli M: Self Starvation: From Individual to Family Therapy in the Treatment of Anorexia Nervosa. New York, Jason Aronson, 1978 [I]

68. Root MPP, Fallon P, Friedrich WN: Bulimia: A Family Systems Approach to Treatment. New York, WW Norton, 1986 [I]

69. Brumberg JJ: Fasting Girls: The Emergence of Anorexia Nervosa as a Modern Disease. Cambridge, MA, Harvard University Press, 1988 [I]

70. Striegel-Moore RH, Silberstein LR, Rodin J: Toward an understanding of risk factors for bulimia. Am Psychol 1986; 41:246–263 [I]

71. Orbach S: Hunger Strike: The Anorectic's Struggle as a Metaphor for Our Age. New York, WW Norton, 1986 [I]

72. Casper RC: Personality features of women with good outcome from restricting anorexia nervosa. Psychosom Med 1990; 52: 156–170 [B]

73. Dolan B: Cross-cultural aspects of anorexia nervosa and bulimia: a review. Int J Eating Disorders 1991; 10:67–80 [I]

74. DiNicola VF: Anorexia multiforme: self starvation in historical and cultural context. Transcultural Psychiatr Research Rev 1990; 27:245–286 [I]

75. Thompson JK: Body Image Disturbance: Assessment and Treatment. Elmsford, NY, Pergamon Press, 1990 [I]

76. Kaye WH, Gwirtsman HE, Obarzanek E, George DT: Relative importance of calorie intake needed to gain weight and level of physical activity in anorexia nervosa. Am J Clin Nutr 1988; 47:989–994 [C]

77. Frisch RE: The right weight: body fat, menarche and ovulation. Baillieres Clin Obstet Gynaecol 1990; 4:419–439 [G]

78. Frisch RE, McArthur JW: Menstrual cycles: fatness as a determinant of minimum weight for height necessary for their maintenance or onset. Science 1974; 185:949–951 [G]

79. Treasure JL: The ultrasonographic features in anorexia nervosa and bulimia nervosa: a simplified method of monitoring hormonal states during weight gain. J Psychosom Res 1988; 32: 623–634 [E]

80. Prior JC, Vigna YM, Schechter MT, Burgess AE: Spinal bone loss and ovulatory disturbances. N Engl J Med 1990; 323: 1221–1227 [C]

81. 1983 Metropolitan height and weight table. Stat Bull Metrop Life Found 1983; 64:3–9 [H]

82. National Center for Health Statistics: Height and weight of youths 12–17 years, United States. Vital and Health Statistics Series 11, Number 124. Health Services and Mental Health Administration. Washington DC, US Government Printing Office, 1973

83. Beumont P, Al-Alami M, Touyz S: Relevance of a standard measurement of undernutrition to the diagnosis of anorexia nervosa: use of Quetelet's Body Mass Index (BMI). Int J Eating Disorders 1988; 7:399–405 [I]

84. Hammer LD, Kraemer HC, Wilson DM, Ritter PL, Dornbusch SM: Standardized percentile curves of body-mass index for children and adolescents. Am J Dis Child 1991; 145:259–263 [H]

85. Owen W, Halmi KA: Medical evaluation and management of anorexia nervosa, in Treatments of Psychiatric Disorders: A Task Force Report of the American Psychiatric Association, vol 1. Washington, DC, APA, 1989 [I]

86. Andersen AE: Practical Comprehensive Treatment of Anorexia Nervosa and Bulimia. Baltimore, Johns Hopkins University Press, 1985 [I]

87. American Psychiatric Association: Eating disorders, in Treatments of Psychiatric Disorders: A Task Force Report of the American Psychiatric Association, vol 1. Washington, DC, APA, 1989 [I]

88. Maxmen JS, Silberfarb PM, Ferrell RB: Anorexia nervosa: practical initial management in a general hospital. JAMA 1974; 229: 801–803 [E]

89. Piran N, Kaplan AS (eds): A Day Hospital Group Treatment Program for Anorexia Nervosa and Bulimia Nervosa. New York, Brunner/Mazel, 1990 [I]

90. Kaplan AS: Day hospital treatment for anorexia and bulimia nervosa. Eating Disorders Rev 1991; 2:1–3 [I]

91. Andersen AE: Hospital treatment of anorexia nervosa, in Treatments of Psychiatric Disorders: A Task Force Report of the American Psychiatric Association, vol 1. Washington, DC, APA, 1989 [I]

92. Agras WS: Eating Disorders: Management of Obesity, Bulimia and Anorexia Nervosa. Oxford, Pergamon Press, 1987 [I]

93. Touyz SW, Beumont PJ, Glaun D, Phillips T, Cowie I: A comparison of lenient and strict operant conditioning programmes in refeeding patients with anorexia nervosa. Br J Psychiatry 1984; 144:517–520 [I]

94. Nusbaum JG, Drever E: Inpatient survey of nursing care measures for treatment of patients with anorexia nervosa. Issues in Mental Health Nursing 1990; 11:175–184 [J]

95. Halmi KA, Licinio E: Outcome: Hospital program for eating disorders, in CME Syllabus and Scientific Proceedings in Summary Form, 142nd Annual Meeting of the American Psychiatric Association. Washington, DC, APA, 1989 [J]

96. Danziger Y, Carel CA, Tyano S, Mimouni M: Is psychotherapy mandatory during the actual refeeding period in the treatment of anorexia nervosa? J Adolesc Health Care 1989; 10:328–331 [B]

97. Garner DM, Rockert W, Olmsted MP, Johnson C, Coscina DZ: Psychoeducation principles in the treatment of bulimia and anorexia nervosa, in Handbook of Psychotherapy for Anorexia Nervosa and Bulimia. Edited by Garner DM, Garfinkel PE. New York, Guilford Press, 1985 [I]

98. Strober M, Yager J: A developmental perspective on the treatment of anorexia nervosa in adolescents, in Handbook of Psychotherapy for Anorexia Nervosa and Bulimia. Edited by Garner DM, Garfinkel PE. New York, Guilford Press, 1985 [I]

99. Russell GF, Szmukler GI, Dare C, Eisler I: An evaluation of family therapy in anorexia nervosa and bulimia nervosa. Arch Gen Psychiatry 1987; 44:1047–1056 [A]

100. Hornyak LM, Baker EK (eds): Experiential Therapies for Eating Disorders. New York, Guilford Press, 1989 [I]

101. Wilson CP, Mintz IL, Northvale CT (eds): Psychosomatic Symptoms: Psychoanalytic Treatment of the Underlying Personality Disorder. New York, Jason Aronson, 1983, 1989 [I]

102. Garner DM: Individual psychotherapy for anorexia nervosa. J Psychiatr Res 1985; 19:423–433 [I]

103. Hall A, Crisp AH: Brief psychotherapy in the treatment of anorexia nervosa: preliminary findings, in Anorexia Nervosa: Recent Developments in Research. Edited by Darby P, Garner D, Coscina D. New York, Alan R Liss, 1983 [I]

104. Halmi KA, Eckert E, LaDu TJ, Cohen J: Anorexia nervosa: treatment efficacy of cyproheptadine and amitriptyline. Arch Gen Psychiatry 1986; 43:177–181 [A]

105. Gross HA, Ebert MH, Faden VB: A double-blind controlled study of lithium carbonate in primary anorexia nervosa. J Clin Psychopharmacol 1981; 1:376–381 [A]

106. Lacey JH, Crisp AH: Hunger, food intake and weight: the impact of clomipramine on a refeeding anorexia nervosa population. Postgrad Med J (Suppl 1) 1980; 56:79–85 [A]

107. Vandereycken W, Pierloot R: Pimozide combined with behavior therapy in the short-term treatment of anorexia nervosa: a double-blind placebo-controlled cross-over study. Acta Psychiatr Scand 1982; 66:445–450 [A]

108. Physicians' Desk Reference, 46th ed. Montvale, NJ, Medical Economics Data, 1992 [J]

109. Horne RL, Ferguson JM, Pope HG Jr, Hudson JI, Lineberry CG, Ascher J, Cato A: Treatment of bulimia with bupropion: a multicenter controlled trial. J Clin Psychiatry 1988; 49:262–266 [A]

110. Garfinkel PE, Garner DM (eds): The Role of Drug Treatments for Eating Disorders. New York, Brunner/Mazel, 1987 [I]

111. Wells LA, Logan KM: Pharmacologic treatment of eating disorders: a review of selected literature and recommendations. Psychosomatics 1987; 28:470–479 [I]

112. Gwirtsman HE, Guze BH, Yager J, Gainsley B: Fluoxetine treatment of anorexia nervosa: an open clinical trial. J Clin Psychiatry 1990; 51:378–382 [E]

113. Kaye WH, Weltzin TE, Hsu LK, Bulik CM: An open trial of fluoxetine in patients with anorexia nervosa. J Clin Psychiatry 1991; 52:464–471 [E]

114. Bachrach LK, Katzman DK, Litt IF, Guido D, Marcus R: Recovery from osteopenia in adolescent girls with anorexia nervosa. J Clin Endocrinol Metab 1991; 72:602–606 [B]

115. Emans SJ, Goldstein DP: Pediatric and Adolescent Gynecology, 3rd ed. Boston, Little, Brown, 1990 [I]

116. Marcus RN, Katz JL: Inpatient care of substance-abusing patient with a concomitant eating disorder. Hosp Community Psychiatry 1990; 41:59–63 [I]

117. Hsu LKG: Outcome and treatment effects, in Handbook of Eating Disorders, Part I. Edited by Beumont PJV, Burrows BD, Casper RC. Amsterdam, Elsevier, 1987 [I]

118. Hsu LKG: Eating Disorders. New York, Guilford Press, 1990 [I]

119. Theander S: Outcome and prognosis in anorexia nervosa and bulimia: some results of previous investigations, compared with those of a Swedish long-term study. J Psychiatr Res 1985; 19: 493–508 [C]

120. Johnson C, Connors ME: The Etiology and Treatment of Bulimia Nervosa. New York, Basic Books, 1987 [I]

121. Fairburn CG, Kirk J, O'Connor M, Cooper PG: A comparison of two psychological treatments for bulimia nervosa. Behav Res Ther 1986; 24:629–643 [A]

122. Lacey JH: Bulimia nervosa, binge eating, and psychogenic vomiting: a controlled treatment study and long term outcome. Br Med J 1983; 286:1609–1613 [B]

123. Ordman AM, Kirschenbaum DS: Cognitive-behavioral therapy for bulimia: an initial outcome study. J Consult Clin Psychol 1985; 53:305-313 [A]

124. Cox GL, Merkel WT: A qualitative review of psychosocial treatments for bulimia. J Nerv Ment Dis 1989; 177:77–84 [I]

125. Laessle RG, Zoettle C, Pirke KM: Meta-analysis of treatment studies for bulimia. Int J Eating Disorders 1987; 6:647–654 [G]

126. Freeman CP, Barry F, Dunkeld-Turnbull J, Henderson A: Controlled trial of psychotherapy for bulimia nervosa. Br Med J 1988; 296:521–525 [A]

127. Touyz SW, Beumont PJV, Hook S: Exercise anorexia: a new dimension in anorexia nervosa, in Handbook of Eating Disorders, Part 1. Edited by Beumont PJV, Burrows GD, Casper RC. New York, Elsevier, 1987 [I]

128. Vandereycken W: The addiction model in eating disorders: some critical remarks and a selected bibliography. Int J Eating Disorders 1990; 9:95–102 [I]

129. Fairburn CG, Jones R, Peveler RC, Carr SJ, Solomon RA, O'Connor ME, Burton J, Hope RA: Three psychological treatments for bulimia nervosa: a comparative trial. Arch Gen Psychiatry 1991; 48:463–469 [A]

130. Fairburn CG: Cognitive behavioral treatment for bulimia, in Handbook of Psychotherapy for Anorexia Nervosa and Bulimia. Edited by Garner DM, Garfinkel PE. New York, Guilford Press, 1985 [I]

131. Agras WS: Cognitive Behavior Therapy Treatment Manual for Bulimia Nervosa. Department of Psychiatry and Behavioral Sciences, Stanford University School of Medicine, 1991 [I]

132. Mitchell JE and Staff Members of the Eating Disorders Program: Bulimia Nervosa: Individual Treatment Manual. Department of Psychiatry, University of Minnesota Hospital and Clinic, 1989 [I]

133. Mitchell JE and Staff Members of the Eating Disorders Program: Bulimia Nervosa: Group Treatment Manual. Department of Psychiatry, University of Minnesota Hospital and Clinic, 1991 [I]

134. Boutacoff LI, Zollman MR, Mitchell JE: Healthy Eating: A Meal Planning System: Group Treatment Manual. Department of Psychiatry, University of Minnesota Hospital and Clinic, 1989 [I]

135. Root MPP: Persistent, disordered eating as a gender-specific, post-traumatic stress response to sexual assault. Psychotherapy 1991; 28:96–102 [E]

136. Rosen JC, Leitenberg H: Bulimia nervosa: treatment with exposure and response prevention. Behavior Therapy 1982; 13:117–124 [E]

137. Schmidt U, Marks IM: Exposure plus prevention of bingeing vs. exposure plus prevention of vomiting in bulimia nervosa: a crossover study. J Nerv Ment Dis 1989; 177:259–266 [A]

138. Wilson GT, Rossiter E, Kleinfield EI, Lindholm L: Cognitive-behavioral treatment of bulimia nervosa: a controlled evaluation. Behav Res Ther 1986; 24:277–288 [A]

139. Agras WS, Schneider JA, Arnow B, Raeburn SD, Telch CF: Cognitive-behavioral and response-prevention treatments for bulimia nervosa. J Consult Clin Psychol 1989; 57:215–221 [A]

140. Agras WS, Schneider JA, Arnow B, Raeburn SD, Telch CF: Cognitive-behavioral treatment with and without exposure plus response prevention in the treatment of bulimia nervosa: a reply to Leitenberg and Rosen. J Consult Clin Psychol 1989; 57:778–779 [J]

141. Connors ME, Johnson CL, Stuckey MK: Treatment of bulimia with brief psychoeducational group therapy. Am J Psychiatry 1984; 141:1512–1516 [A]

142. Huon GF, Brown LB: Evaluating a group treatment for bulimia. J Psychiatr Res 1985; 19:479–483 [A]

143. Kirkley BG, Schneider JA, Agras WS, Bachman JA: Comparison of two group treatments for bulimia. J Consult Clin Psychol 1985; 53:43–48 [A]

144. Yates AJ, Sambrailo F: Bulimia nervosa: a descriptive and therapeutic study. Behav Res Ther 1984; 22:503–517 [E]

145. Lee NF, Rush AJ: Cognitive-behavioral group therapy for bulimia. Int J Eating Disorders 1986; 5:559–615 [A]

146. Schneider JA, Agras WS: A cognitive-behavioural group treatment of bulimia. Br J Psychiatry 1985; 146:66–69 [E]

147. Wolchik S, Weiss L, Katzman M: An empirically validated, short-term psychoeducational group treatment program for bulimia. Int J Eating Disorders 1986; 5:21–34 [E]
148. Oesterheld JR, McKenna MS, Gould NB: Group psychotherapy of bulimia: a critical review. Int J Group Psychother 1987; 37: 163–184 [I]
149. Fettes PA, Peters JM: A meta-analysis of group treatments for bulimia nervosa. Int J Eating Disorders 1992; 11:97–110 [G]
150. Garner DM, Fairburn CG, Davis R: Cognitive-behavioral treatment of bulimia nervosa: a critical appraisal. Behav Modif 1987; 11:398–401 [I]
151. Laessle RG, Beumont PJ, Butow P, Lennerts W, O'Connor M, Pirke KM, Touyz SW, Waadt S: A comparison of nutritional management with stress management in the treatment of bulimia nervosa. Br J Psychiatry 1991; 159:250–261 [A]
152. Mitchell JE, Pyle RL, Eckert ED, Seim H, Crosby R, Zimmerman R: The importance of logistical variables in the treatment of bulimia nervosa. Int J Eating Disorders 1993 (in press) [A]
153. Schwartz RC, Barrett MJ, Saba G: Family therapy for bulimia, in Handbook of Psychotherapy for Anorexia Nervosa and Bulimia. Edited by Garner DM, Garfinkel PE. New York, Guilford Press, 1985 [I]
154. Malenbaum R, Herzog D, Eisenthal S, Wyshak G: Overeaters Anonymous. Int J Eating Disorders 1988; 7:139–144 [C]
155. Yager J, Landsverk J, Edelstein CK: Help seeking and satisfaction with care in 641 women with eating disorders, I: patterns of utilization, attributed change and perceived efficacy of treatment. J Nerv Ment Dis 1989; 177:632–637 [C]
156. Pope HG Jr, Hudson JI, Jonas JM, Yurgelun-Todd D: Bulimia treated with imipramine: a placebo-controlled, double-blind study. Am J Psychiatry 1983; 140:554–558 [A]
157. Agras WS, Dorian B, Kirkley BG, Arnow B, Bachman J: Imipramine in the treatment of bulimia: a double-blind controlled study. Int J Eating Disorders 1987; 6:29–38 [A]
158. Hughes PL, Wells LA, Cunningham CJ, Ilstrup DM: Treating bulimia with desipramine: a double-blind placebo-controlled study. Arch Gen Psychiatry 1986; 43:182–186 [A]
159. Pope HG Jr, Keck PE Jr, McElroy SL, Hudson JI: A placebo-controlled study of trazodone in bulimia nervosa. J Clin Psychopharmacol 1989; 9:254–259 [A]
160. Fluoxetine Bulimia Nervosa Collaborative Study Group: Fluoxetine in the treatment of bulimia nervosa: a multicenter, placebo-controlled, double blind trial. Arch Gen Psychiatry 1992; 49:139–147 [A]
161. Freeman CP, Morris JE, Cheshire KE, Davies F, Hamson M: A double-blind controlled trial of fluoxetine versus placebo for bulimia nervosa, in Proceedings of the Third International Conference on Eating Disorders, New York, 1988 [J]
162. Walsh BT, Stewart JW, Roose SP, Gladis M, Glassman AH: Treatment of bulimia with phenelzine: a double-blind, placebo-controlled study. Arch Gen Psychiatry 1984; 41:1105–1109 [A]
163. Kennedy SH, Piran N, Warsh JJ, Prendergast P, Mainprize E, Whynot C, Garfinkel PE: A trial of isocarboxazid in the treatment of bulimia nervosa. J Clin Psychopharmacol 1988; 8:391–396 [A]
164. Pope HG Jr, Hudson JI: Antidepressant drug therapy for bulimia: current status. J Clin Psychiatry 1986; 47:339–345 [I]
165. Kaplan AS, Garfinkel PE, Darby PL, Garner DM: Carbamazepine in the treatment of bulimia. Am J Psychiatry 1983; 140:1225–1226 [A]
166. Hsu LK: Treatment of bulimia with lithium. Am J Psychiatry 1984; 141:1260–1262. [E]
167. Hsu LK, Clement L, Santhouse R, Ju ES: Treatment of bulimia nervosa with lithium carbonate: a controlled study. J Nerv Ment Dis 1991; 179:351–355 [A]

168. Mitchell JE, Pyle RL, Eckert ED, Hatsukami D, Pomeroy C, Zimmerman R: Response to alternative antidepressants in imipramine nonresponders with bulimia nervosa. J Clin Psychopharmacol 1989; 9:291–293 [E]

169. Pope HG Jr, McElroy SL, Keck PE Jr, Hudson JI: Long-term pharmacotherapy of bulimia nervosa (letter). J Clin Psychopharmacol 1989; 9:385–386 [J]

170. Mitchell JE, Pyle RL, Eckert ED, Hatsukami D, Pomeroy C, Zimmerman R: A comparison study of antidepressants and structured intensive group psychotherapy in the treatment of bulimia nervosa. Arch Gen Psychiatry 1990; 47:149–157 [A]

171. Agras WS, Rossiter EM, Arnow B, Schneider JA, Telch CF, Raeburn SD, Bruce B, Perl M, Koran LM: Pharmacologic and cognitive-behavioral treatment for bulimia nervosa: a controlled comparison. Am J Psychiatry 1992; 149:82–87 [A]

172. Luka LP, Agras WS, Schneider JA: Thirty month follow-up of cognitive behavioural group therapy for bulimia (letter). Br J Psychiatry 1986; 148:614–615 [B]

173. Hsu LK, Sobkiewicz TA: Bulimia nervosa: a four- to six-year follow-up study. Psychol Med 1989; 19:1035–1038 [B]

174. Swift WJ, Ritholz M, Kalin NH, Kaslow N: A follow-up study of thirty hospitalized bulimics. Psychosom Med 1987; 49:45–55 [B]

175. Russell G: Bulimia nervosa: an ominous variant of anorexia nervosa. Psychol Med 1979; 9:429–448 [E]

176. Yager J, Landsverk J, Edelstein CK: A 20-month follow-up study of 628 women with eating disorders, I: course and severity. Am J Psychiatry 1987; 144:1172–1177 [B]

177. Drewnowski A, Yee DK, Krahn DD: Dieting and bulimia: a continuum of behaviors, in CME Syllabus and Scientific Proceedings in Summary Form, 142nd Annual Meeting of the American Psychiatric Association. Washington, DC, APA, 1989 [J]

178. Cooper Z, Fairburn CG: The Eating Disorders Examination: a semi-structured interview for the assessment of the specific psychopathology of eating disorders. Int J Eating Disorders 1987; 6:1–8 [J]

179. Mitchell JE, Hatsukami D, Eckert E, Pyle R: Eating Disorders Questionnaire. Psychopharmacol Bull 1985; 21:1025–1043 [J]

180. Johnson C: Diagnostic Survey for Eating Disorders, in Initial consultation for patients with bulimia and anorexia nervosa, in Handbook for Psychotherapy for Anorexia Nervosa and Bulimia. Edited by Garner DM, Garfinkel PE. New York, Guilford Press, 1985 [J]

181. Agras WS: Stanford Eating Disorders Questionnaire, in Eating Disorders: Management of Obesity, Bulimia and Anorexia Nervosa. Oxford, Pergamon Press, 1987 [J]

182. Garner DM, Olmstead MP, Polivy J: Development and validation of a multidimensional inventory for anorexia nervosa and bulimia. Int J Eating Disorders 1983; 2:15–34 [J]

PRACTICE GUIDELINE

FOR

MAJOR DEPRESSIVE

DISORDER IN ADULTS

WORK GROUP ON MAJOR DEPRESSIVE DISORDER

T. Byram Karasu, M.D., Chair

John Patrick Docherty, M.D.
Alan Gelenberg, M.D.
David J. Kupfer, M.D.
Arnold E. Merriam, M.D.
Richard Shadoan, M.D.

Contents

Major Depressive Disorder in Adults

This practice guideline was published in April 1993 in the *American Journal of Psychiatry*.

Overview

This document is a practical guide to the management of major depression for adults over the age of 18 and represents the consensus of experts in the field regarding current scientific knowledge and rational clinical practice. This guideline strives to be as free as possible of bias toward any theoretical posture, and it aims to represent a practical approach to treatment. Studies were identified through an extensive review of the literature using MEDLARS for the period 1971–1991. The key words used were "affective disorder," "major depression," "depressive disorder," "seasonal affective disorder," "melancholia," "unipolar depression," "endogenous depression," "dysthymic disorder," "postpartum depression," "pseudodementia," "antidepressant drugs," "tricyclic antidepressive agents," "monoamine oxidase inhibitors," "lithium," and "electroconvulsive therapy." Major review articles and standard psychiatric texts were consulted. Review articles and relevant prospective randomized clinical trials were reviewed in their entirety; other studies were selected for review on the basis of their relevance to the particular issues discussed in this guideline. Definitive standards are difficult to achieve, except in narrow circumstances where multiple replicated studies and wide clinical opinion dictate certain forms of treatment. In other areas much is left to the clinical judgment and expertise of the clinician. The recommendations delineated in this guideline are in some instances based on data distilled from randomized prospective clinical trials, while in other areas they are based on individual case reports along with the collective experience and judgment of well-regarded senior psychiatrists. In order that the reader may identify the type of evidence supporting the major recommendations in this practice guide, each is keyed to one or more references and each reference is followed by a letter code in brackets that indicates the nature of the supporting evidence. The codes are defined at the beginning of the reference section, which appears at the end of this document. Minor recommendations not keyed to references may be assumed to be based on expert opinion. This guideline contains a table providing relevant information pertaining to the antidepressant medications described in the body of the document. The summary of treatment recommendations is keyed according to the level of confidence with which each recommendation is made.

Introduction

This guideline seeks to summarize the specific forms of somatic, psychotherapeutic, psychosocial, and educational treatments that have been developed to deal with major depressive disorder and its various subtypes. It begins at the point where the psychiatrist has diagnosed an adult patient as suffering from major depression according to the criteria for this disorder defined in DSM-III-R (1) or DSM-IV (publication anticipated in 1993) and has medically evaluated the patient to ascertain the presence of alcohol or substance abuse or dependence disorder or other somatic factors that may contribute to the disease process (e.g., hypothyroidism, pancreatic carcinoma) or complicate its treatment (e.g., cardiac disorders). The purpose of this guideline is to assist the physician faced with the task of implementing specific antidepressant treatment(s). It should be noted that many patients have coexisting conditions and their difficulties cannot be described with one DSM diagnostic category. The psychiatrist should consider, but not be limited to, the treatment guidelines for a single diagnosis.

This document concerns patients 18 years of age and older. Major depression in children and adolescents will be addressed in a separate guideline because of the complexities of assessment and treatment for this age group.

I.   Disease Definition, Epidemiology, and Natural History

A.   DSM-III-R Criteria

1.   For major depressive episode

A.   At least five of the following symptoms have been present during the same 2-week period and represent a change from previous functioning; at least one of the symptoms is either 1) depressed mood or 2) loss of interest or pleasure. (Do not include symptoms that are clearly due to physical condition, mood-incongruent delusions or hallucinations, incoherence, or marked loosening of associations.)

   1) Depressed mood most of the day, nearly every day, as indicated either by subjective account or observation by others.
   2) Markedly diminished interest or pleasure in all, or almost all, activities most of the day, nearly every day (as indicated either by subjective account or observation by others of apathy most of the time).
   3) Significant weight loss or weight gain when not dieting (e.g., more than 5% of body weight in a month), or decrease or increase in appetite nearly every day.
   4) Insomnia or hypersomnia nearly every day.
   5) Psychomotor agitation or retardation nearly every day (observable by others, not merely subjective feelings of restlessness or being slowed down).
   6) Fatigue or loss of energy nearly every day.
   7) Feelings of worthlessness or excessive or inappropriate guilt (which may be delusional) nearly every day (not merely self-reproach or guilt about being sick).
   8) Diminished ability to think or concentrate, or indecisiveness, nearly every day (either by subjective account or as observed by others).
   9) Recurrent thoughts of death (not just fear of dying), recurrent suicidal ideation without a specific plan, or a suicide attempt or specific plan for committing suicide.

B.   1) It cannot be established that an organic factor initiated and maintained the disturbance.
   2) The disturbance is not a normal reaction to the death of a loved one (uncomplicated bereavement). Note: morbid preoccupation with worthlessness, suicidal ideation, marked functional impairment or psychomotor retardation, or prolonged duration suggests bereavement complicated by major depression.

C.   At no time during the disturbance have there been delusions or hallucinations for as long as 2 weeks in the absence of prominent mood symptoms (i.e., before the mood symptoms developed or after they have remitted).

D.   Not superimposed on schizophrenia, schizophreniform disorder, delusional disorder, or psychotic disorder not otherwise specified.

2. For major depression, single episode

A.   A single major depressive episode.
B.   Has never had a manic episode or an unequivocal hypomanic episode.

3. For major depression, recurrent

A.   Two or more major depressive episodes, each separated by at least 2 months of return to more or less usual functioning. (If there has been a previous major depressive episode, the current episode of depression need not meet the full criteria for a major depressive episode.)
B.   Has never had a manic episode or an unequivocal hypomanic episode.

B.   Specific Features of Diagnosis

1.   Severity

An episode of major depression may be classified as mild, moderate, or severe. Mild episodes are characterized by little in the way of symptoms beyond the minimum required to make the diagnosis and by minor functional impairment. Moderate episodes are characterized by the presence of symptoms in excess of the bare diagnostic requirements and by greater degrees of functional impairment. Severe episodes are characterized by the presence of several symptoms in excess of the minimum requirements and by the symptoms' marked interference with social and/or occupational functioning. In the extreme, the afflicted person may be totally unable to function socially or occupationally or even to feed or clothe himself or herself or to maintain minimal personal hygiene. The nature of the symptoms, such as suicidal ideation and behavior, should also be considered in assessing severity.

2.   Melancholia

The melancholic subtype is a severe form of major depression with characteristic somatic symptoms, and it is believed to be particularly responsive to pharmacotherapy and electroconvulsive therapy.

3. Psychotic features

Major depression may be accompanied by hallucinations and/or delusions; these may be congruent or noncongruent with the depressive mood.

4. Dysthymia

The differential diagnosis of dysthymia and major depression is particularly difficult, since the two disorders share similar symptoms and differ primarily in duration and severity. Usually major depression consists of one or more discrete major depressive episodes that can be distinguished from the person's usual functioning, whereas dysthymia is characterized by a chronic mild depressive syndrome that has been present for at least 2 years. If the initial onset of what appears to be dysthymia directly follows a major depressive episode, the appropriate diagnosis is major depression in partial remission. The diagnosis of dysthymia can be made following major depression only if there has been a full remission of the major depressive episode lasting at least 6 months before the development of dysthymia.

People with dysthymia frequently have a superimposed major depression, and this condition is often referred to as "double depression." Patients with double depression are less likely to have a complete recovery than are patients with major depressive disorder without dysthymia.

C. Natural History and Course

The average age at onset is the late 20s, but the disorder may begin at any age. The symptoms of major depressive disorder typically develop over days to weeks. Prodromal symptoms, including generalized anxiety, panic attacks, phobias, or depressive symptoms that do not meet the diagnostic threshold, may occur over the preceding several months. In some cases, however, a depression may develop suddenly (e.g., when associated with severe psychosocial stress).

The duration of a major depressive episode is also variable. Untreated, the episode typically lasts 6 months or longer. Some patients with major depressive disorder will eventually have a manic or hypomanic episode and will then be diagnosed as having bipolar disorder.

1. Recurrence

While some people have only a single episode of major depression, with full return to premorbid functioning, it is estimated that over 50% of the people who have such an episode will eventually have another episode, at which time the illness will meet the criteria for recurrent major depression. People with major depression superimposed on dysthymia are at greater risk for having a recurrence of major depressive episode than those without dysthymia.

The course of recurrent major depression is variable. Some people have episodes separated by many years of normal functioning; others have clusters of episodes; still others have increasingly frequent episodes as they grow older.

2.   Interepisode status

Functioning usually returns to the premorbid level between episodes. In 20% to 35% of the cases, however, there are persistent residual symptoms and social or occupational impairment. Patients who continue to meet the criteria for a major depressive episode throughout the course of the disturbance are considered to have the chronic type, while those who remain symptomatic are considered to be in partial remission.

3.   Seasonal pattern

A seasonal pattern of depression is characterized by a regular temporal relationship between the onset and remission of symptoms and particular periods of the year (e.g., in the northern hemisphere, regular appearance of symptoms between the beginning of October and the end of November and regular remission from mid-February to mid-April). Patients should not receive this diagnosis if there is an obvious effect of seasonally related psychosocial stressors, e.g., seasonal unemployment.

4.   Complications

The most serious complications of a major depressive episode are suicide and other violent acts. Other complications include marital, parental, social, and vocational difficulties (2). The illness, especially in its recurrent and chronic forms, may cause distress for other individuals in the patient's social network, e.g., children, spouse, and significant others. If the patient is a parent, the disorder may affect his or her ability to fulfill parental role expectations (3). Depressive episodes are associated with occupational dysfunction, including unemployment, absenteeism, and decreased work productivity (4).

D.   Epidemiology

The Epidemiologic Catchment Area study indicates that major depression has a 1-month prevalence of 2.2% and a lifetime prevalence of 5.8% in Americans 18 years and older (5). Other studies estimate the lifetime prevalence to be as high as 26% for females and 12% for males. The illness is 1.5 to 3 times as common among those with a first-degree biological relative affected with the disorder as among the general population. Chronic general medical illness and substance abuse, particularly abuse of alcohol or cocaine, predispose to the development of major depression. Frequently a major depressive episode follows a psychosocial stressor, particularly death of a loved one, marital separation, or the ending of an important relationship. Childbirth sometimes precipitates a major depressive episode. Patients with major depressive disorder identified in psychiatric settings tend to have episodes of greater severity and to have recurrent forms of depression and also are more likely to have other mental disorders than are subjects from the community and primary care settings.

II. Treatment Principles and Alternatives

A. General Issues in Planning and Instituting Treatment

Successful treatment of patients with major depression is promoted by a thorough assessment of the patient's symptoms; past general medical and psychiatric history; psychological makeup and conflicts; life stressors; family, psychosocial, and cultural environment; and preference for specific treatments or approaches.

The psychiatrist's task is both to effect and to maintain improvement. Treatment consists of an *acute phase,* during which remission is induced, a *continuation phase,* during which remission is preserved, and a *maintenance phase,* during which the susceptible patient is protected against the recurrence of subsequent depressive episodes. Psychiatrists initiating treatment of a major depressive episode have at their disposal a variety of psychotherapeutic approaches, a number of medications, electroconvulsive therapy, and light therapy. These various interventions may be used alone or in combination. Furthermore, the psychiatrist must decide whether to conduct treatment on an outpatient, partial hospitalization, or inpatient basis.

B. Psychotherapeutic Interventions

There are a range of psychotherapeutic interventions that may be useful in major depressive disorder. Although various therapies are discussed here and in the literature as distinct entities, such separate categorizations are primarily useful for heuristic or research purposes. In practice, psychiatrists use a combination or synthesis of various approaches and strategies; these in turn are determined by and individually tailored to each patient on the basis of that person's particular conditions and coping capacities. Furthermore, in actual application the techniques and the therapist-patient relationship are powerfully intertwined.

1. Psychotherapeutic management

Psychotherapeutic management (sometimes referred to as "supportive psychotherapy") consists of a number of complex activities that are essential in the treatment of depression.

The establishment and maintenance of a supportive therapeutic relationship, wherein the therapist empathically obtains information and gains the confidence of the patient and is available in times of crisis, are crucial in the treatment of depression. Other essential features include maintaining vigilance toward the emergence of destructive impulses directed toward the self or others; providing a therapeutic rationale or explanation for the patient's symptoms and illness and a prescription for relief that is acceptable and mutually agreed on; providing ongoing education, knowledge, and feedback in regard to the patient's illness, prognosis, and treatment; guiding the patient in reference to the patient's environment—including interpersonal relationships, work, living conditions, and other medical or health related needs; assisting the patient in scheduling absences from work or other responsibilities as required; discouraging the patient from instituting major life changes that might be predicated on the depressive state; helping to bolster the patient's morale by strengthening expectations of help and hope for the future; enlisting the support of others in the patient's social network and supporting them as well if need be; setting realistic, attainable, and tangible goals; and encouraging the patient to seek new success experiences, however small, including greater engagement with the outside world (e.g., vocational, social, and religious activities). The actual delivery of psychotherapeutic management must be skillfully improvised and individually tailored within the framework of a helpful and trusting doctor-patient relationship (6).

2. Psychodynamic psychotherapy and psychoanalysis

A number of psychotherapeutic interventions are now subsumed under the terms "psychodynamic psychotherapy" and "psychoanalysis."

These therapies acknowledge some debt to Freud's original conceptualization of the psychodynamics of depression, in which central importance was ascribed to a relationship with a lost object that is highly ambivalent, resulting in repressed self-directed rage, increased self-criticism, and self-destructive impulses (7–9).

This formulation has subsequently been modified to take into account other factors that experts find play a role in the etiology of depression, such as psychological vulnerability, dependency on external sources to maintain self-esteem, an early lack of love, care, warmth, and protection, and a depressive disposition marked by guilt, helplessness, and fear regarding the loss of love. Most psychodynamic theoreticians share a thesis regarding the etiologic nature of deficits related to early deprivations of love and affection, conflicts related to guilt based on a harsh conscience and repressed fantasies of childhood wishes and transgressions, and/or frustrations related to having excessively high ego ideals (10–29). These deficits and conflicts are seen as engendering in the depressed individual pathological self-punitiveness, self-rejection, depleted self-esteem, and overt depressive manifestations (30).

Psychodynamic theory affirms that the intrapsychic processes underlying depression are perpetuated unless the relevant unconscious forces are brought into consciousness and under the ego's control. Once these forces are made conscious, difficulties can be anticipated and mastered, or conflicts can be neutralized, through the process of insight. Mastery and insight are experienced in the supportive or interpretive relationship with the therapist, permitting the patient not only to overcome ongoing depressive affects but to ward off recurrent depressive episodes. The transference relationship can be used to allow close examination and modification of basic, long-standing, previously unrecognized patterns of thought, emotion, and behavior. In vulnerable individuals who are excessively sensitive to loss and who use reaction formation and turning inward of aggression as defense mechanisms to control the aggressive impulse, the detection and alteration of these psychodynamic mechanisms are of central importance in the treatment of depression. In its more supportive version, the psychodynamic approach seeks to alleviate ongoing symptoms, reduce secondary gains, and help the patient adapt to life circumstances.

The efficacy of long-term psychodynamic psychotherapy or psychoanalysis in either the acute or maintenance phase of major depression, either in conjunction with pharmacotherapy or alone, has not been subjected to controlled studies.

3. Brief therapy

Brief psychodynamic psychotherapy may be used in the acute-phase treatment of depression, especially as an adjunct to pharmacologic treatment. The efficacy of brief psychodynamic psychotherapy as a single modality in the treatment of major depression has not been conclusively demonstrated by controlled studies; although it has been shown to be more effective than a waiting list control (31), the latter is considered a less than satisfactory control condition. Its effectiveness in comparison to other psychotherapeutic approaches requires further research. Research on combined pharmacotherapy and brief psychodynamic psychotherapy (32, 33) is equally sparse and inconclusive. The efficacy of brief therapy in the continuation or maintenance phase is not known.

4. Interpersonal therapy

Interpersonal therapy seeks to recognize and explore depressive precipitants that involve interpersonal losses, role disputes and transitions, social isolation, or deficits in social skills (34). It maintains that losses must be mourned and related affects appreciated, that role disputes and transitions must be recognized and resolved, and that deficits in social skills must be overcome in order to permit the acquisition of social supports. There is some evidence in controlled studies that interpersonal therapy as a single agent is effective in reducing depressive symptoms in the acute phase of nonmelancholic major depressive episodes of lesser severity (35, 36) and that it is especially effective in ameliorating vocational and social aspects of the patient's dysfunction (37). For the pharmacotherapy-responsive patient, the role of added interpersonal therapy as a maintenance treatment is still under study (38, 39). Nevertheless, there is evidence that interpersonal therapy during the maintenance phase can have a useful effect, especially for patients with recent psychosocial conflicts or with work or marital difficulties. Interpersonal therapy alone is an alternative maintenance treatment for patients who are clearly nonresponsive to or intolerant of trials of various medications.

5.   Behavior therapy

Behavior therapy of depression is based on a functional analysis of behavior theory (40) and/or social learning theory (41). The techniques involve activity scheduling (42, 43), self-control therapy (44), social skills training (45), and problem solving (46).

Behavior therapy has been reported to be effective in the acute treatment of patients with mild to moderately severe depressions, especially when combined with pharmacotherapy (31, 47–50). Studies of the prophylactic value of behavior therapy in the acute phase, once discontinued, have been inconclusive (48, 51, 52). The utility of behavior therapy in continuation- and maintenance-phase treatment of depression has not been subjected to controlled studies.

6.   Cognitive behavior therapy

The cognitive approach to psychotherapy maintains that irrational beliefs and distorted attitudes toward the self, the environment, and the future perpetuate depressive affects and that these may be reversed through cognitive behavior therapy (53). There is some evidence that cognitive therapy reduces depressive symptoms during the acute phase of less severe, nonmelancholic forms of major depression (54) but not significantly differently from pill placebo coupled with clinical management (36). Studies of the prophylactic effect of acute-phase cognitive behavior therapy, once discontinued, have had mixed results, and so no firm conclusions can be reached at this time (52, 55–58). The use of cognitive behavior therapy in the continuation- and maintenance-phase treatment of depression has not been studied.

7.   Marital therapy and family therapy

Marital and family problems are common in the course of mood disorders: comprehensive treatment demands that these problems be assessed and addressed. Marital and family problems may be a consequence of depression but may also increase vulnerability to depression and in some instances retard recovery (59, 60).

Techniques for using marital/family approaches for the treatment of depression have been developed. These include behavioral approaches (59), a psychoeducational approach, and a "strategic marital therapy" approach (61). In addition, the use of family therapy in the inpatient treatment of depressed patients has been studied (62).

Research suggests that marital and family therapy may reduce depressive symptoms and the risk of relapse in patients with marital and family problems (58, 63). The role of these treatments for depressed patients without specific family or marital discord is less clear.

8.   Group therapy

The role of group therapy in the treatment of depression is based on clinical experience rather than on systematic controlled studies. It is particularly useful in the treatment of depression in the context of bereavement or such common stressors as chronic illness. Individuals in such circumstances particularly benefit from the example of others who have successfully dealt with the same or similar challenges. Survivors are offered the opportunity to gain enhanced self-esteem by making themselves models for others, and they offer newer patients successful role models.

Medication maintenance support groups, such as those comprising lithium-treated patients, offer similar benefits. In addition, such groups provide information to the patient and to family members regarding prognosis and medication issues, thereby providing a psychoeducational forum that makes a chronic mental illness understandable in the context of a medical model.

Consumer-oriented support groups comprising individuals with depression can serve a useful role by enhancing the support network and self-esteem of participating patients and their families.

9. Selection and implementation of specific therapies

Patient preference plays a large role in the choice of a particular form of psychotherapy. In guiding the choice of individual therapy, the psychiatrist should consider that an interpersonal approach may be most useful for patients who are in the midst of recent conflicts with significant others and for those having difficulty adjusting to an altered career or social role or other life transition; a cognitive approach can be helpful for patients who seek and are able to tolerate explicit, structured guidance from another party. A psychodynamic or psychoanalytic therapeutic approach may best help those with a chronic sense of emptiness; harsh self-expectations and self-underestimation; a history of childhood abuses, losses, or separations; chronic interpersonal conflicts; or coexisting axis II disorders or traits. Factors contributing to the success of a psychodynamic or psychoanalytic modality include motivation, the capacity for insight, psychological mindedness, a capacity to form a relationship, mild to moderate illness, and a stable environment.

Another factor influencing the selection of psychotherapeutic treatment is the stage and severity of the depressive episode. During the initial phase of a severe depression, depending on the patient's personality, social network, and other factors, the focus may have to include support and psychoeducation for the patient and the family, permission for the patient to excuse himself or herself from duties impossible to perform, and assistance regarding the making or postponing of major personal and business decisions. Some patients at this stage may not have the emotional energy or cognitive ability required for insight-oriented treatment. If indicated, this may be initiated later in the course of recovery.

The impact of the frequency of psychotherapeutic treatment on treatment outcome has not received the same scrutiny in controlled studies as have specific aspects of pharmacologic treatment (e.g., dosing); multiple considerations apply to the practice of psychotherapy that have little counterpart in the sphere of psychopharmacology. The psychiatrist must take into account not only the minimum frequency at which contact is required for a particular psychotherapeutic treatment but also other management factors, such as the frequency of visits required to ensure medication compliance, to monitor suicide risk, and to create and maintain a therapeutic relationship. Also affecting the frequency of psychotherapeutic contact are the severity of illness, presence and intensity of suicidal intent, the patient's cooperation with treatment, availability of social supports, and presence of coexistent general medical problems. The frequency of outpatient visits during the acute phase may therefore vary from once a week or every other week in routine cases to as often as several times a week. Treatments that aim at developing insight through free association and analysis of the transference tend to require more frequent and regular visits. During the continuation and maintenance phases, the frequency of visits may vary from once every several months, if the visits are for the purpose of providing psychotherapeutic management for stable patients, to once or more per week, if active psychotherapy is to be maintained. Psychodynamic psychotherapy requires greater frequency, and if psychoanalysis is indicated, the frequency will be three to five times a week. Some patients with depression of mild severity can be treated with psychotherapeutic management or with psychotherapy alone; in such cases, the data indicate no difference in benefit between medication (in this case, imipramine) coupled with clinical management versus interpersonal psychotherapy, cognitive behavior therapy, or clinical management and pill placebo (36). Psychotherapy alone may be similarly sufficient and effective for those with primarily situational forms of depression (64). Even in cases of mild depression, if the symptoms do not respond to psychotherapy, somatic treatment should be considered. Optimal treatment of major depression that is chronic or is moderate to severe generally requires some form of somatic intervention, in the form of medication or electroconvulsive therapy, coupled with psychotherapeutic management or psychotherapy.

C.   Somatic Interventions

1.   Antidepressant medications

a. General considerations.   For cases of first-episode major depression uncomplicated by coexistent general medical illness or by special features such as atypical, psychotic, or bipolar symptoms, many equally effective agents are available. Antidepressant medications can be grouped as follows: 1) *cyclic antidepressants,* which include the tricyclic antidepressants as well as amoxapine, maprotiline, bupropion, and trazodone; 2) *selective serotonin-reuptake inhibiting antidepressants,* which currently include fluoxetine and sertraline but are likely to increase in the near future; and 3) *monoamine oxidase (MAO) inhibitors,* which include the commonly used phenelzine, isocarboxazid, and tranylcypromine.

Before the initiation of pharmacologic treatment, it is important to be aware of the possibilities of coexisting substance use disorders and of the existence of and treatments for general medical conditions, because of the danger of drug interaction upon initiation of antidepressant medication treatment. In the first 3 weeks 10%–15% of patients drop out of medication trials. For those who continue through this initial period, the rate of response to antidepressants is reported to be as high as 60%–70% for all currently available agents;

however, the rate of complete remission may be substantially lower. Patients may show some improvement by the end of the first week (65) but may not fully respond for more than 4 to 6 weeks (66, 67). Therefore, adequacy of response cannot be judged until after this period of time.

In nonselected cases of major depression, the data indicate similar rates of response to all antidepressant drugs; therefore, the choice must be predicated on other factors. These include the drug's tendency to evoke a particular constellation of side effects, as well as specific factors related to the patient's psychiatric and medical history, family history of psychiatric disorder, and response to specific treatments. Some patients may wish to take into account the costs of the various agents considered. Fluoxetine, sertraline, and bupropion have certain advantages given these agents' relative safety in overdose and their equivalent therapeutic efficacy compared to older agents. No one medication can be recommended as optimal for all patients because of the substantial heterogeneity among patients in their likelihood of beneficial response to these medications and the nature, likelihood, and severity of side effects. Furthermore, patients vary in the degree to which particular side effects and other inconveniences of taking medications (e.g., cost and dietary restrictions) affect their preferences.

b. Side effects.   Adherence to a pharmacotherapeutic regimen is in most cases a prerequisite for the effective treatment of major depression. Antidepressant medications are capable of inducing unpleasant or even intolerable side effects; careful attention to the emergence of such complications enables the physician to effectively treat them or to select an alternative agent, thereby maximizing compliance with treatment. An overview of some potential side effects of antidepressant medication follows.

"Dizziness," sedation, and "feeling medicated."   These complaints are grouped together because patients tend to use these terms generically to describe a number of unpleasant side effects. Many patients complain of feeling "dizzy," "foggy," or absent-minded and attribute this to effects of the antidepressant.

All patients who complain of "dizziness" should have their blood pressures checked for orthostatic effects. If orthostasis is pronounced, an agent less likely to induce this effect should be substituted; if orthostasis is present but less severe, the patient should be urged to allow several weeks to acclimate to the effects of the drug.

Alternatively, patients complaining of "feeling foggy" may be experiencing anticholinergic-induced cognitive disruption. Subclinical memory impairment has been documented even in nondemented psychiatric outpatients given psychotropic medications with anticholinergic properties (68). If the patient displays peripheral anticholinergic signs (see the next section) and reports or displays mental confusion or forgetfulness, it is best to switch to an antidepressant free of muscarinic blockade (see table 1).

Some patients who say they feel "overly medicated" are actually overly sedated. Many antidepressants are prone to induce this symptom. Amitriptyline, doxepin, and trazodone are experienced as most sedating, nortriptyline and amoxapine as less sedating, and fluoxetine, sertraline, bupropion, protriptyline, and desipramine as least sedating. Sedation often attenuates in the first weeks of treatment, and patients experiencing only minor difficulty from this side effect should be encouraged to allow some time to pass before changing antidepressant agents, all other factors being equal. Some patients tolerate their medication better when it is given as a single dose before bedtime.

Peripheral anticholinergic side effects.   All tricyclic antidepressants have some degree of antimuscarinic action; desipramine has the lowest potency in this regard (see table 1). While MAO inhibitors are not anticholinergic, their side effects may resemble anticholinergic symptoms. The most common undesirable consequences of muscarinic blockade are dry mouth, impaired ability to focus at close range, constipation, and urinary hesitation. Patients often develop some degree of tolerance to anticholinergic symptoms, but these symp-

TABLE 1.   Drugs Used for Patients With Major Depressive Disorder

Generic (Trade) Name	Starting Dose (mg/day)[a]	Usual Adult Dose (mg/day)[a]	Usual Serum Level	Degree of Muscarinic Blockade
Cyclic antidepressants				
Amitriptyline (Elavil, Endep)	25–50	100–300	—	+++
Doxepin (Adapin, Sinequan)	25–50	100–300	—	++
Imipramine (SK-Pramine, Tofranil)	25–50	100–300	—	+
Trimipramine (Surmontil)	25–50	100–300	—	+
Desipramine (Norpramin, Pertofrane)	25–50	100–300	—	+
Nortriptyline (Pamelor, Aventyl)	25	50–200	—	+
Protriptyline (Vivactil)	10	15–60	—	+++
Clomipramine (Anafranil)	25	100–250	—	+++
Amoxapine (Asendin)	50	100–400	—	+
Maprotiline (Ludiomil)	50	100–225	—	+
Trazodone (Desyrel)	50	150–500	—	0
Bupropion (Wellbutrin)	200	300–450	—	0
Selective serotonin-reuptake inhibitors				
Fluoxetine (Prozac)	5–20	20–80	—	0
Sertraline (Zoloft)	50–100	50–200	—	0
Paroxetine (Paxil)	10–20	20–50	—	0
MAO inhibitors				
Isocarboxazid (Marplan)	10–30	10–50	—	0
Phenelzine (Nardil)	15	15–90	—	0
Tranylcypromine (Parnate)	10	10–40	—	0
Selegiline (Eldepryl)	5	10	—	0
Lithium	600–900	—	0.8–1.0 meq/liter	0
Anticonvulsants				
Carbamazepine (Tegretol)	200–400	—	4–12 µg/ml	0
Valproic acid (Depakene)	750	—	50–100 µg/ml	0
Divalproex sodium (Depakote)	750	—	50–100 µg/ml	0

[a]All doses in this table may require alteration in either direction, depending on the patient's tolerance and response.

toms nevertheless should be treated if they cause substantial dysfunction or interfere with compliance. Impaired visual accommodation may be counteracted through the use of pilocarpine eye drops. Urinary hesitation may be treated by prescribing bethanechol, 30–200 mg/day in divided doses; the clinician should adjust the dose to avoid symptoms of cholinergic excess, principally abdominal cramps, nausea, and diarrhea. Dry mouth may be counteracted by advising the patient to use sugarless gum or candy or by prescribing an oral rinse of 1% pilocarpine used three or four times daily; oral bethanecol may also be effective. Constipation is best dealt with through adequate hydration and the use of bulk laxatives. Side effects of this nature may be avoided entirely if an antidepressant without anticholinergic activity (e.g., bupropion, fluoxetine, sertraline, or trazodone) is used.

Weight gain. Tricyclic antidepressants, MAO inhibitors, and lithium all have the capacity to induce weight gain. Bupropion, fluoxetine, sertraline, and trazodone do not usually induce weight gain, and bupropion and fluoxetine (and perhaps sertraline) may actually cause some (usually transient) degree of appetite and weight loss.

Sexual dysfunction. While loss of erectile or ejaculatory function in men and loss of libido and anorgasmia in both sexes may be complications of virtually any antidepressant agent, these side effects appear to be most common with the MAO inhibitors, fluoxetine, and probably sertraline and to be least common with bupropion. The psychiatrist must ascertain whether the sexual dysfunction is a result of the antidepressant agent or the underlying depression. Neostigmine, 7.5–15.0 mg taken 30 minutes before intercourse, has been reported to enhance libido and reverse retarded or painful ejaculation, and cyproheptadine, 4 mg/day orally, may reverse anorgasmia (69). Alternatively, the clinician may continue treatment to assess whether the dysfunction will disappear with time, may lower the dose, or may select another agent. Trazodone has been reported to induce priapism, a condition that, although rare, may result in impotence.

Neurological side effects. Some antidepressants carry the risk of inducing seizures even in individuals without a history of epilepsy. It is methodologically difficult to accurately compare the various agents in regard to their epileptogenic propensities, since a number of confounding factors influence seizure risk. These include antidepressant blood level, personal and family history of seizures, organic brain disease, alcohol or sedative drug use or withdrawal, and concurrent exposure to other medications. Overall, for most agents and for patients without specific risk factors who receive antidepressants administered within the recommended dose range, the risk of seizures is most often reported to be less than 1% (70, 71). Fluoxetine, sertraline, trazodone, and MAO inhibitors carry a lower risk of inducing seizures. Risk increases with dose for all offending agents.

A patient who develops a first seizure while receiving antidepressant therapy should be neurologically evaluated in the same way as a patient whose first seizure occurs in the absence of medication.

Tricyclic antidepressants sometimes induce mild myoclonus (72). Since this may be a sign of toxicity, the clinician may wish to check the blood level, if available for that agent, to ensure that it is not excessive. If the level is nontoxic and the myoclonus is not symptomatic, the agent may be continued without a change in dose. If the myoclonus is symptomatic and the blood level is within the recommended range, the patient may be treated with clonazepam at a dose of 0.25 mg t.i.d. Alternatively, the antidepressant agent may be changed.

A toxic confusional state has been identified in some patients with high blood levels of tricyclic antidepressant drugs, and it responds to simply lowering the dose (73).

Cardiovascular effects.   Orthostatic hypotension is a common side effect of tricyclic antidepressants, trazodone, and MAO inhibitors. It may be minimized by slow dose increases; tolerance to this effect sometimes develops. While it is little more than a nuisance to most patients, some individuals, especially the elderly, are prone to become faint, fall, and sustain a fracture or head injury. In addition, orthostatic hypotension can be dangerous in patients with impaired cardiac function. Nortriptyline has been reported to induce less orthostatic hypotension than imipramine (74); desipramine may offer similar advantages. Of the newer agents, fluoxetine, sertraline, and bupropion are free of this property altogether. Salt depletion, whether voluntary or a result of diuretic treatment, may contribute to orthostatic hypotension. If there is no medical contraindication, patients with symptomatic orthostatic hypotension should be cautioned against extreme dietary salt restriction.

Tricyclic antidepressants act similarly to such class I antiarrhythmic agents as quinidine, disopyramide, and procainamide in prolonging cardiac repolarization and in depressing fast Na+ channels (75). Consonant with these physiologic properties, both imipramine and nortriptyline have been documented to suppress ventricular premature depolarizations (76, 77). Patients with ventricular arrhythmia who are already taking another class I antiarrhythmic agent and who require tricyclic drug therapy should be under careful medical supervision, as combinations of tricyclic agents and other class I antiarrhythmic agents may exert an additive toxic effect on cardiac conduction. The same properties that make tricyclics class I antiarrhythmic agents may actually provoke arrhythmia in patients with subclinical sinus node dysfunction. In such patients, who may present with tachyrhythmia, treatment with tricyclics may on occasion provoke bradyarrhythmias (78). It has been reported that even patients with normal pretreatment ECGs may develop AV block that reverts to normal after discontinuation of antidepressant treatment (74).

Among patients with preexisting but asymptomatic conduction defects, such as interventricular conduction delay and bundle-branch block, tricyclic treatment may induce symptomatic conduction defects and symptomatic orthostatic hypotension (74). These complications are more likely to develop in patients with more severe forms of pretreatment conduction disturbance. Therapeutic concentrations of tricyclic antidepressants may lengthen the QT interval. Individuals with prolonged QT intervals, whether preexistent or drug-induced, are predisposed to the development of ventricular tachycardia (79).

For the most part, tricyclic agents have been found usually to exert no appreciable effect on ventricular ejection fraction (80) and therefore can usually be prescribed without adversely affecting hemodynamic function. However, on occasion, tricyclics exert a deleterious effect on ejection fraction (81). Patients with marked baseline disturbances of myocardial function should be closely observed during tricyclic antidepressant treatment for further decompensation or for the development of orthostatic hypotension, for which they are particularly at risk (82).

Insomnia and anxiety. Fluoxetine may precipitate or exacerbate anxiety and sleep disturbance in some patients. Anxiety may be minimized by introducing the agent at a low dose; insomnia may be effectively treated by the addition of trazodone, up to 100 mg at bedtime. Other antidepressants, including desipramine and bupropion, may also increase anxiety in some patients.

c. Implementing a medication regimen. The selection and adjustment of the antidepressant dose takes into consideration the medication's side effect profile and typically effective dose range and the patient's age and health status. The initial dose should be incrementally raised as tolerated until a presumably therapeutic dose is reached. The rate of increase and the total daily dose vary from individual to individual. Older adults generally require lower doses than do younger adults.

Blood drug levels have been shown to correlate with both the beneficial and toxic effects of many antidepressants, most notably nortriptyline, desipramine, and imipramine. Although drug level monitoring is not a mandatory component of antidepressant medication treatment, it may be useful when a patient is thought to be particularly vulnerable to the toxic effects of a medication; when a patient is prescribed multiple agents that may interfere with each other's metabolism, potentially causing particularly high or low drug levels; when a patient has displayed an inadequate response to a medication and a decision regarding discontinuation versus addition of another agent must be made; or when the patient's compliance is uncertain.

Antidepressant medications, especially tricyclics, are potentially lethal in overdose. Ingestion of a 10-day supply of a tricyclic agent administered at a dose of 200 mg/day is often lethal, and ingestion of lesser amounts can be quite dangerous. Early on in treatment it is prudent to dispense only small quantities of antidepressant medications, while keeping in mind the possibility that patients can hoard medication over time. Some of the newer antidepressants (notably trazodone, bupropion, sertraline, and fluoxetine) are substantially safer in overdose than the tricyclic agents.

Although some patients may become suicidal after the initiation of antidepressant treatment, the vast majority of studies suggest that all available antidepressants decrease, rather than increase, suicidal thoughts and indicate no predilection on the part of a particular agent to either ameliorate or aggravate suicidal tendencies (83, 84). The prescription of antidepressant medication is accompanied either by a specific program of psychotherapy or by a program of psychotherapeutic management. Whatever therapeutic approach is chosen, the psychiatrist should be observant for possible worsening as well as for improvement, as it may be necessary to change the nature or the site of treatment.

The coadministration of specific forms of psychotherapy with medication has the advantage, particularly in more chronic forms of depression and in those associated with marked psychosocial disabilities, of specifically addressing marital relationships and vocational conflicts and depressive cognitive dispositions. Psychotherapy or psychoanalysis can assist the patient in reversing the negative self-estimations and feelings about the future that are such ubiquitous features of depression. An ongoing psychotherapeutic relationship may help the patient to maintain therapeutic gains, however won, and may, in selected cases, be useful in delaying or preventing relapse.

2.   Electroconvulsive therapy

Electroconvulsive therapy (ECT) has a high rate of therapeutic success, relative speed in inducing improvement in depressive symptoms, and an excellent safety profile. Nevertheless, except in special circumstances, ECT is not generally regarded as a first-line treatment for uncomplicated major depression. This is in part a result of an undeserved reputation among the lay public that the treatment is "dangerous" and induces "brain damage." Alterations in the delivery of the electrical stimulus, the selected use of unilateral treatment, and advanced cardiopulmonary monitoring have made the treatment better tolerated and have increased the number of higher-risk patients who may be safely treated. At this time no absolute contraindications to ECT are recognized. The reader is referred to the 1990 report of the APA Task Force on Electroconvulsive Therapy (85) as the best available summary regarding this treatment's indications, technical considerations, and complications.

The evaluation preceding ECT should consist of a psychiatric history and examination to verify the indication for this treatment, a general medical evaluation to define risk factors (including medical history and physical examination, vital signs, hemogram, serum electrolyte measurements, and ECG), anesthesia evaluation addressing the nature and extent of anesthetic risk and the need for modification of medications or anesthetic technique, the obtaining of informed consent, and, finally, an evaluation that summarizes treatment indications and risks and suggests any indicated additional evaluative procedures, alterations in treatment, or modifications in ECT technique. Recent myocardial infarction, some cardiac arrhythmias, and some intracranial-space-occupying lesions are indications for caution and consultation, since ECT causes a transient rise in heart rate, cardiac workload, blood pressure, intracranial pressure, and blood-brain barrier permeability, which may not be tolerated by some patients with these conditions (85). In assessing such a case for treatment, the relative risks and benefits should be carefully weighed in collaboration with an anesthesiologist and a cardiologist or neurologist, as the case requires.

The chief side effects of ECT are cognitive. Treatment is associated with a transient postictal confusional state and with a longer period of anterograde and retrograde memory interference. The memory impairment, which has been difficult to disentangle from the memory deficits accompanying depression itself, typically resolves in a few weeks after cessation of treatment, except for some recent autobiographical memories (at least with bilateral ECT) (86). Rarely, patients report more pervasive and persistent cognitive disruption, the basis of which is uncertain.

ECT may be administered either bilaterally or unilaterally. Compared to bilateral treatment, unilateral placement induces less cognitive interference in most patients, but in some cases it is also less effective. Some patients who have not responded to unilateral treatment do respond to bilateral placement. When unilateral treatment is used, stimuli that are only marginally above seizure threshold exhibit a less satisfactory antidepressant effect than those of higher intensity, although this effect must be balanced against the cognitive interference evoked by grossly suprathreshold stimulation. In the event that unilateral treatment is initiated and the patient does not respond satisfactorily to the initial six treatments, bilateral treatment should be considered. Stimulus parameters vary from patient to patient but should be titrated to induce a generalized seizure of 25 seconds or more. The total course of treatment should be such that maximal remission of symptoms is achieved, i.e., the patient fully recovers or reaches a plateau.

ECT should be considered as an initial treatment for severe major depression when it is coupled with psychotic features, catatonic stupor, severe suicidality, or food refusal leading to nutritional compromise, as well as in other situations where for particular reasons a rapid antidepressant response is required. ECT is also indicated as a first-line treatment for patients who have previously shown a preferential response to this treatment modality or who prefer it. It should be considered for all patients with functional impairment whose illness has not responded to medication or who have a medical condition that precludes the use of an antidepressant medication.

3. Light therapy

In some patients with seasonal affective disorder, depressive manifestations respond to supplementation of environmental light by means of exposure to bright white artificial light in the morning and/or evening hours, for 30 minutes or more (87). Possible side effects include headache, eyestrain, irritability, and insomnia. Cautions have been raised about possible adverse ocular effects of phototherapy (88). No adverse interactions between light therapy and pharmacotherapy have been identified.

D. Continuation Treatment

Continuation treatment is based on the premise that there is a period of time following symptomatic recovery during which discontinuation of the treatment would likely result in relapse. The available data indicate that patients treated for a first episode of uncomplicated depression who exhibit a satisfactory response to an antidepressant agent should continue to receive a full therapeutic dose of that agent for at least 16–20 weeks after achieving full remission (89). The first 8 weeks after symptom resolution is a period of particularly high vulnerability to relapse. When medication is ultimately tapered and discontinued, patients should be carefully monitored during and immediately after discontinuation to ensure that remission is stable. Patients who have had multiple prior episodes of depression should be considered for maintenance medication treatment. Specific forms of psychotherapy, psychoanalysis, or psychotherapeutic management may be used during the continuation period to attenuate stresses and conflicts that might reexacerbate the depressive disorder or undermine medication compliance.

E. Maintenance Treatment

Depression is, for many, a recurrent disorder. Among those suffering an episode of major depression, between 50% and 85% will go on to have at least one lifetime recurrence, usually within 2 or 3 years. For patients prone to recurrences, continuous prophylactic drug treatment during periods of remission should be considered. Factors include the frequency and severity of past episodes, the efficacy and side effects of continuous treatment, and the potential effects of a recurrent episode in the patient's current life context. Factors increasing the risk of recurrence are the persistence of dysthymic symptoms after recovery from a depressive episode, presence of an additional nonaffective psychiatric diagnosis, presence of a chronic general medical disorder, and prior history of multiple episodes of depression (90). Increased severity of subsequent episodes is predicted by a history of a prior episode complicated by serious suicide attempts, psychotic features, or severe functional impairment. Drug side effects or monitoring requirements are themselves rarely the limiting factor in deciding for or against continuous drug treatment: the decision is most often based on factors related to the illness and to the patient's attitudes toward taking medication.

The therapeutic options for maintenance treatment include the various antidepressants and lithium (91, 92). In a study in which imipramine at full therapeutic dose was continued as maintenance therapy in unipolar depression, a significant benefit of active drug treatment was still evident at the conclusion of a 5-year period of investigation (38, 39). However, data are limited with regard to the full range of clinical decisions regarding medication use in the maintenance phase. For example, it is not yet clear whether lower doses, which are less likely to produce side effects, would be as effective as full doses (2). A reasonable strategy, therefore, is to continue the antidepressant medication at the full dose used to exert the initial therapeutic effect, unless this is not well tolerated, and to adjust the duration of maintenance treatment according to the factors already enumerated. For some patients with frequent depressive episodes, maintenance treatment may be required indefinitely. In the presence of a comorbid alcohol or substance abuse or dependence disorder, it is important to continue the appropriate treatment of the alcoholism or other substance dependence.

The timing and method of discontinuing maintenance treatment has not been systematically studied. Tapering, rather than abrupt discontinuation, is generally recommended because of the risk of cholinergic rebound with some medications (93) and theoretical concerns about depressive recurrences after the discontinuation of any antidepressant.

Patients stabilized with ECT who require maintenance therapy may first be given a trial of antidepressant medication according to the principles already outlined. Whether initially stabilized with medication or with ECT, patients who exhibit repeated episodes of moderate or severe depression despite maintenance with a combination of an antidepressant and lithium or patients who are medically ineligible for such treatment may be maintained with periodic ECT. Maintenance ECT is usually administered monthly; individuals for whom this is insufficient may find treatment at more frequent intervals to be beneficial. The benefits and optimal duration of maintenance ECT have not been well studied.

The decision to recommend continuing psychotherapy and the choice of which psychotherapy during the maintenance phase depend on a variety of factors; these include the degree of response to medication and the presence of unresolved intrapsychic or interpersonal conflicts that are distressing and that are thought to predispose the patient to depressive episodes. One report suggests that interpersonal psychotherapy during the maintenance phase may be effective in lengthening the interepisode interval in some less severely ill patients not receiving medication (38); its additive role in patients receiving medication is less well established (37).

F. Management of Medication-Resistant Depression

Initial treatment with antidepressant medication fails to achieve a satisfactory response in approximately 20%–30% of patients with major depressive disorder; in some cases the apparent lack of treatment response is actually a result of faulty diagnosis, inadequate treatment, or failure to appreciate and remedy coexisting general medical and psychiatric disorders or other complicating psychosocial factors (94). Adequate treatment for at least 6–8 weeks is necessary before concluding that a patient is not responsive to a particular medication (67). Some clinicians require two successive trials of medication of different categories for adequate durations before they consider a patient treatment resistant. The sequential use of antidepressants may subject patients to toxic interactions because of the persistence of the discontinued drug and its metabolites. If the clinician chooses to discontinue a monoamine uptake blocking antidepressant and substitute an MAO inhibitor, toxic interactions can best be avoided by allowing a 1- to 2-week washout period between drug trials. The long half-life of fluoxetine and its metabolites necessitates a 5-week washout period before the use of an MAO inhibitor.

1. Review of diagnosis

The first step in the care of a patient who has not responded to medication should be a review and reappraisal of the psychosocial and biological information base, aimed at re-verifying the diagnosis and identifying and remedying any neglected and possibly contributing factors, including general medical problems, alcohol or substance abuse or dependence, other psychiatric disorders, and general psychosocial issues impeding recovery. When the latter conditions are prominent, psychotherapy, if not already a part of the treatment approach, may prove to be effective in enhancing response (95).

2. Addition of an adjunct to an antidepressant

Lithium is the drug primarily used as an adjunct; other agents in use are thyroid hormone and stimulants. Data indicating the relative efficacies of the various adjunctive treatments are also lacking; opinion differs as to the relative benefits of lithium and thyroid supplementation. Lithium is felt by many experienced clinicians to be the most effective adjunct; it is reported useful in over 50% of antidepressant nonresponders and is usually well tolerated (96). The interval before full response to adjunctive lithium is said to be in the range of several days to 3 weeks. The blood level required in this context has not yet been determined. If effective and well tolerated, lithium should be continued for the duration of treatment of the acute episode. Thyroid hormone supplementation, even in euthyroid patients, may also increase the effectiveness of antidepressant treatment (97). The dose proposed for this purpose is 25 µg/day of triiodothyronine (T_3), increased to 50 µg/day in a week or so in the event of continued nonresponse. The duration of treatment required has not been well studied. Case reports suggest that stimulant medications may be effective adjuncts to antidepressant therapy (98, 99). There are no clear guidelines regarding the length of time stimulants should be coadministered.

3. Simultaneous use of multiple antidepressants

It is generally desirable to use the fewest medications possible, in order to minimize the risk of undesirable drug-drug interaction and to maximize compliance. Nonetheless, depression, especially if severe or unresponsive to simple or common regimens, is a serious, disabling, and potentially fatal illness; experienced clinicians sometimes find it necessary to combine various pharmacologic agents in their attempts to alleviate their patients' suffering. Antidepressant coadministration most commonly consists of the use of multiple non-MAO inhibitor antidepressants. Combinations of antidepressants carry a risk of adverse interaction and sometimes require dose adjustments. A selective serotonin-reuptake inhibitor in combination with a tricyclic agent, such as desipramine, has been reported to induce a particularly rapid antidepressant response (100). However, fluoxetine added to a tricyclic antidepressant causes an increased blood level and delayed elimination of the tricyclic drug, predisposing the patient to tricyclic drug toxicity unless the dose of the tricyclic is reduced (101). Another strategy is the combined use of a tricyclic antidepressant and an MAO inhibitor, a combination that is sometimes effective in alleviating severe medication-resistant depression, but the risk of toxic interactions necessitates careful monitoring (102, 103). The combined use of MAO inhibitors and other antidepressants has in some circumstances led to serious untoward reactions characterized by delirium, hyperthermia, hyperreflexia, and myoclonus; the reaction is sometimes referred to as the "serotonin syndrome" and is thought to be the result of overly enhanced serotonergic transmission. Tranylcypromine, clomipramine, and fluoxetine figure most prominently in reports of this interaction. Sertraline, because of its serotonin-uptake inhibiting properties, may be able to elicit the same toxic interaction. Psychiatrists choosing to use an MAO inhibitor in combination with another antidepressant should be well acquainted with the hazards of so doing, should carefully weigh the relative risks and benefits, and should avoid the agents most often implicated in toxic interactions.

4. Electroconvulsive therapy

ECT has the highest rate of response of any form of antidepressant treatment and should be considered in virtually all cases of moderate or severe major depression not responsive to pharmacologic intervention. ECT is considered safer than many forms of combination antidepressant treatment, although hard data are lacking. Approximately 50% of medication-resistant patients exhibit a satisfactory response to ECT (104). Lithium should be discontinued before initiation of ECT, as it has been reported to prolong postictal delirium (105) and delay recovery from neuromuscular blockade (106).

5. Anticonvulsants

Although their use in this context has not been extensively evaluated, carbamazepine and valproic acid have demonstrated some benefit in the treatment of medication-resistant depression (107, 108). Lithium may also increase the antidepressant effectiveness of carbamazepine (109).

G. Clinical Features Influencing Treatment

1. Suicide risk

Patients with major depression are at increased risk for suicide. Suicide risk should be assessed initially and over the course of treatment. If the patient has suicidal ideation, intention, and/or a plan, close surveillance is necessary. Factors to be considered in determining the nature and intensity of treatment include (but are not limited to) the nature of the doctor-patient alliance, the availability and adequacy of social supports, access to and lethality of suicide means, and past history of suicidal behavior. The risk of suicide in some patients recovering from depression increases transiently as they develop the energy and capacity to act on self-destructive plans made earlier in the course of their illness. Clinicians must be aware of the risk of suicide throughout the course of treatment of a depressive episode. However, it is not possible to predict with certainty whether a given patient will kill himself or herself. Therefore, even with the best possible care, a small proportion of depressed patients are likely to die by suicide.

2. Melancholia

The presence of melancholic features increases the likelihood of response to somatic intervention. While the most severe forms of major depression often fit the melancholic subtype, the presence of melancholic features and the severity of depression are to some degree independent phenomena.

3.   Severity

Patients with mild depression may be treated with psychotherapy alone or with a combination of medication and psychotherapy. Even mild depression, if unresponsive to nonsomatic treatment, should be considered for antidepressant medication therapy. As severity increases, somatic intervention, usually in the form of antidepressant medication, becomes progressively indicated; in the most severe cases, ECT plays a greater role as a primary treatment. In general, the rate of response of very severe depression, even to somatic treatment, is less satisfactory than that of moderate depression (110), although some quite severe cases exhibit virtually total remission after somatic treatment.

4.   Recurrent depression

Depression is often a recurrent disorder. Although the data do not indicate a preferential response to any particular form of antidepressant treatment simply on the basis of a history of multiple prior episodes, patients who have sustained repetitive bouts of major depression should be carefully considered for maintenance therapy after the remediation of the current episode. When deciding on a course of treatment for individuals who have been treated for prior episodes, the psychiatrist should carefully ascertain the degree of response to and tolerance of the prior treatment modalities.

5.   Prior mania or hypomania

All antidepressant treatments, including ECT, may provoke manic or hypomanic episodes in some patients treated for depression (111). Individuals with a history of mania or hypomania are at particular risk for this untoward effect, although it may occur even in patients with no such history; this complication is estimated to occur in 5%–20% of depressed patients treated with antidepressants (112, 113). Patients who display a switch from depression to hypomania or mania provoked by antidepressant drugs may have underlying bipolar disorder, in that such individuals are likely to subsequently develop spontaneous mania and frequently have family histories of bipolar disorder (113).

A related untoward effect of antidepressant treatment, especially with tricyclic agents and especially in bipolar patients, is the precipitation of rapid cycling between depression and mania. Individuals who have developed rapid cycling could be treated by withdrawing the tricyclic antidepressant and instituting treatment with lithium, either alone or in conjunction with an MAO inhibitor or another antidepressant, such as bupropion (114, 115). ECT is also effective for this condition and may be used if medications are ineffective. For most patients with major depression and no history of manic or hypomanic episodes, the risk of antidepressant medication precipitating either rapid cycling or a switch into mania is small (112).

6. Depression with psychotic features

Depression with psychotic features carries a higher risk of suicide than does major depression uncomplicated by psychosis (116), and it constitutes a risk factor for recurrent depression. Depression with psychotic features responds better to treatment with a combination of a neuroleptic and an antidepressant than to treatment with either component alone (117). Some clinicians prefer to use amoxapine, an antidepressant with neuroleptic activity, in order to confine treatment to a single agent (118). Lithium augmentation is helpful in some cases refractory to combined antidepressant-neuroleptic treatment (119). ECT is highly effective in depression with psychotic features and may be considered a first-line treatment for this disorder (120).

7. Depression with catatonic features

Catatonic features may occur in the context of mood disorders and are characterized by at least two of the following manifestations: motoric immobility as evidenced by catalepsy or stupor; extreme agitation; extreme negativism; peculiarities of voluntary movement as evidenced by posturing, stereotyped movements, mannerisms, or grimacing; and echolalia or echopraxia (121). Catatonia often dominates the presentation and may be so severe as to be life-threatening, compelling the consideration of urgent biological treatment. Immediate relief may often be obtained by the intravenous administration of amobarbital or lorazepam. For patients who show some relief, continued oral administration of amobarbital, lorazepam, or diazepam may be helpful. Concurrent antidepressant drug treatments should be considered. When relief is not immediately obtained by administering barbiturates or benzodiazepine, the urgent provision of ECT should be considered. The efficacy of ECT, usually apparent after a few treatments, is well documented; ECT may initially be administered daily. After the catatonic manifestations are relieved, treatment may be continued with antidepressants, lithium, neuroleptics, or a combination of these compounds, as determined by the patient's condition.

8. Depression with atypical features

Atypical depressive features include severe anxiety, vegetative symptoms of reversed polarity (i.e., increased rather than decreased sleep, appetite, and weight), marked mood reactivity, sensitivity to emotional rejection, phobic symptoms, and a sense of severe fatigue that creates a sensation of "leaden paralysis" or extreme heaviness of the arms or legs (122). Patients need not have all of these features to be diagnosed as having atypical depression. In some patients symptoms of anxiety predominate, while others have predominantly vegetative symptoms (123). There is some overlap between patients with atypical depression and patients with anergic bipolar depression. Tricyclic antidepressants yield response rates of only 35%–50% in patients with atypical depression; in contrast, MAO inhibitors yield response rates of 55%–75% in patients with atypical depression, comparable to the rate of response of typical forms of major depression to tricyclic therapy (124, 125). If it is determined that the patient does not wish to, cannot, or is unlikely to adhere to the dietary and drug precautions associated with MAO inhibitor treatment, the use of an alternative antidepressant is indicated. Many clinicians claim considerable success with fluoxetine and sertraline in this disorder, and some studies suggest a role for bupropion (126, 127), although this agent may be anxiogenic and is not preferred in cases where anxiety predominates.

9. Alcohol and/or substance abuse or dependence

Because of the frequent comorbidity of depression and alcohol or other substance abuse, the psychiatrist should make every effort to obtain a detailed history of the patient's substance use. If there is suspicion that there is a problem in this area, the clinician should consider questioning a collateral for confirmation. If the patient is found to have a substance use disorder, a program to secure abstinence should be regarded as a principal priority in the treatment. A patient suffering from major depression with comorbid addiction is more likely to require hospitalization, more likely to attempt suicide, and less likely to comply with treatment than is a patient with depression of similar severity not complicated by this factor. Some alcohol- and/or chemical-abusing patients reduce their consumption of these substances upon remediation of an underlying depressive disorder, making the recognition and treatment of depression doubly important for such individuals. Among depressed patients with habitual alcohol or other substance abuse, however, the majority of depressive symptoms remit simply with abstinence (128), but sometimes only after a period of 6 weeks. It is likewise advisable, if other factors permit, to detoxify such a patient before initiating antidepressant therapy. Identifying which patients should be started on a regimen of antidepressant therapy earlier, after initiation of abstinence, is difficult. A positive family history of depression, a history of depression preceding alcohol or other substance abuse, or a history of major depression during periods of sobriety raises the likelihood that the patient would benefit from antidepressant treatment, which may then be started earlier in treatment.

Concurrent drug abuse, especially with stimulant drugs, predisposes the patient to toxic interactions with MAO inhibitors, although there have been few reports of such events (129). Benzodiazepines and other sedative hypnotics carry the potential for abuse or dependence and should be used cautiously except as part of a detoxification regimen. Benzodiazepines have also been reported to contribute to depressive symptoms. Hepatic dysfunction and hepatic enzyme induction frequently complicate pharmacotherapy of patients with alcoholism and other substance abuse; these conditions require careful monitoring of blood levels, if available, therapeutic effects, and side effects to avoid either psychotropic drug intoxication or inadequate treatment.

10. Depression with features of obsessive-compulsive disorder

Depressive episodes have a higher than chance likelihood of occurring in obsessive-compulsive disorder. Clomipramine and the selective serotonin-reuptake blockers have demonstrated efficacy in the management of obsessive-compulsive disorder (130, 131); these agents are also effective antidepressants and may be used to good effect when obsessive symptoms accompany an episode of major depression.

11. Depression with panic and/or other anxiety disorders

Panic disorder complicates major depression in 15%–30% of the cases (132). Individuals with symptoms of both disorders manifest greater degrees of impairment than do patients with major depression only. Depression with coexistent anxiety or panic disorder generally responds less well to non-MAO antidepressants than do other forms of depression; despite the somewhat greater efficacy of MAO inhibitors (132), therapy should first be initiated with another agent because of the somewhat greater complications associated with MAO inhibitors. Imipramine has been shown to be effective in this context (133). Tricyclic antidepressants and selective serotonin-reuptake inhibitors may initially worsen rather than alleviate anxiety and panic symptoms; these medications should therefore be introduced at a low dose and slowly increased when used to treat such patients. Bupropion has been reported as ineffective in the treatment of panic disorder (134). Alprazolam may sometimes be used with benefit either in conjunction with antidepressants or as the sole pharmacologic agent for anxiety, with or without panic, coupled with milder forms of depression. However, the efficacy of alprazolam in the treatment of depression of greater severity is inferior to that of most antidepressants.

12. Depression-related cognitive dysfunction (pseudodementia)

Major depression is routinely accompanied by signs and symptoms of cognitive inefficiency. Some patients have both depression and dementia, while others have depression that causes cognitive impairment (i.e., pseudodementia). In the latter case, the treatment of the depression should reverse the signs and symptoms of cognitive dysfunction. Many patients complain that their thoughts are slowed and their capacity to process information is reduced, and they display diminished attention to their self-care and to their environment. Transient cognitive impairments, especially involving attention, concentration, and memory storage and retrieval, are demonstrable through neuropsychological testing (135). In extreme examples, especially in the elderly, these complaints and deficits are so prominent that patients may appear demented. Depression-related cognitive dysfunction is a reversible condition that resolves with treatment of the underlying depression. Several clinical features help differentiate depressive pseudodementia from true dementia. When performing cognitive tasks, pseudodemented patients generally exert relatively less effort but report more incapacity than do demented patients. The latter group, especially in more advanced stages, typically neither recognize nor complain of their cognitive failures, since insight is impaired; in comparison, pseudodemented patients characteristically complain bitterly that they "can't think" or "can't remember." Depressive pseudodementia lacks the signs of cortical dysfunction (i.e., aphasia, apraxia, agnosia) encountered in degenerative dementia, such as Alzheimer's disease (136). It is vital that individuals with depression-related cognitive disturbance not be misdiagnosed and thereby denied vigorous antidepressant treatment or ECT.

13.   Postpsychotic depression

Depressive symptoms complicate the course of schizophrenia in as many as 25% of the cases (137). The depressive symptoms may coexist with the manifestations of the schizophrenic illness or may emerge after the resolution of the acute schizophrenic psychosis, a pattern referred to as "postpsychotic depression." The recognition of this syndrome is complicated by an overlap with the negative symptoms of schizophrenia (138), the akinetic effects of antipsychotic medications (139), or inaccurately diagnosed bipolar and schizoaffective syndromes. The depressive manifestations are severe enough to represent the equivalent of major depression in only a minority of cases of true postpsychotic depression, but when they are present they result in accrued and prolonged disability and may increase the risk of suicide. Postpsychotic depression has been effectively treated by adding an antidepressant agent to the patient's neuroleptic regimen (140).

14.   Depression during pregnancy or following childbirth

Major depression occurring during pregnancy is a difficult therapeutic problem. Women of childbearing potential in psychiatric treatment should be carefully counseled as to the risks of becoming pregnant while taking psychotropic medications. Whenever possible, a pregnancy should be planned in consultation with the psychiatrist so that medication may be discontinued before conception if feasible. The clinician must carefully weigh the risks and benefits of prescribing psychotropic agents to the pregnant patient, taking into consideration the possibilities of physical (especially during the first trimester) and behavioral teratogenesis. The latter concern is based in part on the documentation in experimental animals exposed prenatally to psychotropic medications of abnormalities of behavioral and neurochemical development (141). This effect has not yet been demonstrated in human beings but remains a theoretical consideration. Although tricyclic antidepressants, MAO inhibitors, and the newer antidepressant medications have not been specifically incriminated as causing physical birth defects, this issue too remains open (142). Benzodiazepines have been inconclusively implicated in the development of cleft lip and palate when used in the first trimester. Although lithium exposure in the first trimester has been associated with an increased risk of cardiac malformations (143), the only prospective study of this issue indicated that the risks associated with lithium may not be as high as was previously believed (144).

The relative risks and benefits of prescribing antidepressants must be particularly carefully weighed in the treatment of a pregnant woman. In patients whose safety and well-being require antidepressant medications, a tricyclic or any of the newer antidepressant compounds may be justifiably used, after the first trimester if possible. In selected cases refractory to or unsuitable for medication, for patients with depression with psychotic features, or for individuals electing to use this modality as a matter of preference after having weighed the relative risks and benefits, ECT may be used as an alternative treatment; the current literature supports the safety for mother and fetus, as well as the efficacy of ECT during pregnancy (145).

Several depressive conditions may follow childbirth (146). The transient 7- to 10-day depressive condition referred to as "postpartum blues" typically is too mild to meet the criteria for major depressive disorder and does not require medication. It is optimally treated by reassuring the patient of its brief nature and favorable outcome. Puerperal psychosis is a more severe disorder complicating 1–2 per 1,000 births; more than one-half of the episodes of this type meet the criteria for major depression (147), and many patients who have had episodes of this type ultimately prove to have bipolar disorder. Women whose maintenance antidepressant treatment was discontinued during pregnancy appear to be particularly at risk for recurrence of depression; such individuals should have their medications restored after delivery, in the absence of a contraindication. Postpartum depressive illness should be treated according to the same principles delineated for other depressive conditions. Nursing mothers ideally should not receive antidepressants or lithium in order not to pass metabolically active compounds to their infants; mothers should be counseled regarding the relative risks and benefits of so doing (148).

15.   Depression superimposed on dysthymia

"Double depression" is the term used to describe the condition of a patient with chronic dysthymia who suffers the additional burden of a more severe and pervasive major depressive episode. Patients with this syndrome should not be denied specific antidepressant treatment on the basis of the chronicity of dysfunction. Antidepressant treatment may reverse not only the acute depressive episode but also the underlying chronic dysthymia (149). A variety of antidepressant agents have proven useful in the treatment of chronic dysthymia (150); the selective serotonin-reuptake inhibitors and MAO inhibitors may be the most effective (151). It is suggested that MAO inhibitors be reserved for patients who are not responding to other agents. Individuals with this syndrome should be carefully considered for psychodynamic psychotherapy or psychoanalysis in order to examine psychological factors that maintain the depressed disposition.

16.   Depression superimposed on a personality disorder

People with any of a variety of personality disorders, including obsessive-compulsive, avoidant, dependent, and borderline disorders, are prone to episodes of major depression (152). Clinical experience indicates that patients with narcissistic personality disorder are also particularly vulnerable to episodes of major depressive disorder. Depression in patients meeting the criteria for borderline personality disorder frequently exhibits atypical features, including mood reactivity, and may be more likely to respond to MAO inhibitors and to selective serotonin-uptake inhibitors than to tricyclics (153). Patients with virtually any form of personality disorder exhibit less satisfactory antidepressant treatment response, in terms of both social functioning and residual depressive symptoms, than do individuals without personality disorders (154). However, psychodynamic psychotherapy or psycho-analysis may be beneficial in modifying the personality disorder in selected patients. Antisocial personality traits tend to interfere with treatment compliance and particularly with a psychotherapeutic relationship.

17. Seasonal depression

Some individuals suffer annual episodes of depression whose onset is in the fall or early winter, usually at the same time each year. Some of these patients suffer manic or hypomanic episodes as well. The depressive episodes frequently have atypical features such as hyper-somnia and overeating. The entire range of treatments for depression may also be used to treat seasonal affective disorder, either in combination with or as an alternative to light therapy. As a sole form of treatment, light therapy may be recommended as a time-limited trial (87), primarily in outpatients with clear seasonal patterns. In patients with more severe forms of seasonal depression, its use is considered adjunctive to psychopharmacologic intervention.

H.   Treatment Implications of Concurrent General Medical Disorders

1.   Asthma

Individuals with asthma who receive MAO inhibitors should be cautioned regarding interactions with sympathomimetic bronchodilators, although other antiasthma agents appear to be safe. Other antidepressants may be used for patients with asthma without fear of interaction.

2.   Cardiac disease

The presence of specific cardiac conditions complicates or contraindicates certain forms of antidepressant therapy, notably use of tricyclic agents; the cardiac history should therefore be carefully explored before the initiation of drug treatment. Psychiatrists should take particular care in using tricyclics for patients with a history of ventricular arrhythmia, subclinical sinus node dysfunction, conduction defects (including asymptomatic conduction defects), prolonged QT intervals, or a recent history of myocardial infarction (74, 76–79, 81, 82).

Bupropion, fluoxetine, sertraline, and ECT appear to be safe for patients with preexisting cardiac disease (155, 156). MAO inhibitors do not adversely affect cardiac conduction, rhythm, or contraction but may induce orthostatic hypotension and also run the risk of interacting adversely with other medications that may be taken by such patients. There is anecdotal evidence that trazodone may induce ventricular arrhythmias, but the agent appears to be safe for the overwhelming majority of patients.

A depressed patient with a history of any cardiac problem should be monitored for the emergence of cardiac symptoms, ECG changes, or orthostatic blood pressure decrements. Consultation with the patient's cardiologist before and during antidepressant treatment may be advisable and is especially advisable during any treatment for a patient who has recently had a myocardial infarction.

3. Dementia

Treatment of depression in the cognitively impaired patient requires the involvement of care providers in the patient's pharmacotherapy, supervision, and monitoring: this may entail education of home health aides, nursing home providers, and others.

Individuals with dementia are particularly susceptible to the toxic effects of muscarinic blockade on memory and attention. Therefore, individuals suffering from dementia generally do best when given antidepressant medications with the lowest possible degree of anticholinergic effect, e.g., bupropion, fluoxetine, sertraline, trazodone, and, of the tricyclic agents, desipramine or nortriptyline. Alternatively, some patients do well given stimulants in small doses. ECT is also effective in depression superimposed on dementia, and it should be used if medications are contraindicated or are not tolerated or if immediate resolution of the depressive episode is medically indicated, as when it interferes with the patient's acceptance of food.

4. Epilepsy

Although many antidepressants lower the seizure threshold and theoretically exert an adverse effect on seizure control in depressed patients with epilepsy, major depression in patients with seizure disorders can usually be safely and effectively managed according to the same principles outlined for patients without this condition. Likewise, epilepsy is not a contraindication to ECT, which actually exerts a transient suppressive effect on seizure frequency (157).

5. Glaucoma

Drugs with anticholinergic potency may precipitate acute narrow-angle glaucoma in susceptible individuals (i.e., those with shallow anterior chambers) (158). Patients with glaucoma receiving local miotic therapy may be treated with antidepressants, including those possessing anticholinergic properties, provided that their intraocular pressure is monitored during antidepressant treatment. Agents lacking anticholinergic activity (bupropion, sertraline, fluoxetine, and trazodone) avoid this liability.

6. Hypertension

Antihypertensive agents and tricyclic antidepressants may interact to either intensify or counteract the effect of the antihypertensive therapy. The action of antihypertensive agents that block alpha receptors (e.g., prazosin) may be intensified by tricyclic antidepressants that block these same receptors, notably the tricyclic antidepressants and trazodone. Tricyclic antidepressants may antagonize the therapeutic actions of guanethidine, clonidine, or α-methyldopa. Concurrent antihypertensive treatment, especially with diuretics, increases the likelihood that tricyclic antidepressants, trazodone, or MAO inhibitors will induce symptomatic orthostatic hypotension. Beta blockers, especially propranolol, may be a cause of depression in some patients; individuals who have become depressed after initiation of treatment with one of these drugs should be changed to another antihypertensive regimen.

7. Obstructive uropathy

Prostatism and other forms of bladder outlet obstruction are relative contraindications to the use of antidepressant compounds with antimuscarinic effects. Benzodiazepines, trazodone, and MAO inhibitors may also retard bladder emptying. The antidepressant medications with the least propensity to do this are fluoxetine, sertraline, bupropion, and desipramine.

8. Parkinson's disease

Amoxapine, an antidepressant with dopamine-receptor blocking properties, should be avoided for patients who have Parkinson's disease. Lithium may in some instances induce or exacerbate parkinsonian symptoms. Bupropion, in contrast, exerts a beneficial effect on the symptoms of Parkinson's disease in some patients but may also induce psychotic symptoms, perhaps because of its agonistic action in the dopaminergic system (159). MAO inhibitors (other than selegiline, also known as L-deprenyl, a selective type B MAO inhibitor recommended in the treatment of Parkinson's disease) may adversely interact with L-dopa products (160). Selegiline loses its specificity for MAO-B in doses greater than 10 mg/day and may induce the serotonin syndrome when given in higher doses in conjunction with serotonin-enhancing antidepressants. Depression, which occurs to some degree in 40%–50% of the patients with Parkinson's disease, may be related to the alterations of serotonergic and noradrenergic systems that occur in this disorder. There is no evidence favoring any particular antidepressant from the standpoint of therapeutic efficacy in depression complicating Parkinson's disease. The theoretical benefits of the antimuscarinic effects of some of the tricyclic agents in the treatment of depressed patients with Parkinson's disease are offset by the memory impairment that may result. ECT exerts a transient beneficial effect on the symptoms of idiopathic Parkinson's disease in many patients (161).

I. Influence of Family History on Treatment

1. Family history of depression

The presence of a positive family history of recurrent depression increases the chances that the patient's own illness will be recurrent and that the patient will not fully recover between episodes.

2. Family history of bipolar disorder

The presence in a depressed patient of a positive family history of bipolar disorder or acute psychosis probably increases the chances that the patient's own depressive disorder is a manifestation of bipolar rather than unipolar disorder and that antidepressant therapy may incite a switch into mania (113). Patients with such a family history should be particularly closely questioned regarding a prior history of mania or hypomania, since lithium used alone or in conjunction with another antidepressant is particularly likely to exert a beneficial effect in depressed patients with bipolar disorder. Depressed patients with a family history of bipolar disorder should be carefully observed for signs of a switch to mania during antidepressant treatment.

J.   Treatment Implications of Various Demographic and Psychosocial Variables

1.   Major stressors

Major depression may follow a substantial adverse life event, especially one that involves the loss of an important human relationship or life role. Major depressive episodes following life stresses are no less likely than others either to require or to benefit from antidepressant medication treatment. Nonetheless, attention to the relationship of both prior and concurrent life events to the onset, exacerbation, or maintenance of depressive symptoms is an important aspect of the overall treatment approach. A close relationship between a life stressor and major depression suggests the potential utility of a psychotherapeutic intervention, coupled, as indicated, with somatic treatment.

2.   Bereavement

Bereavement is a particularly severe stressor and is commonly accompanied by the signs and symptoms of major depression. Historically, such depressive manifestations have been regarded as normative, and presentations otherwise diagnosable as major depression are therefore diagnosed in DSM-III-R as "uncomplicated bereavement" when they begin within the first 3 months of the loss (1). Data indicate that almost one-quarter of bereaved individuals meet the criteria for major depression at 2 months and again at 7 months and that many of these people continue to do so at 13 months (162). Individuals with more prolonged depressive manifestations tend to be younger and to have a history of prior episodes of major depression. Although psychiatrists formerly believed that in most cases there is little reason to treat the depressive symptoms of bereavement with antidepressants or psychotherapy, it is now recognized that these treatments should be used when the reaction to a loss is particularly prolonged and psychopathology and functional impairment persist.

3. Family distress

The recognition of a problem in the family setting is important in that such a situation constitutes an ongoing stressor that may hamper the patient's response to treatment. Ambivalent, abusive, rejecting, or highly dependent family relationships may particularly predispose to depression. Such families should be evaluated for family therapy, which may be used in conjunction with individual and pharmacologic therapies. In some cases the stresses imposed on the patient by the family conflict may be so severe that hospitalization is indicated as a means of removing the patient from an otherwise unavoidable stressor. Even in instances where there is no apparent family dysfunction it is important to provide the family with education about the nature of the illness and to enlist the family's support and cooperation.

4. Older age

Indications for psychotherapy for the elderly are essentially the same as for younger patients. The elderly typically display more vegetative signs and cognitive disturbance and complain less of subjective dysphoria than do their younger counterparts; depression may consequently be misattributed to physical illness, dementia, or the aging process itself. It is recognized, however, that depression and general medical illness frequently coexist in this age group, and those undergoing their first major depressive episode in old age should be regarded as possibly harboring an as yet undiagnosed neurological or other general medical disorder that is responsible for the depressive condition. Some medications commonly prescribed for the elderly (e.g., beta blockers) are thought to be risk factors for the development of major depression. The clinician should carefully assess whether a given agent contributed to the depression before prematurely altering what may be a valuable medication regimen. Major depression is a common complication of cerebral infarction, especially in the anterior left hemisphere (163).

While elderly patients typically require a lower oral dose than younger patients to yield a particular blood level and tolerate a given blood level less well, the blood levels at which antidepressant agents are maximally effective appear to be the same as for younger patients (164). Elderly patients are particularly prone to orthostatic hypotension and cholinergic blockade, discussed elsewhere; for this reason, fluoxetine, sertraline, bupropion, desipramine, and nortriptyline are frequently chosen rather than amitriptyline, imipramine, and doxepin. Although the role of stimulants for antidepressant monotherapy is very limited, these compounds have some role in apathetic depression in elderly patients with complicating general medical conditions.

5. Gender

The diagnostic assessment for women, in particular, should include a detailed inquiry regarding sexual and physical abuse and reproductive life history, including menstruation, menopause, birth control, and abortion.

Some women who are taking birth control pills require higher doses of tricyclic anti-depressants because of the induction of the hepatic enzymes responsible for drug metabolism. While newly menopausal women may exhibit depressive symptoms, there is no established role for estrogen replacement in the treatment of full-blown major depression in this group of patients.

Caution is advised in the prescription of trazodone to men because of the risk of priapism. Older men are at risk for prostatic hypertrophy, making them particularly sensitive to drug effects on the bladder outlet.

6. Cultural factors

Specific cultural variables may hamper the accurate assessment of depressive symptoms. An appreciation by the therapist of cultural variables is critical in the accurate diagnosis of depression and in the selection and conduct of psychotherapy and pharmacotherapy. There is evidence that the expression of depressive symptoms may vary among cultures, especially the tendency to manifest somatic and psychomotor symptoms (165). Ethnic groups may also differ in their pharmacotherapeutic responses to antidepressant agents (166, 167). The language barrier has also been shown to severely impede accurate psychiatric diagnosis and effective treatment (168). These issues are extensively reviewed in *Culture and Depression* (169).

K. Assessment of the Need for Hospitalization

1. The patient lacking the capacity to cooperate with treatment

Depressed patients who, along with any available social supports, are unable to adequately care for themselves, cooperate with outpatient treatment of their depression, and/or provide reliable feedback to their psychiatrist regarding their clinical status are candidates for hospitalization, full or partial, even in the absence of a tendency toward intentional self-harm.

2. The patient at risk for suicide and/or homicide

Patients with suicidal or homicidal ideation, intention, and/or a plan require close monitoring. Patients at particularly high risk may benefit from hospitalization, where close observation, restricted access to violent means, and more intensive treatment are possible.

3. The patient lacking psychosocial supports

Recovery from major depression is aided by an environment that encourages safety, constructive activity, positive interpersonal interactions, and compliance with treatment. If the environment lacks these features or exposes the patient to undesirable or dangerous activities, such as alcohol or drug abuse, admission to a hospital or an intensive day program should be considered.

4. Other factors influencing the need for hospitalization

Hospitalization may be necessary for patients with complicating psychiatric or general medical conditions that make outpatient treatment unsafe. Detoxification and/or withdrawal from psychoactive substances may necessitate hospitalization. Depressed patients, especially those with psychotic symptoms, may engage in bizarre or imprudent behavior that may endanger their important relationships, reputation, or assets; hospitalization may be necessary to protect the patient and others. Patients who have not responded to outpatient treatment may need to be hospitalized in order to receive the type or intensity of treatment that is deemed necessary.

III. Summary of Recommendations

A. Coding System

Each recommendation is identified as falling into one of three categories of endorsement, by a bracketed Roman numeral following the statement. The three categories represent varying levels of clinical confidence regarding the efficacy of the treatment for the disorder and conditions described.

[I]   indicates recommended with substantial clinical confidence.
[II]   indicates recommended with moderate clinical confidence.
[III] indicates options that may be recommended on the basis of individual circumstances.

B. General Considerations

Each patient treated for major depression requires an individually tailored therapeutic program. Other mental disorders, including alcohol or substance abuse and dependence, and general medical comorbidities must be assessed and treated appropriately. The presence and degree of suicidal ideation and/or behaviors are important factors in the choice and intensity of treatment throughout the course of the disorder. Effective treatments for major depression include psychotherapy, antidepressant medications, and ECT [I]. Most patients are best treated with antidepressant medication coupled with psychotherapeutic management or psychotherapy [II]. Some patients with mild to moderate degrees of impairment may be treated with psychotherapeutic management or psychotherapy alone, provided that it is not prolonged without distinct improvement before a trial of antidepressants is initiated (unless there is a specific therapeutic contraindication) [II].

The psychiatrist must also decide on the site of treatment. Hospitalization may be indicated for patients who lack the capacity to cooperate with treatment, are at risk for suicide or other violent behavior, lack psychosocial supports, require detoxification or withdrawal, have other psychiatric or general medical problems that make outpatient treatment unsafe, or are judged to need a hospital environment to safely receive the treatment that is required [I].

C. Acute Phase

The *psychosocial therapeutic program* may range from psychotherapeutic management to one of a number of forms of systematic psychotherapy. The approach most congruent with the patient's needs should be chosen. The differential efficacies of and the indications for the various psychotherapies have not been fully established by formal studies. Interpersonal therapy may be suited for individuals who have experienced recent interpersonal conflicts or difficult role transitions [II]. Cognitive therapy may be used for those who desire and/or tolerate structured guidance to correct their distorted concepts of themselves and others [II]. The psychodynamic approach or psychoanalysis may be used in the presence of chronic self-underestimation, excessive self-expectations, chronic interpersonal conflicts, or unresolved early losses or separations, if the patient is inclined to be introspective, psychologically minded, and motivated and has a stable environment [II]. Marital, family, behavior, and group therapies may also be used [II]. Alcohol or substance abuse and dependence must be treated when they coexist with major depressive disorder [I].

The *somatic therapeutic program* consists of antidepressant medications or ECT [I]. Any one of a number of antidepressant agents may be rationally selected, according to principles outlined in the body of this guideline. Except in specific circumstances that will be enumerated, antidepressant medication treatment may begin with any non-MAO antidepressant compound [I].

Depression with atypical features responds more frequently to MAO inhibitors than to tricyclic agents; there are some positive data on the response to selective serotonin-reuptake blockers. Given the possible complications of MAO inhibitor use, the clinician must weigh the risks and benefits of prescribing MAO inhibitors before a trial of another agent [II].

Patients with various general medical problems, especially cardiac dysfunction or conditions contraindicating exposure to anticholinergic side effects, may tolerate bupropion, fluoxetine, sertraline, trazodone, or ECT better than they do the tricyclic antidepressants [I]. Patients suffering from depression with psychotic features usually require treatment with a combination of an antidepressant and a neuroleptic [I] or with ECT [I] or, alternatively, with amoxapine [II]. The presence of food refusal and nutritional compromise, suicidal actions from which the patient cannot be protected, and severe withdrawal are indications for considering ECT in preference to medication [I]. The use of sedative-hypnotics and coexisting alcohol or drug use disorders must be closely monitored during treatment with antidepressant medication.

Patients not responding after 6–8 weeks of antidepressant treatment at an adequate dose may be considered medication resistant. Others reserve this category for patients who do not respond to successive courses of treatment with two different agents given at adequate doses. Before a patient is considered medication resistant, the general medical and psychiatric evaluation should be reviewed to confirm the diagnosis. If the patient is considered medication resistant on the basis of unsatisfactory response to an antidepressant agent for 6–8 weeks, the preferred treatment option is a trial of an alternative non-MAO inhibitor antidepressant with a different biochemical profile [II], coadministration of the original antidepressant plus lithium [II] or thyroid hormone [II], or the coadministration of a second antidepressant. Other alternatives include changing the medication to an MAO inhibitor or an anticonvulsant [II] or the use of adjunctive stimulants [III].

ECT is highly efficacious in moderate or severe major depression and in major depression with melancholic features, and it should be considered as an initial treatment in patients with psychotic features, catatonic stupor, severe suicidality, or food refusal [I]. Also, it should be offered to all moderately or severely depressed patients who do not respond to adequate trials of medication [I]. It is important that the clinician discuss the possibility of ECT with a patient before pursuing a prolonged series of medication trials.

D.   Continuation Phase

Patients with a first episode of uncomplicated major depression who respond satisfactorily to an antidepressant agent should be maintained with a full therapeutic dose of that medication for a minimum of 16–20 weeks after remission has been achieved, in combination with an appropriate psychotherapeutic program [I].

E.   Maintenance Phase

For many patients with recurrent unipolar depression of sufficient severity and frequency, maintenance therapy using the medication effective in inducing remission may be best continued for a prolonged period of time, in some cases indefinitely [II]. In cases where there has been a long period of stability with maintenance treatment, the physician and patient may wish to discuss the pros and cons of a trial without medication [II]. In medication-compliant depressed patients receiving adequate doses of maintenance antidepressants who manifest breakthrough depressive episodes, lithium may be substituted or used in combination [II]. Psychological and interpersonal factors often play a substantive role in increasing the risk of recurrence, and psychotherapy may be very productive during the maintenance phase. The specific therapeutic approach, frequency of contact, and duration of treatment are selected according to the factors outlined in the text [II].

IV. Research Directions

It is necessary that the very components and nature of the psychotherapeutic processes be better understood in order to define the specific indications for various forms of therapy and their differential utility for various subtypes and stages of depression. The precise roles and degrees of efficacy of these therapies in the acute, continuation, and maintenance phases of treatment require further investigation. Which treatments are most efficacious in the initial phase of treatment? Which treatments are most effective in preventing relapse? Should multiple forms of therapy be used, and, if so, should they be given conjunctively or sequentially? What is the optimal frequency of psychotherapeutic contacts, for the various forms of treatment, in the acute, continuation, and maintenance phases?

Despite notable clinical progress in predicting a beneficial response to antidepressant medication treatment, many issues continue to require clarification. While something is known of the specific clinical indications for the various antidepressant agents, this area is still relatively unclear. For example, what is the utility of the newer antidepressants in atypical depression? The duration of treatment before a patient is considered medication resistant and whether or not this varies among agents require clarification. The relationship between blood level and response for older medications continues to be controversial; there is still less information in this regard for the newer antidepressants. Specific indications for each of the various adjunctive treatments for nonresponders and the duration of treatment required for these adjunctive treatments continue to be unknown. The cardiotoxic effects of the newer agents in comparison to older-generation antidepressants require further study. In the maintenance phase, the comparative efficacy of newer antidepressants requires study. The required duration of maintenance treatment, indications for its trial discontinuation, and possible risks of so doing vis-à-vis the long-term prognosis of the disorder are unknown and should be elucidated. Little is known about the treatment of depression in patients over age 80.

Regarding ECT, the indications for initial treatment with bilateral electrode placement and the optimal number of unilateral treatments without satisfactory response before a switch from unilateral to bilateral electrode placement require elucidation. Methods of avoiding cognitive interference require exploration. The indications for and best methods of providing maintenance ECT require study.

There is a relative void in our ability to offer patients and their families a firm prognosis specific to individual circumstances in regard to expected course of illness, date of return to routine responsibilities, and the likelihood of further episodes with and without maintenance treatment.

V. Major Depression Guideline Reviewers and Consultants

Sigurd H. Ackerman, M.D.
Hagop S. Akiskal, M.D.
Thomas E. Allen, M.D.
Paul J. Ambrosini, M.D.
Gregory M. Asnis, M.D.
Henry Bachrach, Ph.D.
Ross J. Baldessarini, M.D.
Donald Banzhaf, M.D.
Aaron T. Beck, M.D.
Jerome S. Beigler, M.D.
Richard Belitsky, M.D.
Jules R. Bemporad, M.D.
Roger Bland, M.D.
Dan G. Blazer, M.D.
Peter Blos, Jr., M.D.
Charles Lee Bowden, M.D.
Martin Brenner, M.D.
Walter A. Brown, M.D.
Anna Burton, M.D.
Robert P. Cabaj, M.D.
Oliver G. Cameron, M.D., Ph.D.
Magda Campbell, M.D.
Robert Cancro, M.D.
Barry Chaitin, M.D.
Robert M. Chalfin, M.D.
Dennis S. Charney, M.D.
James L. Claghorn, M.D.
Paula J. Clayton, M.D.
Norman A. Clemens, M.D.
Irvin Myron Cohen, M.D.
Jonathan O. Cole, M.D.
Joseph T. Coyle, M.D.
Kenneth L. Davis, M.D.
Barbara G. Deutsch, M.D.
Leah Dickstein, M.D.
William R. Dubin, M.D.
David Dunner, M.D.

Irene Elkin, Ph.D.
Max Fink, M.D.
Richard J. Frances, M.D.
Richard A. Friedman, M.D.
Glen O. Gabbard, M.D.
Marc Galanter, M.D.
Max L. Gardner, M.D.
T.B. Ghosh, M.D.
Michael J. Gitlin, M.D.
Alexander H. Glassman, M.D.
Marion Goldstein, M.D.
Alberto Goldwater, M.D.
Paul J. Goodnick, M.D.
Sheila Gray, M.D.
John F. Greden, M.D.
Blaine S. Greenwald, M.D.
Donald E. Greydanus, M.D.
Ezra E.H. Griffith, M.D.
Frederick G. Guggenheim, M.D.
Moses Herrera, M.D.
Alfred Herzog, M.D.
Kenneth Jaffe, M.D.
James W. Jefferson, M.D.
Michael A. Jenike, M.D.
John M. Kane, M.D.
Sylvia R. Karasu, M.D.
Martin B. Keller, M.D.
Charles H. Kellner, M.D.
Hugo S. Kierszenbaum, M.D.
Martha Kirkpatrick, M.D.
Donald F. Klein, M.D.
Harvey J. Klein, M.D.
Gerald L. Klerman, M.D.
Lawrence Y. Kline, M.D.
James H. Kocsis, M.D.
Margaret Kordylewska, M.D.
George Kowallis, M.D.

Douglas J. Lanska, M.D.
Y.D. Lapierre, M.D.
Kevin Leehey, M.D.
Laurent Lehmann, M.D.
A.L. Lesser, M.D.
Stewart Levine, M.D.
Lawrence B. Lurie, M.D.
K. Roy MacKenzie, M.D.
Velandy Manohar, M.D.
Luis R. Marcos, M.D.
Philip M. Margolis, M.D.
Rick A. Martinez, M.D.
Thomas H. McGlashan, M.D.
Herbert Y. Meltzer, M.D.
Robert Michels, M.D.
Kevin Miller, M.D.
Robert M. Morse, M.D.
Rodrigo A. Munoz, M.D.
J. Craig Nelson, M.D.
Charles B. Nemeroff, M.D.
John C. Nemiah, M.D.
James Edward Nininger, M.D.
Judith Nowak, M.D.
Ned Nunes, M.D.
Frederick Petty, Ph.D., M.D.
Herbert S. Peyser, M.D.
Cynthia R. Pfeffer, M.D.
Kelley Phillips, M.D.
Gilbert Pinard, M.D.
Theodore M. Pinkert, M.D., J.D.
Robert Post, M.D.
William Z. Potter, M.D., Ph.D.
Sheldon Preskorn, M.D.
Fred Quitkin, M.D.

Maurice Rappaport, M.D., Ph.D.
Burton V. Reifler, M.D., M.P.H.
Mario I. Rendon, M.D.
Elliott Richelson, M.D.
Arthur Rifkin, M.D.
Bertram Rosen, M.D.
Barbara Rosenfeld, M.D.
Norman E. Rosenthal, M.D.
A. John Rush, M.D.
Harold A. Sackeim, Ph.D.
Marc A. Schuckit, M.D.
Theodore Shapiro, M.D.
Stewart Shevitz, M.D.
Moisy Shopper, M.D.
R. Bruce Sloane, M.D.
Edmund H. Sonnenblick, M.D.
Nada L. Stotland, M.D.
David M. Tobolowsky, M.D.
Gary J. Tucker, M.D.
John Chapman Urbaitis, M.D.
Herman M. van Praag, M.D., Ph.D.
Herman Vergara, M.D.
Milton Viederman, M.D.
Ramaswamy Viswanathan, M.D.
Steven G. Wager, M.D.
Raymond W. Waggoner, Sr., M.D.
R. Dale Walker, M.D.
Richard D. Weiner, M.D., Ph.D.
Myrna Weissman, Ph.D.
Elizabeth Weller, M.D.
Peter Whybrow, M.D.
Thomas N. Wise, M.D.
Lyman Wynne, M.D., Ph.D.
Sidney Zisook, M.D.

VI. Organizations That Submitted Comments

Academy of Psychosomatic Medicine
Alcohol, Drug Abuse, and Mental Health Administration
American Academy of Child and Adolescent Psychiatry
American Academy of Clinical Psychiatrists
American Academy of Family Physicians
American Academy of Neurology
American Academy of Pediatrics
American Academy of Psychiatrists in Alcoholism and Addiction
American Academy of Psychiatry and the Law
American Association for Geriatric Psychiatry
American Association for Marriage and Family Therapy
American Association of Community Psychiatrists
American Association of Psychiatric Administrators
American Association of Psychiatric Services for Children
American Association of Psychiatrists from India
American Board of Forensic Psychiatry, Inc.
American College of Psychoanalysts
American Group Psychotherapy Association, Inc.
American Nurses' Association
American Psychoanalytic Association
American Psychological Association
American Society for Adolescent Psychiatry
Association for Academic Psychiatry
Association for Child Analysis
Association for Medical Education and Research in Substance Abuse
Committee on Problems of Drug Dependence, Inc.
Joint Commission on Accreditation of Healthcare Organizations
National Association of State Mental Health Program Directors
National Depressive and Manic-Depressive Association
National Guild of Catholic Psychiatrists
National Institute of Mental Health
National Institute on Alcohol Abuse and Alcoholism
National Mental Health Association
Society for Adolescent Medicine
Society of Biological Psychiatry
U.S. Veterans Administration, Mental Health Section

VII.   References

The bracketed letter following each reference indicates the nature of the supporting evidence, as follows:

[A]   Randomized controlled clinical trial
[B]   Nonrandomized case-control study
[C]   Nonrandomized cohort study
[D]   Clinical report with nonrandomized historical comparison groups
[E]   Case report or series
[F]   Expert consensus
[G]   Subject review subsuming multiple categories A–E

1.   American Psychiatric Association: Diagnostic and Statistical Manual of Mental Disorders, 3rd ed, revised. Washington, DC, APA, 1987 [F]
2.   Klerman GL, Weissman MM: The course, morbidity, and costs of depression. Arch Gen Psychiatry 1992; 49:831–834 [G]
3.   Keller MB, Beardslee WR, Dorer DJ, Lavori PW, Samuelson H, Klerman GR: Impact of severity and chronicity of parental affective illness on adaptive functioning and psychopathology in children. Arch Gen Psychiatry 1986; 43:930–937 [B]
4.   Mintz J, Mintz LI, Arruda MJ, Hwang SS: Treatments of depression and the functional capacity to work. Arch Gen Psychiatry 1992; 49:761–768 [G]
5.   Regier DA, Boyd JH, Burke JD Jr, Rae DS, Myers JK, Kramer M, Robins LN, George LK, Karno M, Locke BZ: One-month prevalence of mental disorders in the United States: based on five Epidemiologic Catchment Area sites. Arch Gen Psychiatry 1988; 45:977–986 [A]
6.   Akiskal HS: The clinical management of affective disorders, in Psychiatry, vol 1. Edited by Michels R, Cooper AM, Guze SB, Judd LL, Klerman GL, Solnit AJ. Philadelphia, JB Lippincott, 1985 [G]
7.   Jacobson E: Contribution to the metapsychology of cyclothymic depression, in Affective Disorders. Edited by Greenacre P. New York, International Universities Press, 1953 [G]
8.   Jacobson E: Depression. New York, International Universities Press, 1964 [F]
9.   Jacobson E: The Self and the Object World. New York, International Universities Press, 1964 [F]
10. Rado S: The problem of melancholia (1927), in Collected Papers, vol 1. New York, Grune & Stratton, 1956 [G]
11. Rado S: The problem of melancholia. Int J Psychoanal 1928; 9:420–438 [G]
12. Klein MA: Contribution to the psychogenesis of manic-depressive states (1934), in Contributions to Psycho-Analysis 1921–1945. London, Hogarth Press, 1945 [G]
13. Gero G: The construction of depression. Int J Psychoanal 1936; 17:423–461 [G]
14. Bibring E: The mechanism of depression, in Affective Disorders. Edited by Greenacre P. New York, International Universities Press, 1953 [G]
15. Sandler J, Joffee WG: Notes on childhood depression. Int J Psychoanal 1965; 46:88–96 [G]
16. Kohut H: The Analysis of the Self. New York, International Universities Press, 1971 [G]
17. Kohut H: The Restoration of the Self. New York, International Universities Press, 1977 [G]
18. Bowlby J: Attachment and Loss. London, Hogarth Press, 1969 [G]

19. Bowlby J: The making and breaking of affectional bonds II: some principles of psychotherapy. Br J Psychiatry 1977; 130: 421–431 [G]
20. Rutter M: Maternal Deprivation Reassessed. London, Penguin, 1972 [G]
21. Paykel ES, Myers JK, Deinelt MN, Klerman GL, Lindenthal JJ, Pepper MP: Life events and depression: a controlled study. Arch Gen Psychiatry 1969; 21:753–760 [B]
22. Brown GW, Harris T, Copeland JR: Depression and loss. Br J Psychiatry 1977; 130:1–18 [G]
23. Henderson S: A development in social psychiatry; the systematic study of social bonds. J Nerv Ment Dis 1980; 168:63–69 [G]
24. Henderson S, Byrne DG, Duncan P: Neurosis and the Social Environment. San Diego, Academic Press, 1982 [G]
25. Miller P, Ingham JG: Friends, confidants and symptoms. Soc Psychiatry 1976; 11:51–58 [G]
26. Roy A: Vulnerability factors and depression in women. Br J Psychiatry 1978; 133:106–110 [C]
27. Holmes TH, Rahe RH: The Social Readjustment Rating Scale. J Psychosom Res 1967; 11:213–218 [G]
28. Paykel E: Recent life events in the development of depressive disorders, in The Psychobiology of Depressive Disorders: Implications for the Effects of Stress. Edited by Defue EA. New York, Academic Press, 1978 [G]
29. Brenner C: Psychoanalytic Technique and Psychic Conflict. New York, International Universities Press, 1976 [F]
30. Karasu TB: Developmentalist metatheory of depression and psychotherapy. Am J Psychother 1992; 46:37–49 [G]
31. Thompson LW, Gallagher D, Breckenridge JS: Comparative effectiveness of psychotherapies for depressed elders. J Geriatr Psychiatry 1987; 21:133–146 [A]
32. Daneman EA: Imipramine in office management of depressive reactions (a double-blind study). Dis Nerv Syst 1961; 22:213–217 [A]
33. Covi L, Lipman RS, Derogatis LR, Smith JE III, Pattison JH: Drugs and group psychotherapy in neurotic depression. Am J Psychiatry 1974; 131:191–198 [A]
34. Klerman GL, Weissman MM, Rounsaville BJ, Chevron ES: Interpersonal Psychotherapy of Depression. New York, Basic Books, 1984 [G]
35. DiMascio A, Weissman MM, Prusoff BA, Neu C, Zwilling M, Klerman GL: Differential symptom reduction by drugs and psychotherapy in acute depression. Arch Gen Psychiatry 1979; 36: 1450–1456 [A]
36. Elkin I, Shea T, Watkins JT, Imber SD, Sotsky SM, Collins JF, Glass DR, Pilkonis PA, Leber WR, Docherty JP, Fiester SJ, Parloff MB: National Institute of Mental Health Treatment of Depression Collaborative Research Program: general effectiveness of treatments. Arch Gen Psychiatry 1989; 46:971–982 [A]
37. Klerman GL, DiMascio A, Weissman MM, Prusoff B, Paykel ES: Treatment of depression by drugs and psychotherapy. Am J Psychiatry 1974; 131:186–191 [A]
38. Frank E, Kupfer DJ, Perel JM, Cornes C, Jarrett DB, Mallinger AG, Thase ME, McEachran AB, Grochocinski VJ: Three-year outcomes for maintenance therapies in recurrent depression. Arch Gen Psychiatry 1990; 47:1093–1099 [A]
39. Kupfer DJ, Frank E, Perel JM, Cornes C, Mallinger AG, Thase ME, McEachran AB, Grochocinski VJ: Five-year outcome for maintenance therapies in recurrent depression. Arch Gen Psychiatry 1992; 49:769–773 [A]
40. Ferster CB: A functional analysis of depression. Am Psychol 1973; 10:857–870 [F]
41. Bandura A: Social Learning Theory. Englewood Cliffs, NJ, Prentice Hall, 1977 [F]
42. Lewinsohn PM, Antonuccio DA, Steinmetz-Breckinridge J, Teri L: The Coping With Depression Course: A Psychoeducational Intervention for Unipolar Depression. Eugene, OR, Castalia Publishing, 1984 [F]

43. Lewinsohn P, Clarke G: Group treatment of depressed individuals: the "Coping With Depression" course. Advances in Behaviour Res Therapy 1984; 6:99–114 [F]

44. Rehm LP: Behavior Therapy for Depression. New York, Academic Press, 1979 [F]

45. Bellack AS, Hersen M, Himmelhoch JM: A comparison of social-skills training, pharmacotherapy and psychotherapy for depression. Behav Res Ther 1983; 21:101–107 [A]

46. Nezu AM: Efficacy of a social problem-solving therapy for unipolar depression. J Consult Clin Psychol 1986; 54:196–202 [A]

47. McLean PD, Hakstian AR: Clinical depression: comparative efficacy of outpatient treatments. J Consult Clin Psychol 1979; 47:818–836 [A]

48. Brown RA, Lewinsohn PM: A psychoeducational approach to the treatment of depression: comparison of group, individual, and minimal contact procedures. J Consult Clin Psychol 1990; 52:774–783 [A]

49. Usaf SO, Kavanagh DJ: Mechanisms of improvement in treatment for depression: test of self-efficacy and performance model. J Cognitive Psychother 1990; 4:51–70 [A]

50. Nezu AM, Perri MG: Social problem-solving therapy for unipolar depression: an initial dismantling investigation. J Consult Clin Psychol 1989; 57:408–413 [B]

51. Gallagher DE, Thompson LW: Treatment of major depressive disorder in older adult outpatients with brief psychotherapies. Psychotherapy: Theory, Research, and Practice 1982; 19:482–490 [A]

52. Gallagher-Thompson D, Hanley-Peterson P, Thompson LW: Maintenance of gains versus relapse following brief psychotherapy for depression. J Consult Clin Psychol 1990; 58:371–374 [A]

53. Beck AT, Rush AJ, Shaw BF, Emery G: Cognitive Therapy of Depression. New York, Guilford Press, 1979 [G]

54. Rush AJ, Beck AT, Kovacs M, Hollon SD: Comparative efficacy of cognitive therapy and pharmacotherapy in the treatments of depressed outpatients. Cognitive Therapy Res 1977; 1:17–37 [A]

55. Hollon SD, DeRubeis RJ, Seligman MEP: Cognitive therapy and the prevention of depression. Applied Preventive Psychology 1992; 1:89–95 [G]

56. Shea MT, Elkin I, Imber SD, Sotsky SM, Watkins JT, Collins JF, Pilkonis PA, Beckham E, Glass DR, Dolan RT, Parloff MB: Course of depressive symptoms over follow-up: findings from the National Institute of Mental Health Treatment of Depression Collaborative Research Program. Arch Gen Psychiatry 1992; 49:782–787 [A]

57. Ross M, Scott M: An evaluation of the effectiveness of individual and group cognitive therapy in the treatment of depressed patients in an inner city health centre. J R Coll Gen Pract 1985; 35:239–242 [A]

58. O'Leary KD, Beach SRH: Marital therapy: a viable treatment for depression and marital discord. Am J Psychiatry 1990; 147: 183–186 [A]

59. Beach SRH, Sandeen EE, O'Leary KD: Depression in Marriage. New York, Guilford Press, 1990 [G]

60. Yager J: Patients with mood disorders and marital/family problems, in Annual Review of Psychiatry, vol 11. Edited by Tasman A. Washington, DC, American Psychiatric Press, 1992 [G]

61. Coyne JC, in Affective Disorders and the Family: Assessment and Treatment. Edited by Clarkin JF, Haas GL, Glick ID. New York, Guilford Press, 1988 [F]

62. Coyne JC, Kessler RC, Tal M, Turnbull J, Wortman CB, Greden JF: Living with a depressed person. J Consult Clin Psychol 1987; 55:347–352 [F]

63. Jacobson NS, Dobson K, Fruzzetti AE, Schmaling KB, Salusky S: Marital therapy as a treatment for depression. J Consult Clin Psychol 1991; 59:547–557 [A]

64. Prusoff BA, Weissman MM, Klerman GL, Rounsaville BJ: Research diagnostic criteria subtypes of depression: their role as predictors of differential response to psychotherapy and drug treatment. Arch Gen Psychiatry 1980; 37:796–801 [A]

65. Katz MM, Koslow SH, Maas JW, Frazer A, Bowden CL, Casper R, Croughan J, Kocsis J, Redmond E Jr: The timing, specificity and clinical prediction of tricyclic drug effects in depression. Psychol Med 1987; 17:297–309 [C]

66. Quitkin FM, Rabkin JG, Markowitz JM, Stewart JW, McGrath PJ, Harrison W: Use of pattern analysis to identify true drug response. Arch Gen Psychiatry 1987; 44:259–264 [A]

67. Quitkin FM, Rabkin JG, Ross D, McGrath PJ: Duration of antidepressant drug treatment: what is an adequate trial? Arch Gen Psychiatry 1984; 41:238–245 [G]

68. Tune LE, Strauss ME, Lew MF, Breitlinger E, Coyle JT: Serum levels of anticholinergic drugs and impaired recent memory in chronic schizophrenic patients. Am J Psychiatry 1982; 139: 1460–1462 [C]

69. Pollack MH, Rosenbaum JF: Management of antidepressant-induced side effects: a practical guide for the clinician. J Clin Psychiatry 1987; 48:3–8 [G]

70. Davidson J: Seizures and bupropion: a review. J Clin Psychiatry 1989; 50:256–261 [G]

71. Johnston JA, Lineberry CG, Ascher JA, Davidson J, Khayrallah MA, Feighner JP, Stark P: A 102-center prospective study of seizure in association with bupropion. J Clin Psychiatry 1991; 52:450–456 [C]

72. Garvey MJ, Tollefson GD: Occurrence of myoclonus in patients treated with cyclic antidepressants. Arch Gen Psychiatry 1987; 44:269–272 [E]

73. Preskorn SH, Jerkovich GS: Central nervous system toxicity of tricyclic antidepressants: phenomenology, course, risk factors, and role of therapeutic drug monitoring. J Clin Psychopharmacol 1990; 10:88–95 [E]

74. Roose SP, Glassman AH, Giardina EG, Walsh BT, Woodring S, Bigger JT: Tricyclic antidepressants in depressed patients with cardiac conduction disease. Arch Gen Psychiatry 1987; 44:273–275 [A]

75. Stoudemire A, Atkinson P: Use of cyclic antidepressants in patients with cardiac conduction disturbance. Gen Hosp Psychiatry 1988; 10:389–397 [G]

76. Bigger JT, Giardina EG, Perel JM, Kantor SJ, Glassman AH: Cardiac antiarrhythmic effect of imipramine hydrochloride. N Engl J Med 1977; 296:206–208 [E]

77. Giardina EG, Barnard T, Johnson L, Saroff AL, Bigger JT Jr, Louie M: The antiarrhythmic effect of nortriptyline in cardiac patients with ventricular premature depolarizations. J Am Coll Cardiol 1986; 7:1363–1369 [E]

78. Connolly SJ, Mitchell LB, Swerdlow CD, Mason JW, Winkle RA: Clinical efficacy and electrophysiology of imipramine for ventricular tachycardia. Am J Cardiol 1984; 53:516–521 [E]

79. Schwartz P, Wolf S: QT interval prolongation as predictor of sudden death in patients with myocardial infarction. Circulation 1978; 57:1074–1077 [E]

80. Veith RC, Raskind MA, Caldwell JH, Barnes RF, Gumbrecht G, Ritchie JL: Cardiovascular effects of tricyclic antidepressants in depressed patients with chronic heart disease. N Engl J Med 1982; 306:954–959 [A]

81. Dalack GW, Roose SP, Glassman AH: Tricyclics and heart failure (letter). Am J Psychiatry 1991; 148:1601 [E]

82. Glassman AH, Johnson LL, Giardina EG, Walsh BT, Roose SP, Cooper TB, Bigger JT Jr: The use of imipramine in depressed patients with congestive heart failure. JAMA 1983; 250:1997–2001 [C]

83. Fava M, Rosenbaum JE: Suicidality and fluoxetine: is there a relationship? J Clin Psychiatry 1991; 52:108–111 [G]

84. Mann JJ, Kapur S: The emergence of suicidal ideation and behavior during antidepressant pharmacotherapy. Arch Gen Psychiatry 1991; 48:1027–1033 [G]

85. American Psychiatric Association Task Force on Electroconvulsive Therapy: The Practice of Electroconvulsive Therapy. Washington, DC, APA, 1990 [F]

86. Weiner RD, Rogers HJ, Davidson JR, Kahn EM: Effects of electroconvulsive therapy upon brain electrical activity. Ann NY Acad Sci 1986; 462:270–281 [C]

87. Rosenthal NE, Sack DA, Carpenter CJ, Parry BL, Mendelson WB, Wehr TA: Antidepressant effects of light in seasonal affective disorder. Am J Psychiatry 1985; 142:163–170 [C]

88. Vanselow W, Dennerstein L, Armstrong S, Lockie P: Retinopathy and bright light therapy (letter). Am J Psychiatry 1991; 148: 1266–1267 [E]

89. Prien RF, Kupfer DJ: Continuation drug therapy for major depressive episodes: how long should it be maintained? Am J Psychiatry 1986; 143:18–23 [A]

90. Mood Disorders: Pharmacologic Prevention of Recurrences. Natl Inst Health Consensus Dev Conf Consensus Statement 1984; 5(4) [F]

91. Prien RF, Kupfer DJ, Mansky PA, Small JG, Tuason VB, Voss CB, Johnson WE: Drug therapy in the prevention of recurrences in unipolar and bipolar affective disorders: report of the NIMH Collaborative Study Group comparing lithium carbonate, imipramine, and a lithium carbonate-imipramine combination. Arch Gen Psychiatry 1984; 41:1096–1104 [A]

92. Greenhouse JB, Stangl D, Kupfer DJ, Prien RF: Methodologic issues in maintenance therapy clinical trials. Arch Gen Psychiatry 1991; 48:313–318 [G]

93. Dilsaver SC, Kronfol Z, Sackellares JC, Greden JF: Antidepressant withdrawal syndromes: evidence supporting the cholinergic overdrive hypothesis. J Clin Psychopharmacol 1983; 3:157–164 [E]

94. Guscott R, Grof P: The clinical meaning of refractory depression: a review for the clinician. Am J Psychiatry 1991; 148:695–704 [G]

95. Marcus ER, Bradley SS: Combination of psychotherapy and psychopharmacotherapy with treatment-resistant inpatients with dual diagnoses. Psych Clin N Am 1990; 13:209–214 [E]

96. Price LH, Charney DS, Heninger GR: Variability of response to lithium augmentation in refractory depression. Am J Psychiatry 1986; 143:1387–1392 [C]

97. Prange AJ Jr, Loosen PT, Wilson IC, Lipton MA: The therapeutic use of hormones of the thyroid axis in depression, in The Neurobiology of Mood Disorders, vol 1. Edited by Post R, Ballenger J. Baltimore, Williams & Wilkins, 1984 [E]

98. Wharton RN, Perel JM, Dayton PG, Malitz S: A potential clinical use for methylphenidate with tricyclic antidepressants. Am J Psychiatry 1971; 127:1619–1625 [E]

99. Feighner JP, Herbstein J, Damlouji N: Combined MAOI, TCA, and direct stimulant therapy of treatment-resistant depression. J Clin Psychiatry 1985; 46:206–209 [G]

100. Nelson JC, Mazure CM, Bowers MB Jr, Jatlow PI: A preliminary, open study of the combination of fluoxetine and desipramine for rapid treatment of major depression. Arch Gen Psychiatry 1991; 48:303–307 [C]

101. Rosenstein DL, Takeshita J, Nelson JC: Fluoxetine-induced elevation and prolongation of tricyclic levels in overdose (letter). Am J Psychiatry 1991; 148:807 [E]

102. Razani J, White KL, White J, Simpson G, Sloane RB, Rebal R, Palmer R: The safety and efficacy of combined amitriptyline and tranylcypromine antidepressant treatment: a controlled trial. Arch Gen Psychiatry 1983; 40:657–661 [A]

103. Young JPR, Lader MH, Hughes WC: Controlled trial of trimipramine, monoamine oxidase inhibitors, and combined treatment in depressed outpatients. BMJ 1979; 2:1315–1317 [A]

104. Prudic J, Sackeim HA: Refractory depression and electroconvulsive therapy, in Treatment Strategies for Refractory Depression. Edited by Roose SP, Glassman AH. Washington, DC, American Psychiatric Press, 1990 [G]

105. Penney JF, Dinwiddie SH, Zorumski CF, Wetzel RD: Concurrent and close temporal administration of lithium and ECT. Convulsive Therapy 1990; 6:139–145 [D]

106. Hill GE, Wong KC, Hodges MR: Potentiation of succinylcholine neuromuscular blockade by lithium carbonate. Anesthesiology 1976; 44:439–442 [E]

107. Cullen M, Mitchell P, Brodaty H, Boyce P, Parker G, Hickie I, Wilhelm K: Carbamazepine for treatment-resistant melancholia. J Clin Psychiatry 1991; 52:472–476 [C]

108. Hayes SG: Long-term use of valproate in primary psychiatric disorders. J Clin Psychiatry 1989; 50(3 suppl):35–39 [E]

109. Kramlinger KG, Post RM: The addition of lithium to carbamazepine: antidepressant efficacy in treatment-resistant depression. Arch Gen Psychiatry 1989; 46:794–800 [C]

110. Kocsis JH, Croughan JL, Katz MM, Butker TP, Secunda S, Bowden CL, Davis JM: Response to treatment with antidepressants of patients with severe or moderate nonpsychotic depression and of patients with psychotic depression. Am J Psychiatry 1990; 147:621–624 [A]

111. Bunney WE Jr: Psychopharmacology of the switch process in affective disorders, in Psychopharmacology: A Generation of Progress. Edited by Lipton MA, DiMascio A, Killam KF. New York, Raven Press, 1978 [E]

112. Wehr TA, Goodwin FK: Can antidepressants cause mania and worsen the course of affective illness? Am J Psychiatry 1987; 144:1403–1411 [G]

113. Akiskal HS, Walker P, Puzantian VR, King D, Rosenthal TL, Dranon M: Bipolar outcome in the course of depressive illness: phenomenologic, familial, and pharmacologic predictors. J Affective Disord 1983; 5:115–128 [A]

114. Wehr TA, Sack DA, Rosenthal NE, Cowdry RW: Rapid cycling affective disorder: contributing factors and treatment responses in 51 patients. Am J Psychiatry 1988; 145:179–184 [A]

115. Haykal RF, Akiskal HS: Bupropion as a promising approach to rapid cycling bipolar II patients. J Clin Psychiatry 1990; 51: 450–455 [C]

116. Glassman AH, Roose SP: Delusional depression. Arch Gen Psychiatry 1981; 38:424–427 [E]

117. Spiker DG, Weiss JC, Dealy RS, Griffin SJ, Hanin I, Neil JF, Perel JM, Rossi AJ, Soloff PH: The pharmacological treatment of delusional depression. Am J Psychiatry 1985; 142:430–436 [A]

118. Anton RF Jr, Burch EA Jr: Amoxapine versus amitriptyline combined with perphenazine in the treatment of psychotic depression. Am J Psychiatry 1990; 147:1203–1208 [A]

119. Price LH, Conwell Y, Nelson JC: Lithium augmentation of combined neuroleptic-tricyclic treatment in delusional depression. Am J Psychiatry 1983; 140:318–322 [E]

120. Kantor SJ, Glassman AH: Delusional depression: natural history and response to treatment. Br J Psychiatry 1977; 131:351–360 [E]

121. Fink M, Taylor MA: Catatonia: a separate category for DSM-IV? Integrative Psychiatry 1991; 7:2–10 [G]

122. Liebowitz MR, Quitkin FM, Stewart JW, McGrath PJ, Harrison WM, Markowitz JS, Rabkin JG, Tricamo E, Goetz DM, Klein DF: Antidepressant specificity in atypical depression. Arch Gen Psychiatry 1988; 45:129–137 [A]

123. Davidson JR, Miller R, Turnbull CD, Sullivan JL: Atypical depression. Arch Gen Psychiatry 1982; 39:527–534 [G]

124. Quitkin FM, Stewart JW, McGrath PJ, Liebowitz MR, Harrison WM, Tricamo E, Klein DF, Rabkin JG, Markowitz JS, Wager SG: Phenelzine versus imipramine in the treatment of probable atypical depression: defining syndrome boundaries of selective MAOI responders. Am J Psychiatry 1988; 145:306–311 [A]

125. Quitkin FM, Harrison W, Stewart JW, McGrath PJ, Tricamo E, Ocepek-Welikson K, Rabkin JG, Wager SG, Nunes E, Klein DF: Response to phenelzine and imipramine in placebo nonresponders with atypical depression: a new application of the crossover design. Arch Gen Psychiatry 1991; 48:319–323 [A]

126. Goodnick PJ, Extein I: Bupropion and fluoxetine in depressive subtypes. Ann Clin Psychiatry 1989; 1:119–122 [C]

127. Goodnick PJ: Acute and long-term bupropion therapy: response and side effects. Ann Clin Psychiatry 1991; 3:311–313 [C]

128. Brown SA, Schuckit MA: Changes in depression among abstinent alcoholics. J Stud Alcohol 1988; 49:412–417 [C]

129. Sands BF, Ciraulo DA: Cocaine drug-drug interactions. J Clin Psychopharmacol 1992; 12:49–55 [G]

130. Clomipramine Collaborative Study Group: Clomipramine in the treatment of patients with obsessive-compulsive disorder. Arch Gen Psychiatry 1991; 48:730–738 [A]

131. Jenike MA, Buttolph L, Baer L, Ricciardi J, Holland A: Open trial of fluoxetine in obsessive-compulsive disorder. Am J Psychiatry 1989; 146:909–911 [A]

132. Grunhaus L: Clinical and psychobiological characteristics of simultaneous panic disorder and major depression. Am J Psychiatry 1988; 145:1214–1221 [G]

133. Schatzberg AF, Ballenger JC: Decisions for the clinician in the treatment of panic disorder: when to treat, which treatment to use, and how long to treat. J Clin Psychiatry 1991; 52(2 suppl): 26–31 [G]

134. Sheehan DV, Davidson J, Manschreck T, Van Wyck Fleet J: Lack of efficacy of a new antidepressant (bupropion) in the treatment of panic disorder with phobias. J Clin Psychopharmacol 1983; 3:28–31 [C]

135. Stoudemire A, Hill C. Gulley L-R. Morris R: Neuropsychological and biomedical assessment of depression-dementia syndromes. J Neuropsychiatry Clin Neurosci 1989; 1:347–361 [G]

136. Caine ED: Pseudodementia: current concepts and future directions. Arch Gen Psychiatry 1981; 38:1359–1364 [G]

137. McGlashan TH, Carpenter WT Jr: Postpsychotic depression in schizophrenia. Arch Gen Psychiatry 1976; 33:231–239 [C]

138. Siris SG, Adan F, Cohen M, Mandeli J, Aronson A, Casey E: Postpsychotic depression and negative symptoms: an investigation of syndromal overlap. Am J Psychiatry 1988; 145:1532–1537 [A]

139. Van Putten T, May PRA: "Akinetic depression" in schizophrenia. Arch Gen Psychiatry 1978; 35:1101–1107 [C]

140. Siris SG, Morgan V, Fagerstrom R, Rifkin A, Cooper TB: Adjunctive imipramine in the treatment of postpsychotic depression: a controlled trial. Arch Gen Psychiatry 1987; 44:533–539 [A]

141. Vorhees CV, Brunner RL, Butcher RE: Psychotropic drugs as behavioral teratogens. Science 1979; 205:1220–1225 [C]

142. Elia J, Simpson GM: Antidepressant medication during pregnancy and lactation: fetal teratogenic and toxic effects, in Pharmacotherapy of Depression. Edited by Amsterdam JD. New York, Marcel Dekker, 1990 [G]

143. Nora JJ, Nora HA, Toews WH: Lithium, Ebstein's anomaly, and other congenital heart defects. Lancet 1974; 2:594–595 [D]

144. Jacobson SJ, Jones K, Johnson K, Ceolin L, Kaur P, Sahn D, Donnenfeld AE, Rieder M, Santelli R, Smythe J, Pastuszak A, Einarson T, Koren G: Prospective multicentre study of pregnancy outcome after lithium exposure during first trimester. Lancet 1992; 339:530–533 [C]

145. Nurnberg HG: An overview of somatic treatment of psychosis during pregnancy and post-partum. Gen Hosp Psychiatry 1989; 11:328–338 [G]

146. Gitlin MJ, Pasnau RO: Psychiatric syndromes linked to reproductive function in women: a review of current knowledge. Am J Psychiatry 1989; 146:1413–1422 [G]

147. Brockington IF, Cernik KF, Schofield EM, Downing AR, Francis AF, Keelan C: Puerperal psychosis: phenomena and diagnosis. Arch Gen Psychiatry 1981; 38:829–833 [C]

148. Ananth J: Side effects in the neonate from psychotropic agents excreted through breast feeding. Am J Psychiatry 1978; 135: 801–805 [E]

149. Kocsis JH, Frances AJ, Voss C, Mann JJ, Mason BJ, Sweeney J: Imipramine treatment for chronic depression. Arch Gen Psychiatry 1988; 45:253–257 [A]

150. Akiskal HS, Rosenthal TL, Haykal RF, Lemmi H, Rosenthal RH: Characterological depressions: clinical and sleep EEG findings separating "subaffective dysthymias" from "character spectrum disorders." Arch Gen Psychiatry 1980; 37:777–783 [B]

151. Howland RH: Pharmacotherapy of dysthymia: a review. J Clin Psychopharmacol 1991; 11:83–92 [G]

152. Shea MT, Glass DR, Pilkonis PA, Watkins J, Docherty JP: Frequency and implications of personality disorders in a sample of depressed outpatients. J Personality Disord 1987; 1:27–42 [C]

153. Parsons B, Quitkin FM, McGrath PJ, Stewart JW, Tricamo E, Ocepek-Welikson K, Harrison W, Rabkin JG, Wager SG, Nunes E: Phenelzine, imipramine, and placebo in borderline patients meeting criteria for atypical depression. Psychopharmacol Bull 1989; 25:524–534 [A]

154. Shea MT, Pilkonis PA, Beckham E, Collins JF, Elkin I, Sotsky SM, Docherty JP: Personality disorders and treatment outcome in the NIMH Treatment of Depression Collaborative Research Program. Am J Psychiatry 1990; 147:711–718 [A]

155. Roose SP, Dalack GW, Glassman AH, Woodring S, Walsh BT, Giardina EGV: Cardiovascular effects of bupropion in depressed patients with heart disease. Am J Psychiatry 1991; 148:512–516 [C]

156. Roose SP, Glassman AH, Giardina EG, Johnson LL, Walsh BT, Bigger JT Jr: Cardiovascular effects of imipramine and bupropion in depressed patients with congestive heart failure. J Clin Psychopharmacol 1987; 7:247–251 [A]

157. Sackeim HA, Decina P, Prohovnik I, Malitz S, Resor SR: Anticonvulsant and antidepressant properties of electroconvulsive therapy: a proposed mechanism of action. Biol Psychiatry 1983; 18:1301–1310 [G]

158. Lieberman E, Stoudemire A: Use of tricyclic antidepressants in patients with glaucoma. Psychosomatics 1987; 28:145–148 [G]

159. Goetz CG, Tanner CM, Klawans HL: Bupropion in Parkinson's disease. Neurology 1984; 34:1092–1094 [C]

160. Monoamine oxidase inhibitors for depression. Med Lett Drugs Ther 1980; 22:58–60 [G]

161. Andersen K, Balldin J, Gottfries CG, Granerus AK, Modigh K, Svennerholm L, Wallin A: A double-blind evaluation of electroconvulsive therapy in Parkinson's disease with "on-off" phenomena. Acta Neurol Scand 1987; 76:191–199 [A]

162. Zisook S, Shuchter SR: Depression through the first year after the death of a spouse. Am J Psychiatry 1991; 148:1346–1352 [C]

163. Robinson RG, Starkstein SE: Current research in affective disorders following stroke. J Neuropsychiatry Clin Neurosci 1990; 2:1–14 [F]

164. Nelson JC, Jatlow PI, Mazure C: Rapid desipramine dose adjustment using 24-hour levels. J Clin Psychopharmacol 1987; 7:72–77 [C]

165. Escobar JI, Gomez J, Tuason VB: Depressive phenomenology in North and South American patients. Am J Psychiatry 1983; 140:47–51 [C]

166. Marcos LR, Cancro R: Psychopharmacotherapy of Hispanic depressed patients: clinical observations. Am J Psychother 1982; 36:505–512 [E]

167. Escobar JI, Tuason VB: Antidepressant agents: a cross-cultural study. Psychopharmacol Bull 1980; 16:49–52 [C]

168. Marcos LR, Uruyo L, Kesselman M, Alpert M: The language barrier in evaluating Spanish-American patients. Arch Gen Psychiatry 1973; 29:655–659 [C]

169. Kleinman A, Good B: Culture and Depression. Berkeley, University of California Press, 1985 [G]

PRACTICE GUIDELINE

FOR

TREATMENT OF

PATIENTS WITH

BIPOLAR DISORDER

WORK GROUP ON BIPOLAR DISORDER

Robert M.A. Hirschfeld, M.D., Chair

Paula J. Clayton, M.D.
Irvin Cohen, M.D.
Jan Fawcett, M.D.
Paul Keck, M.D.
Jon McClellan, M.D.
Susan McElroy, M.D.
Robert Post, M.D.
Aaron Satloff, M.D.

Contents

Treatment of Patients With Bipolar Disorder

This practice guideline was published in December 1994 in the *American Journal of Psychiatry*.

Development Process

This practice guideline was developed under the auspices of the Steering Committee on Practice Guidelines. The development process is detailed in a document available from the APA Office of Research entitled "APA Practice Guideline Development Process." Key features of the process included: 1) initial drafting by a work group consisting of psychiatrists with clinical and research expertise in bipolar disorder; 2) a comprehensive literature review; 3) the production of multiple drafts, each of which received widespread review, with over 120 individuals and 40 organizations submitting comments (see sections V and VI); 4) approval by the APA Assembly and Board of Trustees; and 5) planned revisions at 3- to 5-year intervals.

Computerized searches of the relevant literature were conducted using MEDLINE. The key words used were "bipolar disorder–treatment" for the period January 1987 through October 1993; "bipolar disorder–psychological treatments" for the period January 1981 through December 1986 and "psychotic depression–treatment" for the period January 1987 through November 1993.

Papers selected from these searches for further review included those published in English in peer-reviewed journals. Preference was given to those articles based on randomized, placebo-controlled clinical trials. Clinical reports involving descriptions of patients or groups of patients were reviewed when data from controlled trials were not available. Review articles, especially those published in well-regarded peer-reviewed journals, and book chapters were reviewed.

Introduction

This guideline seeks to provide guidance to psychiatrists who treat patients with bipolar I disorder (manic-depressive illness). The pharmacologic, other somatic, and psychotherapeutic treatments that are used for patients with bipolar I disorder are summarized. Although many of the treatments discussed in this guideline may be effective for patients with bipolar II disorder or for patients with schizoaffective disorder, bipolar type, the focus is to guide the treatment of patients with bipolar I disorder. It should be assumed that the use of the term "bipolar disorder" in this document refers to bipolar I disorder, as defined in DSM-IV, unless a broader meaning is specified (e.g., "to include bipolar II disorder"). The guideline begins at the point where the psychiatrist has established the diagnosis of bipolar I disorder and has evaluated the patient for the presence of comorbid psychiatric conditions (e.g., alcohol and/or substance abuse or dependence disorder, personality disorders) as well as general medical conditions (e.g., thyroid disease, Cushing's disease, cerebral neoplasms) that could mimic bipolar disorder or be important to its treatment.

The purpose of this guideline is to assist the physician faced with the task of managing patients with bipolar disorder. This may involve different treatment strategies at different points in time. Because the needs of individual patients vary substantially during the course of this long-term disorder and because patients may have comorbid disorders, the psychiatrist should consider, but not be limited to, the recommendations in this treatment guideline.

I. Disease Definition, Epidemiology, and Natural History

A. Diagnosis of Bipolar Disorder

By DSM-IV definition, patients with bipolar I disorder have had at least one episode of mania. Some patients have had previous depressive episodes, and most patients will have subsequent episodes that can be either manic or depressive. In addition, hypomanic and mixed episodes can occur, as well as significant subthreshold mood lability between episodes.

B. Specific Features of Diagnosis

The assessment of a patient with bipolar disorder includes both cross-sectional (i.e., current or recent features of the patient's condition) and longitudinal (i.e., past and ongoing course of the disorder) issues.

1. Cross-sectional issues

There are a number of important clinical and psychosocial issues to consider in the cross-sectional evaluation of a patient with bipolar disorder. First, the psychiatrist should determine whether the patient meets DSM-IV criteria for a manic, hypomanic, depressive, or mixed episode.

Cross-sectional issues include assessment for the presence of psychotic features, cognitive impairment, risk of suicide, risk of violence to persons or property, risk-taking behavior (including financial extravagance), sexually inappropriate behavior, and substance abuse, as well as the DSM-IV specifiers for current or most recent episode. Assessment of the individual's ability to care for himself or herself, childbearing status or plans, and supports, including family and friends, housing, and financial resources, is important. The degree of distress and disability is also important. Careful attention to these factors will enable the psychiatrist to make a recommendation as to the site of treatment (e.g., inpatient, outpatient, partial hospitalization) and to formulate well-reasoned and appropriate clinical approaches to the patient and family.

2. Longitudinal issues

Bipolar disorder is an episodic, long-term illness with a variable course. In evaluating the individual patient in order to make immediate clinical recommendations and decisions, as well as in beginning to formulate a long-term treatment plan, a number of longitudinal issues must be considered. These include the number of prior episodes, the average length of episodes and average interepisode duration, the interval since the last episode of mania or depression, the level of psychosocial and symptomatic functioning between episodes of illness, and the response to prior treatment.

Bipolar disorder should always be considered in the differential diagnosis of patients with depression. Very often patients do not report prior episodes of mania and hypomania. Therefore, the psychiatrist needs to ask explicitly about such prior manic episodes because knowledge of their presence can influence treatment recommendations and decisions. The psychiatrist should also ask about a family history of mood disorders, including mania and hypomania. Consultation with family members and significant others may be extremely useful in establishing family history. DSM-IV specifiers describing the course of recurrent episodes include rapid cycling, seasonal pattern, and longitudinal course (with or without full interepisode recovery). Some patients switch rapidly and frequently between manic and depressive symptoms without experiencing an intervening period of euthymia. Although these patients are sometimes referred to as rapid cyclers, in this guideline we will refer to these patients as ultrarapid cyclers and reserve the term "rapid cycling" for those patients who have four or more episodes per year (i.e., the DSM-IV definition).

C. Natural History and Course

The first episode of bipolar disorder may be manic, hypomanic, mixed, or depressive and may be followed by several years during which the patient is symptom-free. Because the illness may be associated with substance-related disorders, recklessness, impulsivity, truancy, and other antisocial behavior, the diagnosis of bipolar disorder must be carefully differentiated from substance-related disorders, antisocial behavior, or personality disorders. In children and adolescents, the diagnoses of attention deficit hyperactivity disorder and conduct disorder must also be considered.

Untreated patients with bipolar disorder may have more than 10 total episodes of mania and depression during their lifetime, with the duration of episodes and interepisode periods stabilizing after the fourth or fifth episode (1). Often 5 years or more may elapse between the first and second episode, but the time periods between subsequent episodes usually narrow. However, it must be emphasized that variability is the hallmark of this illness.

Bipolar disorder causes substantial psychosocial morbidity that frequently affects the patient's marriage, children, occupation, and other aspects of the patient's life. Divorce rates are substantially higher in patients with bipolar disorder, approaching two to three times the rate of normal comparison subjects (2). The occupational status of patients with bipolar disorder is twice as likely to deteriorate as that of comparison subjects (2).

In a review of studies of depressive and manic-depressive illnesses conducted between 1937 and 1988 involving over 9,000 patients, the mean suicide completion rate was 19% (1). The rate for bipolar disorder alone was not reported. Suicide occurs more often among males than females and is most likely during a depressive episode. Comorbid substance abuse and anxiety disorders substantially increase the risk of suicide.

Pharmacotherapy may substantially reduce the risk of suicide (3). For example, in an 11-year follow-up of 103 bipolar patients taking lithium, death rates were well below that expected for this group based on age and sex (4). Mortality in general is higher in those with mania in late life compared to those with depression alone (5).

D. Epidemiology

Bipolar I disorder affects approximately 0.8% of the adult population (estimates from community samples range between 0.4% and 1.6%) and bipolar II disorder affects approximately 0.5% over the course of a lifetime (6). Bipolar I disorder affects men and women fairly equally, although bipolar II disorder is more common in women. There are no known significant differences among racial groups in the prevalence of either bipolar I or bipolar II disorder.

The Epidemiologic Catchment Area study reported a mean age at onset of 21 years for bipolar disorder (7). When studies examining age at onset are stratified into 5-year intervals, the peak age at onset of first symptoms falls between ages 15–19, followed closely by ages 20–24. There is often a 5- to 10-year interval, however, between age at onset of illness and age at first treatment or first hospitalization. Onset of mania before age 15 has been less well studied. Clinical experience suggests that onset of bipolar disorder prior to age 12 is uncommon (8).

The first episode in males is more likely to be a manic episode. The first episode in females is more likely to be a depressive episode. Frequently, a patient will experience several episodes of depression before a manic episode occurs (9–15).

Onset of mania after age 60 is less likely to be associated with a positive family history of bipolar disorder and is more likely to be associated with identifiable general medical factors, including cerebral vascular problems. Morbidity and mortality rates are especially high in patients over age 60 (5, 16).

Evidence from epidemiologic and twin studies strongly suggests that bipolar disorder is a heritable illness (17, 18). First-degree relatives of patients with bipolar disorder have significantly higher rates of mood disorder compared with relatives of nonpsychiatrically ill control populations. However, the mode of inheritance remains unknown, and the magnitude of the role played by environmental stressors, particularly early in the course of the illness, also remains uncertain. In clinical practice, a family history of mood disorder, especially of bipolar disorder, provides strong corroborative evidence of the existence of a mood disorder in a patient with otherwise predominantly psychotic features.

II. Treatment Principles and Alternatives

The development of a treatment plan for patients with bipolar disorder requires the consideration of many issues. The cross-sectional (e.g., current clinical status) and longitudinal (e.g., frequency, severity, and consequences of past episodes) context of the treatment decision should guide the psychiatrist and patient in choosing from among various possible treatments and treatment settings. These decisions must be based on knowledge of the beneficial and adverse effects of available options, along with information about patient preferences. In addition, treatment decisions should be continually reassessed as new information becomes available and/or the patient's clinical status changes. It should also be kept in mind that denial is often a prominent part of this disorder and may at times interfere with the patient's ability to make reasoned treatment decisions.

At this time there is no cure for bipolar disorder; however, treatment can decrease the associated morbidity and mortality. The specific goals of treatment are to decrease the frequency, severity, and psychosocial consequences of episodes and to improve psychosocial functioning between episodes. Some patients with severe and chronic impairments will need specific rehabilitative services.

This section is organized as follows. First, treatment options for patients with bipolar disorder, including psychiatric management, pharmacologic treatments, and electroconvulsive therapy (ECT), are reviewed along with the evidence for their efficacy. Second, issues to be considered in choosing and implementing these treatment options (including the factors that underlie the choice of treatment setting) are discussed in the context of specific phases of the illness. Finally, the ways in which particular clinical features of the patient's illness alter the general treatment recommendations are elucidated.

A. Psychiatric Management

Psychiatric management includes a specific set of interventions, some of which have been included in the concept of "supportive psychotherapy" and/or "insight-oriented psychotherapy" and others in the concept of "clinical management." The general goals are to assess and treat acute exacerbations, prevent recurrences, improve interepisode functioning, and provide assistance, insight, and support to the patient and family.

Specific goals of psychiatric management include establishing and maintaining a therapeutic alliance, monitoring the patient's psychiatric status, providing education regarding bipolar disorder, enhancing treatment compliance, promoting regular patterns of activity and wakefulness, promoting understanding of and adaptation to the psychosocial effects of bipolar disorder, identifying new episodes early, and reducing the morbidity and sequelae of bipolar disorder (19).

1.   Establishing and maintaining a therapeutic alliance

Bipolar disorder is a long-term illness that manifests itself in different ways at different points during its course. Establishing and maintaining a supportive therapeutic relationship is critical to the proper understanding and management of an individual patient. A crucial element of this alliance is the knowledge gained about the course of the patient's illness that allows new episodes to be identified as early as possible.

2.   Monitoring the patient's psychiatric status

The psychiatrist should remain vigilant for changes in psychiatric status. While this is true for all mental disorders, it is especially important in bipolar disorder because lack of insight on the part of the patient is so frequent, especially during manic episodes, and because small changes in mood or behavior may herald the onset of an episode with potentially devastating consequences. Such monitoring may be enhanced by knowledge gained over time about particular characteristics of the patient's illness, including typical sequence (e.g., mania is usually followed by depression) and typical duration and severity of episodes (e.g., depressions are mild and often self-limiting).

3.   Providing education regarding bipolar disorder

Patients with bipolar disorder often benefit from education and feedback regarding their illness, prognosis, and treatment. Frequently, their ability to understand and retain this information will vary over time and may be impeded by a tendency to deny the existence and consequences of the illness. Education should therefore be an ongoing process in which the psychiatrist gradually but persistently introduces facts about the illness, with adequate therapeutic attention to the psychological forces promoting denial and to the patient's stage of adaptation to the chronic illness. Importantly, patient education over an extended period of time will assist in reinforcing the patient's role as collaborator in the treatment of this persistent illness. In this capacity, the patient will know when to report subsyndromal symptoms and gradually learn to increase or decrease medications with the waxing and waning of the illness. Printed material on cross-sectional and longitudinal aspects of bipolar illness and its treatment can be helpful (20–23). Family members may also deny the illness and its consequences, and similar educational approaches by the psychiatrist may be important with family members.

4.   Enhancing treatment compliance

Bipolar disorder is a long-term illness in which adherence to carefully designed treatment plans can improve the patient's health status. However, patients with this disorder are frequently ambivalent about treatment. This ambivalence often takes the form of non-compliance with medication and other treatments (24, 25). Noncompliance with mood-stabilizing medications is a major cause of relapse (26, 27).

Ambivalence about treatment stems from many factors. One is denial. Patients who do not believe that they have a serious illness are not likely to be willing to adhere to long-term treatment regimens. Patients with this disorder may minimize or deny the reality of a prior episode, their own behavior, and often the consequences of their behavior. Denial may be especially pronounced during a manic episode.

Another important factor for some patients is their reluctance to give up the experience of mania (24). The increased energy, euphoria, heightened self-esteem, and ability to focus may be very desirable and enjoyable. Patients often recall this experience and minimize or deny entirely the subsequent devastating features of full-blown mania or the extended demoralization of a depressive episode. They are therefore often reluctant to take medication that prevents mania.

Medication side effects and other demands of long-term treatment may be burdensome and need to be discussed realistically with the patient and family members. Many side effects can be corrected with careful attention to dosing, scheduling, and preparation. Troublesome side effects that remain must be discussed in the context of an informed assessment of the risks and benefits of the current treatment and its potential alternatives.

5. Promoting regular patterns of activity and wakefulness

Patients with bipolar disorder may benefit from regular patterns of daily activities, including sleeping, eating, physical activity, and social and/or emotional stimulation. The psychiatrist should help the patient determine the degree to which these factors affect mood states and to develop methods to monitor and modulate daily activities. Many patients find that if they establish regular patterns of sleeping, other important aspects of life fall into regular patterns as well.

6. Promoting understanding of and adaption to the psychosocial effects of bipolar disorder

All patients with bipolar disorder have had at least one manic episode. Many patients have had several episodes of mania and depression. Typically, such a history leaves patients with emotional, social, family, academic, occupational, and financial issues that require therapeutic help to address and deal with effectively.

During the episode itself, the psychiatrist should assist the patient with issues related to his or her environment, including interpersonal relationships, work and living conditions, and other medical or health-related needs. Examples of this assistance include helping the patient to avoid engaging in embarrassing behavior during manic episodes, assisting the patient in scheduling absences from work or other responsibilities as required, discouraging the patient from instituting major life changes that might be predicated on the depressed or manic state, helping to bolster the patient's morale by strengthening expectations of help and hope for the future, enlisting the support of others in the patient's social network and supporting them as necessary, and setting realistic, attainable, and tangible goals. Patients who have children may need help assessing their children's needs, both during and in the wake of the parent's episodes, and making appropriate plans to meet those needs. At times, it may be important to help the parent with bipolar disorder obtain a psychiatric evaluation for the child (e.g., if the parent reports that the child or adolescent is showing early signs of mood instability). Bipolar patients who are considering having children may benefit from genetic counseling (27).

7.   Identifying new episodes early

The psychiatrist should help the patient and family members to identify early signs and symptoms of manic or depressive episodes. Such identification can help the patient to enhance mastery over his or her illness and can help ensure that adequate treatment is instituted as early as possible in the course of an episode. Early markers of episode onset vary from patient to patient. Many patients experience changes in sleep patterns early in the development of an episode. Other symptoms may be quite subtle and specific to the individual (e.g., participating in religious activities more or less often than usual). The identification of these early, prodromal signs or symptoms is facilitated by the presence of a consistent relationship between the psychiatrist and the patient, as well as the patient's family. The use of a graphic display of life events and mood can be very helpful in this process (28). First conceived by Kraepelin (29) and Meyer (30) and refined and advanced by Post et al. (28), a life chart provides a valuable display of illness course and episode sequence, polarity, severity, frequency, and relationship, if any, to environmental stressors, as well as response to treatment. A graphic display of sleep patterns may be sufficient for some patients to identify early signs of episodes.

8.   Reducing the morbidity and sequelae of bipolar disorder

Through many of the activities already described, psychiatric management helps minimize the sequelae of abnormal mood states by helping the patient respond adaptively on an interpersonal, academic, occupational, social, and financial level.

Psychiatric management should be an ongoing process. Different interventions will be needed at different times as the patient experiences episodes of the illness and as the patient and family develop and grow in their ability to respond adaptively to the demands of the illness.

B.   Pharmacologic Treatments

Pharmacologic treatments are a critical component in the treatment of patients with bipolar disorder. Medications have been shown to be effective in the treatment of acute episodes, as well as in the prevention of future episodes. In addition, many patients benefit between episodes from the mood-stabilizing effects of some medications. The review of efficacy data for bipolar disorder is hampered somewhat by inconsistencies in the measurement and description of patient outcomes, as well as in the terms used to describe changes in the course of the illness.

Medications for patients with bipolar disorder include those that decrease symptoms of mania or depression, those that prevent episodes, and those that may not act primarily on mood but that are helpful at various times during the course of the disorder. These medications have been categorized in a variety of ways. In this guideline, we use the following categories: mood stabilizers (medications with both antimanic and antidepressive actions); antimanic agents; antidepressants; adjunctive medications; and new or atypical medications that have not been fully assessed.

The three mood stabilizers currently available—lithium, valproate, and carbamazepine—have been studied and used in the treatment of all phases of bipolar disorder. The following review of efficacy data for each medication is organized according to phase of disorder and goal of the treatment (e.g., during the manic phase, the goal is to reduce manic symptoms and shorten the episode.)

Traditionally, lithium has been the primary pharmacologic treatment for patients with bipolar disorder. It was first reported to have antimanic effects in 1949 (31) and has been in widespread use in this country for the acute and preventive treatment of bipolar disorder since the mid 1960s (32). Valproate and carbamazepine, on the other hand, have only been reported useful for this disorder since the late 1970s. The total number of patients studied in lithium trials as well as the breadth of clinical experience with lithium far exceeds that for the two newer agents. However, the quality of study design and outcome measures have improved over time, so that some of the soundest studies include the newer agents.

1. Lithium

Lithium is effective in the acute treatment of manic and depressive episodes and in the prevention of recurrent manic and depressive episodes (1). In addition, lithium has been reported to decrease the mood instability that plagues many patients between episodes (1).

a. Acute mania.   Considerable research supports the efficacy of lithium in the treatment of manic episodes. In a review of 10 early uncontrolled trials of 413 patients with bipolar disorder, 81% displayed reduced manic symptoms during acute lithium treatment (33). The overall response rate to lithium in four placebo-controlled studies of 116 patients with acute mania was 78% (34–38). These studies also demonstrated that up to 2 weeks of treatment with lithium may be necessary to reach maximal effectiveness for manic patients. In a recent randomized, double-blind, controlled study of lithium, divalproex, and placebo (39), 49% of the patients taking lithium had at least a 50% reduction in their mania rating scale score at 3 weeks, despite the fact that over half of the patients reported that lithium had not been effective for their most recent prior episode. Lithium was significantly more effective than placebo and was not statistically more or less effective than divalproex. Preliminary, unpublished data from this study suggest that lithium is more effective than divalproex in the treatment of "classic mania" and less effective than divalproex in the treatment of "mixed mania." These hypotheses need further study.

Lithium has also been compared with neuroleptics. While most studies are confounded by having included a wide diagnostic mix of patients, Janicak et al. (40) recently reviewed the available studies that included only patients with acute mania. They found that in these well-designed studies lithium was superior to neuroleptics in the acute treatment of mania.

b. Acute bipolar depression. A review of nine controlled studies comparing lithium with placebo in the treatment of the depressive phase of bipolar disorder (41) showed that 63 (79%) of 80 patients displayed an antidepressant response to lithium (41). Despite controversy over the methodology of some of these studies, it seems clear that many patients in the depressive phase of bipolar disorder can expect a clinically significant response to lithium. The time frame for response for depression is longer than that for mania, however. Many patients require lithium treatment for 6 to 8 weeks before a full response becomes evident. When the patient's clinical status prohibits such a long lag between the onset of treatment and a full response, the addition of psychotherapy, an antidepressant, or other medication may be warranted. These options are discussed in later sections.

c. Maintenance treatment. Open studies in the 1960s and 1970s of the prophylactic efficacy of lithium showed that the use of this drug reduces the frequency, duration, and severity of manic and depressive episodes (1). Many of these studies included patients with high rates of recurrence prior to treatment with lithium. In such patients the results were often dramatic. For example, in one study the average time ill during a 12-month period dropped from 13 weeks to 2 weeks (42).

These results have since been confirmed by 10 double-blind, placebo-controlled studies. A review of these studies found that patients taking lithium had a significantly lower probability of having an episode than those taking placebo (1). Overall, 34% of the patients taking lithium had an episode compared to 81% of those taking placebo, although these summary statistics are confounded by variations in entry criteria, definitions of relapse, and length of follow up.

Lithium appears to be equally effective in preventing episodes of mania and major episodes of depression. Many investigators have found that patients taking lithium prophylactically continue to have minor episodes of depression, however. This asymmetry of response between minor depressive and minor manic episodes may be based, in part, on the fact that patients are more likely to report mild depression than mild hypomania. Many investigators have also reported that lithium decreases the intensity of episodes that do occur and that lithium reduces subsyndromal mood variations between episodes. These two effects are often very valuable to patients and are frequently omitted from summary statistics of lithium's efficacy (1).

Discontinuation of long-term lithium therapy in patients with bipolar disorder has been associated with a significant short-term increase in risk of recurrence. In one study, over 50% of patients with bipolar disorder experienced recurrent mood episodes within 6 months of lithium discontinuation (43). Whether this represents a "lithium withdrawal syndrome" or simply a reemergence of the disorder is not clear (1, 44, 45). It is also possible that in some patients who choose to stop taking lithium, discontinuation itself may be an early manifestation of recurrence. If the decision is made to discontinue previously effective lithium therapy, slow tapering has been reported to reduce the risk of early recurrence (43). Some patients develop a more severe and relatively nonresponsive form of the illness following the discontinuation of effective prophylactic lithium (46). In this instance, switching to a medication with a novel mechanism of action, providing ECT, or discontinuing that medication for a period of time followed by a renewed trial may be successful, at least temporarily, in reinitiating a treatment response (47).

d. Pharmacokinetics and drug–drug interactions.   Lithium is available in tablets or capsules as the carbonate salt or as lithium citrate in syrup form. A 300 mg tablet of lithium carbonate contains 8 meq (or mmol); 5 cc of the citrate syrup also contains 8 meq. Lithium is readily absorbed after oral administration; no parenteral forms are available. Standard preparations lead to peak serum levels in 1½ to 2 hours; slow release forms lead to peak serum levels in 4 to 4½ hours. Lithium is excreted almost entirely by the kidneys, with a half-life between 14 and 30 hours. (Normally the lithium clearance is about one-fourth of the creatinine clearance.) The rate of lithium clearance is faster in younger persons and decreases in association with diminished glomerular function and age.

Therapeutic and toxic effects of lithium are correlated with serum levels, which are correlated, to a lesser extent, with oral dose. Therefore, safe and effective administration of lithium requires that serum levels be monitored. The relatively long half-life of lithium means that steady-state levels after a dosage change will not occur for 5 to 7 days. Trough levels are typically reported, and these are traditionally sampled 12 hours after the last dose. If this procedure is not followed, the results are likely to be unreliable and misleading. The availability of a slow-release form and the practice of switching from a multiple-dose regimen to a once-daily regimen may confuse the interpretation of serum levels. In general, a patient whose lithium regimen changes from twice a day to once a day can expect a 10% to 26% increase in 12-hour lithium levels (32).

Lithium is distributed in total body water, is not protein bound, and is not metabolized. Changes in hydration will affect lithium levels, with episodes of dehydration leading to higher levels. Lithium excretion, and therefore serum levels, can be affected by changes in renal function. Decreases in glomerular filtration rates, due to either age or disease, will decrease lithium clearance. In addition, sodium deficiency (secondary to diet, medication, or other causes) will increase lithium reabsorption and increase lithium levels. Thiazide diuretics increase lithium levels by 30% to 50%. Furosemide appears to have no direct effect on lithium levels, although lithium levels should be monitored in any patient beginning treatment with a diuretic because of potential changes in total body fluid. Many types of medications have been reported to increase lithium levels, including some nonsteroidal anti-inflammatory agents and angiotensin converting enzyme-inhibiting antihypertensive agents (1). Although there have been reports of enhanced neurotoxicity, including the development of neuroleptic malignant syndrome, when lithium was administered in conjunction with a neuroleptic (especially haloperidol), most investigators have found that these medications can be safely combined at standard doses, and are, in fact, used together quite commonly without severe adverse effects (32).

e. Side effects and toxicity. Up to 75% of patients treated with lithium experience some side effects (1, 32). These side effects vary in clinical significance; most are either minor or can be reduced or eliminated by lowering the lithium dose or changing the dosage schedule. For example, Schou (48) has reported a 30% reduction in side effects among patients treated with an average lithium level of 0.68 meq/liter compared to those with an average level of 0.85 meq/liter. Side effects that appear to be related to peak serum levels (e.g., tremor that peaks within 1 to 2 hours of a dose) may be reduced or eliminated by using a slow-release preparation or changing to a single bedtime dose.

Dose-related side effects. Side effects of lithium include polyuria, polydypsia, weight gain, cognitive problems (e.g., dulling, impaired memory, poor concentration, confusion, mental slowness), tremor, sedation or lethargy, impaired coordination, gastrointestinal distress (e.g., nausea, vomiting, dyspepsia, diarrhea), hair loss, benign leukocytosis, acne, and edema. Side effects persisting despite dosage adjustment may be managed with other medications (e.g., β-blockers for tremor; diuretics for polyuria, polydipsia or edema; topical antibiotics or retinoic acid for acne). Gastrointestinal disturbances can be managed by administering lithium with meals or switching lithium preparations (especially to lithium citrate).

Lithium may cause benign ECG changes associated with repolarization. Less commonly, cardiac conduction abnormalities have been associated with lithium treatment. Anecdotal reports have linked lithium with other ECG changes, including the exacerbation of existing arrhythmias and, less commonly, the development of new arrhythmias (32).

The most common renal effect of lithium is impaired concentrating capacity due to reduced renal response to ADH, manifested as polyuria and/or polydipsia. Although the polyuria associated with early lithium treatment may resolve, persistent polyuria (ranging from mild and well tolerated to severe nephrogenic diabetes insipidus) may occur. Polyuria can frequently be managed by changing to a once-daily bedtime dose. If the polyuria persists, management includes ensuring that fluid intake is adequate and that the lithium dose is as low as possible. Some clinicians have found that decreasing the total daily protein intake, in conjunction with a nutritional assessment, is helpful. If these measures do not ameliorate the problem, then concurrent administration of a thiazide diuretic (e.g., hydrochlorothiazide at a dose of 50 mg/day) may be helpful. The dosage of lithium will usually need to be decreased (typically by 50%) to account for the increased reabsorption induced by thiazides (32). In addition, potassium levels will need to be monitored, and potassium replacement may be necessary. Amiloride, a potassium-sparing diuretic, is reported to be effective in treating lithium-induced polyuria and polydipsia; its advantages are that it does not alter lithium levels and does not cause potassium depletion. Amiloride may be started at 5 mg b.i.d. and may be increased to 10 mg b.i.d., as needed (49).

Hypothyroidism occurs in 5% to 35% of patients treated with lithium, is more frequent in women, tends to appear after 6 to 18 months of lithium treatment, and may be associated with rapid cycling (1, 32, 50). Lithium-induced hypothyroidism is generally reversible when lithium is discontinued. However, lithium-induced hypothyroidism is not a contraindication to continuing lithium treatment. When lithium is continued, the associated hypothyroidism is easily treated by administration of levothyroxine (32). In addition to the classic signs and symptoms of hypothyroidism, patients with bipolar disorder are at risk of developing depression and/or rapid cycling as a consequence of suboptimal thyroid functioning. If these symptoms occur in the presence of laboratory evidence of suboptimal thyroid functioning, then thyroid supplementation and/or discontinuation of lithium should be considered (51, 52).

Idiosyncratic side effects. A small number of case reports describe exacerbation or first oc-currences of psoriasis associated with lithium treatment. Some of these patients improved with appropriate dermatologic treatment and/or when the lithium dose was lowered. In some cases, however, lithium seemed to block the effects of dermatologic treatment, and the condition cleared only after lithium was discontinued. In addition, occasionally patients experience severe pustular acne that does not respond well to standard dermatologic treat-ments and only resolves once the lithium has been discontinued. (This is in contrast to the more common mild to moderate acne that can occur with lithium treatment and that is usually responsive to standard treatments [32].)

Much concern has been raised about whether long-term lithium exposure may cause irreversible kidney damage. Approximately 10% to 20% of patients receiving long-term lithium treatment (more than 10 years) display morphological kidney changes—usually interstitial fibrosis, tubular atrophy, and sometimes glomerular sclerosis. These changes may be associated with impairment of water reabsorption, but not with reduction in glomerular filtration rate or development of renal insufficiency (1, 32, 53–55). Although irreversible renal failure due to lithium has not been unequivocally established, there are two case reports of probable lithium-induced renal insufficiency (55, 56). Additionally, several studies show that a small percentage of patients treated with lithium may develop rising serum creatinine concentrations after 10 years or more of treatment (55).

Toxicity/overdose. Toxic effects of lithium become more likely as the serum level rises. Most patients will experience some toxic effects with levels above 1.5 meq/liter; levels above 2.0 meq/liter are commonly associated with life-threatening side effects. For many patients, the therapeutic range within which beneficial effects outweigh toxic effects is quite narrow, so that small changes in serum level may lead to clinically significant altera-tions in the beneficial and harmful effects of lithium. Elderly patients may experience toxic effects at lower levels and have a correspondingly narrower therapeutic window.

Signs and symptoms of early intoxication (with levels above 1.5 meq/liter) include marked tremor, nausea and diarrhea, blurred vision, vertigo, confusion, and increased deep tendon reflexes. With levels above 2.5 meq/liter, patients may experience more severe neurological complications and eventually experience seizures, coma, cardiac dysrhythmia, and permanent neurological impairment. The magnitude of the serum level and the du-ration of exposure to a high level of lithium are both correlated with risk of adverse effects. Therefore, rapid steps to reduce the serum level are essential. In addition, during treatment for severe intoxication, patients may experience "secondary peaks," during which the serum level rises after a period of relative decline; the clinician must therefore continue to monitor serum levels during treatment for severe intoxication. The patient with lithium intoxication should be treated with supportive care (e.g., maintenance of fluid and electrolyte balance), and steps should be taken to prevent further absorption of the medication (e.g., induction of emesis in the alert patient, gastric lavage). Hemodialysis is the only reliable method of rapidly removing excess lithium from the body and is more effective than peritoneal dialysis for this purpose. Criteria for use of hemodialysis in lithium intoxication are not firmly established, and the decision to dialyze must take into account both the patient's clinical status and the serum lithium level. While most authorities agree that dialysis should be used in instances when clinical signs of intoxication are severe, it is not clear that a clinically tolerated high lithium level is, by itself, an indication for dialysis.

f. Implementing lithium treatment. Prior to beginning lithium treatment, the patient's general medical history should be reviewed, with special reference to those systems that might affect, or be affected by, lithium therapy (i.e., renal, thyroid, and cardiac functioning). In addition, pregnancy or the presence of a dermatologic disorder must be ascertained.

In general, laboratory measures and other diagnostic tests are recommended based on knowledge of pathophysiology and anticipated clinical decisions, rather than on evidence from experimental studies that indicate their clinical utility. The decision to recommend a test is based on the probability of detecting a finding that would alter treatment and the expected benefit of the resulting alteration in treatment. Recommended tests fall into three categories: 1) baseline measures that are used to facilitate the later interpretation of laboratory tests (e.g., ECG, CBC); 2) tests to determine whether different or additional treatments are needed (e.g., pregnancy, thyroid-stimulating hormone level); and 3) tests to determine whether the standard dosage regimen of lithium needs to be altered (e.g., creatinine level).

Based on these considerations, the following are generally recommended prior to beginning lithium therapy: general medical history and physical examination; BUN and creatinine levels; pregnancy test; tests of thyroid function; ECG with rhythm strip for patients over age 40; and some authorities suggest a CBC.

There are two methods to initiate lithium treatment and achieve therapeutic serum levels. The first involves administering a single test dose of lithium, obtaining a serum level 24 hours later, and using a nomogram to predict the appropriate daily dose (57). Alternatively, lithium may be started in low divided doses to minimize side effects (e.g., 300 mg t.i.d. or less, depending on the patient's weight and age) and the dose titrated upward (generally to serum concentrations of 0.5 to 1.2 meq/liter) according to response and side effects (58). Lithium levels should be checked after each dosage increase (and prior to the next); steady-state levels are likely to be reached approximately 5 days after a dosage adjustment, but levels may need to be checked sooner if a rapid increase is necessary (e.g., in the treatment of acute mania) or if toxicity is suspected. As levels approach the upper limits of the therapeutic range (i.e., ≥1.0 meq/liter), levels should be checked at shorter intervals after each dosage increase to minimize the risk of toxicity.

Serum concentrations required for prophylaxis may be, in some cases, as high as those required for treatment of the acute episode. A controlled study by Gelenberg et al. (58) found that patients randomly assigned to a "low" lithium level (0.4–0.6 meq/liter) had fewer side effects but more episodes than patients in the "standard" lithium group (0.8–1.0 meq/liter). However, the lithium levels of some of the patients in the "low" group decreased relatively rapidly from their previous treatment levels, which could have increased their risk of relapse. Although the prophylactic efficacy of lithium levels between 0.6–0.8 meq/liter has not been formally studied, this range is commonly chosen by patients and their psychiatrists. Despite the lack of formal study, it is likely that for many patients increases in maintenance lithium levels will result in a trade-off between greater protection from episodes at the cost of increased side effects. The "optimal" maintenance level may therefore vary somewhat from patient to patient. Some patients find that a single daily dose facilitates treatment compliance and reduces or does not change side effects.

The clinical status of patients on lithium needs to be monitored especially closely, with the frequency of monitoring dependent on the individual patient's clinical situation, but generally no less than every 6 months in stable patients. The optimal frequency of serum level monitoring in an individual patient will depend on the following features: the range of therapeutic lithium levels; the stability of lithium levels during the average course of events for that patient; and the degree to which the patient can be relied upon to notice and report symptoms. These features will vary with the phase of the illness.

In general, renal function should be tested every 2 to 3 months during the first 6 months of treatment, and thyroid function should be tested once or twice during the first 6 months of lithium treatment. Subsequently, renal and thyroid function may be checked every 6 months to 1 year in stable patients or whenever clinically indicated (e.g., in the presence of breakthrough affective symptoms, changes in side effects, or new general medical or psychiatric signs or symptoms) (32, 54).

2. Valproate

Valproate has been studied alone and in combination with other mood stabilizers in all phases of bipolar disorder.

a. Acute mania. Janicak et al. (40) reviewed the available data on the use of valproate in the treatment of acute mania. They found that numerous studies, comprising 297 patients, demonstrate an overall "moderate to marked" response rate of 56%. However, these studies had many methodologic problems, including a lack of standard diagnostic information about the patients, nonblind conditions, and the use of valproate in conjunction with other active medications.

Two double-blind, placebo-controlled trials of valproate in the acute treatment of mania have been reported, with a total of 36 patients in one study (59) and 179 patients in the other (39). These studies used careful diagnostic criteria, limited supplemental medications, and employed double-blind conditions. The study by Bowden et al. (39) included three treatment groups: placebo, lithium, and valproate. Taken together, these two studies demonstrate that over a 3-week period, valproate is superior to placebo and is as effective as lithium for patients with acute mania. In addition, as mentioned earlier, preliminary unpublished data suggest that divalproex may be more effective than lithium for patients with mixed mania and less effective than lithium for patients with classic mania. These hypotheses need to be tested in further studies.

Improvement in manic symptoms has been observed within 3 days using oral loading (60, 61) and within 5 days with standard dosing regimens (39). Other studies have demonstrated that certain patients who are resistant to the antimanic effects of a single mood stabilizer may benefit from the combination of valproate with lithium, valproate with carbamazepine, and valproate with neuroleptics, including clozapine (62–64).

b. Acute bipolar depression. There are no controlled studies examining the efficacy of valproate in acute bipolar depression. Open studies have had response rates that are in the range consistent with a placebo mechanism of action; 30% of depressed bipolar patients had "some response" and significantly fewer had a "marked response" to valproate (65–69).

There may be a role for valproate in the treatment of depressed bipolar patients who require an antidepressant but need to be protected from the induction of mania (68).

c. Maintenance treatment. There are no controlled studies of valproate in the maintenance phase of bipolar disorder. Open studies indicate that valproate may reduce the frequency and/or intensity of recurrent episodes over extended periods of time in some patients with bipolar disorder, including those with rapid cycling (65, 67, 69, 70).

d. Pharmacokinetics and drug–drug interactions. Valproate is commercially available in the United States in a wide variety of preparations: valproate (available in capsules and syrup), divalproex sodium (an enteric-coated, stable coordination compound containing equal proportions of valproic acid and sodium valproate), and divalproex sodium sprinkle capsules (containing coated particles of divalproex sodium that can be ingested intact or pulled apart and sprinkled on food). There are only minor differences in the pharmacokinetic properties of these different preparations (71–74), and valproate is the common compound in plasma. Valproate, in both capsules and syrup, is rapidly absorbed after ingestion; peak serum concentrations are reached within 2 hours. Peak serum concentrations of divalproex sodium are attained within 3 to 8 hours. The plasma half-life of both valproate and divalproex sodium ranges from 6 to 16 hours.

The relationship between valproate serum concentrations and mood-stabilizing effects is not fully defined. The range considered therapeutic for epilepsy is 50–100 µg/ml (75). A recent study of the use of valproate in patients with acute mania found that the beneficial effects increased markedly with levels above 45 µg/ml and certain adverse effects increased markedly with levels above 125 µg/ml (unpublished 1994 study of Bowden et al.).

Because valproate is extensively metabolized by the liver and highly protein bound, interactions may occur with other metabolized or protein-bound drugs (71, 72). In addition, valproate weakly inhibits drug oxidation, so serum concentrations of drugs that undergo oxidative metabolization (e.g., phenobarbital, phenytoin, and tricyclics) can be increased when coadministered with valproate. Conversely, valproate serum concentrations can be decreased by coadministration of microsomal enzyme-inducing drugs (e.g., carbamazepine) or increased by drugs that inhibit metabolism (e.g., fluoxetine) (76). Also, serum valproate free fraction concentrations can be increased and valproate toxicity precipitated by coadministration of other highly protein-bound drugs (e.g., aspirin), which can displace valproate from its protein binding sites.

e. Side effects and toxicity.   Minor side effects of valproate, such as sedation or gastrointestinal distress, are common initially and typically resolve with continued treatment or dosage adjustment. In addition, the medication has a wide therapeutic window. Inadvertent overdose is uncommon, and purposeful overdose less likely to be lethal than with lithium. However, the medication can rarely cause life-threatening reactions, and patients must be relied upon to report the often quite subtle symptoms of these reactions promptly.

Dose-related side effects.   Common dose-related side effects of valproate include gastrointestinal distress (e.g., anorexia, nausea, dyspepsia, vomiting, diarrhea), benign hepatic transaminase elevations, tremor, and sedation. Patients with past or current hepatic disease may be at increased risk for hepatotoxicity. Mild, asymptomatic leukopenia and thrombocytopenia (reversible upon drug discontinuation) occur less frequently. Other side effects often bothersome to the patient include hair loss (usually transient), increased appetite, and weight gain. Persistent gastrointestinal distress associated with valproate can be alleviated by dosage reduction, change of preparation (use of the divalproex sodium formulation rather than valproic acid), or administration of a histamine-2-antagonist (e.g., famotidine or cimetidine) (77). Tremor can be managed with dosage reduction or coadministration of β-blockers. If mild, asymptomatic thrombocytopenia occurs, a decrease in valproate dosage will usually restore the platelet count to normal. Similarly, cases of mild, asymptomatic leukopenia (total WBC count above 3000 and polymorphonuclear leukocyte count above 1500) is usually reversible upon dosage reduction or discontinuation.

Idiosyncratic side effects.   One recent uncontrolled report indicated that 80% of women receiving long-term valproate treatment for epilepsy before the age of 20 had polycystic ovaries or hyperandrogenism (78). The implications of this for women who take valproate for bipolar disorder (both for acute and perhaps maintenance treatment) need to be assessed. Rare, idiosyncratic, but potentially fatal adverse events include irreversible hepatic failure, pancreatitis, and agranulocytosis. Patients taking valproate need to be instructed to contact their psychiatrist immediately if they develop symptoms of these conditions.

Toxicity/overdose.   Valproate has a wide therapeutic window, and unintentional overdose is therefore uncommon. Signs of overdose include somnolence, heart block, and eventually coma. Deaths have been reported. Overdose can be treated with hemodialysis and/or naloxone (40, 75).

f. Implementing valproate treatment.   Before initiating valproate treatment, a general medical history should be taken, with special attention to hepatic, hematologic, and bleeding abnormalities. Ideally, liver function and hematologic measures should be obtained at baseline prior to drug administration to evaluate general medical health.

Valproate may be initiated in low, divided doses to minimize gastrointestinal and neurologic toxicity. Dosage should generally be started at 250 mg t.i.d., with the dose increased every few days as side effects allow (49). The dose is then titrated upward by 250–500 mg/day every several days according to response and side effects, generally to a serum concentration between 50–100 μg/ml (with a maximum adult daily dose of 60 mg/kg per day) (75). Patients with acute mania may tolerate larger initial doses of up to 20 mg/kg per day (valproate loading) and more rapid dosage increments than elderly patients and patients who are hypomanic, euthymic, or depressed (60, 61). Once the patient is stable, valproate dosage regimens can be simplified to enhance convenience and compliance.

Asymptomatic hepatic enzyme elevations, leukopenia, and thrombocytopenia do not reliably predict life-threatening hepatic or bone marrow failure. In conjunction with careful monitoring of clinical status, educating patients about the signs and symptoms of hepatic and hematologic dysfunction and instructing them to report these symptoms if they occur is essential. Some investigators believe that routine monitoring of hematologic and hepatic function in otherwise healthy patients with epilepsy receiving long-term valproate treatment is not necessary (79). Nevertheless, most psychiatrists perform clinical assessments, including tests of hematologic and hepatic function, at a minimum of every 6 months for stable patients who are taking valproate (61, 80, 81). Patients who cannot reliably report signs or symptoms of toxicity need to be monitored more frequently.

3. Carbamazepine

Carbamazepine has been studied alone and in combination with other mood stabilizers in the treatment of all phases of bipolar disorder (63, 80–84).

a. Acute mania. Janicak et al. (40) reviewed 16 studies of carbamazepine that included patients with acute mania. The data generally support the conclusion that carbamazepine is effective in the acute treatment of manic episodes. However, precise interpretation of the data is difficult because of inadequate study design, frequent concomitant use of other active medications, and the use of patient samples that are likely to be atypical.

The results of studies comparing carbamazepine to lithium are mixed, with one investigator finding lithium to be superior (85) and one finding the two drugs to be statistically equivalent, with a trend toward greater efficacy of lithium (86). Studies comparing carbamazepine to neuroleptics have generally found the two medications to be equivalent in efficacy (87–89).

b. Acute bipolar depression. There are two double-blind comparisons of carbamazepine with placebo in the treatment of bipolar depression (90, 91). These studies included patients with bipolar I and bipolar II disorder. In total, 10 of 17 patients had a good or partial response. Another double-blind, controlled study of 13 patients with bipolar I disorder who had not responded to carbamazepine alone found that six responded to lithium augmentation (92).

c. Maintenance treatment.   Reviews of the data on carbamazepine in the maintenance phase of bipolar disorder have concluded that carbamazepine may effectively reduce the frequency and severity of episodes for some patients (40, 93). However, the data are limited by such methodologic flaws as lack of a randomized, double-blind, placebo-controlled design; concomitant administration of other active medications; and insufficient doses (40, 94–98).

d. Pharmacokinetics and drug–drug interactions.   Carbamazepine is available in a wide variety of preparations, including solutions, suspensions, syrups, and newly developed chewable and slow-release formulations. All of these preparations appear to have similar bioavailability. Peak plasma carbamazepine concentrations are generally obtained between 4 and 8 hours after ingestion, but peaks as late as 26 hours have been reported. The elimination half-life of carbamazepine ranges from 18 to 55 hours. With maintenance treatment, carbamazepine induces its own metabolism, and its half-life may be decreased to 5 to 26 hours.

Because carbamazepine also induces the metabolism of other drugs metabolized by the liver and is highly protein bound, it can have clinically important interactions with other drugs stemming from changes in protein binding and hepatic metabolism (71, 72, 99, 100). Carbamazepine decreases the plasma levels of many medications metabolized by the liver, including neuroleptics, benzodiazepines (except clonazepam), tricyclic antidepressants, anticonvulsants, sex steroids and hormonal contraceptives, and thyroid hormones. Conversely, carbamazepine serum concentrations can be increased by drugs that inhibit carbamazepine metabolism, including erythromycin, the calcium channel blockers diltiazem and verapamil (but not nifedipine or nimodipine), and serotonin reuptake inhibitors (40, 75).

e. Side effects and toxicity.   Up to 50% of patients receiving carbamazepine experience side effects, and the drug is associated with potentially serious adverse reactions (72, 79, 101).

Dose-related side effects.   The most common side effects of carbamazepine include neurological symptoms, such as diplopia, blurred vision, fatigue, nausea, and ataxia. These effects are usually dose related, transient, and often reversible with dosage reduction. Elderly patients, however, may be more sensitive to the side effects. Less frequent side effects include skin rashes, mild leukopenia, mild thrombocytopenia, hyponatremia and (less commonly) hyposmolality, and mild liver enzyme elevations (occurring in 5%–15% of patients). Mild asymptomatic leukopenia is not related to serious idiopathic dyscrasia and usually resolves with dosage reduction or spontaneously with continuation of carbamazepine treatment. In the event of asymptomatic leukopenia, thrombocytopenia, or elevated liver enzymes, the carbamazepine dosage can be reduced or, with severe changes, the drug discontinued. Hyponatremia may be related to water retention due to carbamazepine's antidiuretic effect. Hyponatremia occurs in 6% to 31% of patients, is rare in children but probably more common in the elderly, occasionally develops many months after the initiation of carbamazepine treatment, and sometimes necessitates carbamazepine discontinuation. In addition, carbamazepine may decrease total and free thyroxine levels and increase free cortisol levels, but these effects are rarely clinically significant.

Idiosyncratic side effects. Rare, idiosyncratic, but serious and potentially fatal side effects of carbamazepine include agranulocytosis, aplastic anemia, hepatic failure, exfoliative dermatitis (e.g., Stevens-Johnson syndrome), and pancreatitis (79, 102). Although these side effects usually occur within the first 3 to 6 months of carbamazepine treatment, in some cases they occurred after more extended periods of treatment. Routine blood monitoring does not reliably predict blood dyscrasias, hepatic failure, or exfoliative dermatitis. Thus, in addition to careful monitoring of clinical status, it is essential to educate patients about the signs and symptoms of hepatic, hematologic, or dermatologic reactions and instruct them to report symptoms if they occur. Other rare side effects include systemic hypersensitivity reactions; cardiac conduction disturbances; psychiatric symptoms, including sporadic cases of mania and psychosis; and, very rarely, renal effects, including renal failure, oliguria, hematuria, and proteinuria.

Toxicity/overdose. Carbamazepine may be fatal in overdose (deaths have been reported with ingestions of more than 6 g). Signs of impending carbamazepine toxicity include dizziness, ataxia, sedation, and diplopia. Acute intoxication can result in hyperirritability, stupor, or coma. The most common symptoms of carbamazepine overdose are nystagmus, ophthalmoplegia, cerebellar and extrapyramidal signs, impairment of consciousness, convulsions, and respiratory dysfunction. Cardiac symptoms may include tachycardia, arrhythmia, conduction disturbances, and hypotension. Gastrointestinal and anticholinergic symptoms may also occur. Management of carbamazepine intoxication includes symptomatic treatment, gastrolavage, and hemoperfusion.

f. Implementing carbamazepine treatment. The pretreatment evaluation for carbamazepine should include a general medical history and physical examination, with special emphasis on prior history of blood dyscrasias or liver disease. Most authorities recommend that the minimum baseline evaluation include a CBC with differential and platelet count, a liver profile (LDH, SGOT, SGPT, bilirubin, alkaline phosphatase), and renal function tests (49). Serum electrolytes may also be obtained, especially in the elderly, who may be at higher risk for hyponatremia.

Although dosages can range from 200–1800 mg/day, the relationships among dose, serum concentration, response, and side effects are variable. Therefore, the dose should be titrated upward according to response and side effects. In patients over the age of 12, carbamazepine is usually begun at a total daily dosage of 200–600 mg, in three to four divided doses. In hospitalized patients with acute mania, the dosage may be increased in increments of 200 mg/day up to 800–1000 mg/day (unless side effects develop), with slower increases thereafter as indicated. In less acutely ill outpatients, dosage adjustments should be slower, as rapid increases may cause patients to develop nausea and vomiting or mild neurologic symptoms such as drowsiness, dizziness, ataxia, clumsiness, or diplopia. Should such side effects occur, the dose can be decreased temporarily and then increased again more slowly once these side effects have passed.

While therapeutic serum levels for bipolar disorder have not been established, levels established for treatment of seizure disorders (serum concentration between 4–15 µg/ml) are generally applied to patients with bipolar disorder. Trough levels are most meaningful for establishing an effective level for a given patient and are conveniently drawn prior to the first morning dose and then 5 days after a dosage change, or sooner if toxicity is suspected. Maintenance doses average about 1000 mg/day, but may range from 200–1600 mg/day in routine clinical practice (49). Doses higher than 1600 mg/day are not recommended. CBC, platelets, and liver function tests should be performed every 2 weeks during the first 2 months of carbamazepine treatment. Thereafter, if laboratory tests remain normal and no symptoms of bone marrow suppression or hepatitis appear, blood counts and liver function tests should be obtained at least every 3 months (49). More frequent monitoring is necessary in patients with laboratory findings, signs, or symptoms consistent with hematologic or hepatic abnormalities. Life-threatening reactions, however, are not always detected by routine monitoring. The psychiatrist should educate patients about signs and symptoms of hepatic, hematologic, or dermatologic reactions and instruct patients to report these symptoms if they occur. More frequent clinical and laboratory assessment is needed for those patients who cannot reliably report symptoms.

The combination of carbamazepine and lithium may be particularly effective for some patients, although it appears to increase their risk of developing an acute confusional state. If this combination is used, it is prudent to attempt to taper one of the medications once the patient is stable. While the majority of patients will not require the continued use of lithium and carbamazepine, the condition of some patients who discontinue combined treatment will worsen and require resumption of both mood stabilizers. During combined treatment, it is important to minimize the use or dose of other medications (e.g., neuroleptics, anticholinergics, benzodiazepines) that may contribute to the development of a confusional state. If the patient's mental status worsens, the possibility of drug toxicity should be considered (49).

4. Neuroleptics

Controlled studies have shown that neuroleptics are superior to placebo in the treatment of acute mania (1) (see section II.B.1.). Studies comparing lithium with neuroleptics (usually chlorpromazine) further suggest that while lithium may be superior to neuroleptics for the specific normalization of mood, neuroleptics may have a quicker onset of action and therefore may be useful, at least initially, in the highly agitated or psychotic patient (103). Neuroleptics may be used in the treatment of mania before a mood stabilizer is started to enhance compliance or in conjunction with a mood stabilizer to reduce symptoms while waiting for the effects of the mood stabilizer to become apparent. However, the use of benzodiazepines should be considered as an alternative to neuroleptics in the adjunctive treatment of mania. Benzodiazepines are frequently as effective as neuroleptics for adjunctive treatment of mania, yet do not pose a risk of extrapyramidal symptoms or tardive dyskinesia (1, 104–108).

Neuroleptics have been shown to be effective in conjunction with antidepressants in the treatment of unipolar and bipolar patients with psychotic depression (109, 110). However, clinical experience suggests that some patients with psychotic depression in the context of bipolar disorder may respond to the combination of a mood stabilizer and an antidepressant alone and therefore may not inevitably require a neuroleptic.

Little research supports the routine use of neuroleptics alone as a maintenance treatment for bipolar disorder. Some investigators believe that neuroleptics may exacerbate postmanic major depressive episodes and induce rapid cycling in some bipolar patients (111). However, use of neuroleptics, either intermittently or long term in conjunction with other mood-stabilizing agents, may be necessary in those patients whose psychotic symptoms have inadequately responded to standard mood-stabilizing agents (112).

Depot neuroleptics may be the only treatment option in those patients with seriously disruptive manic and/or psychotic symptoms who are noncompliant with oral medication regimens. In such cases, the risk of tardive dyskinesia should be balanced against the consequences of repeated manic episodes or chronic manic symptoms.

It is possible that clozapine and other newer antipsychotic agents will be effective alternatives for some patients with bipolar disorder (see section II.B.7.).

5.   Benzodiazepines

Clonazepam and lorazepam have been studied alone and in combination with lithium in the treatment of acute mania. The interpretation of many of these studies is confounded by small sample sizes, short durations of treatment, concomitant use of neuroleptics, and difficulties in distinguishing putative specific antimanic effects from nonspecific sedative effects (104, 113–117). Taken together, these studies suggest that benzodiazepines are effective, in place of or in conjunction with a neuroleptic, in sedating the acutely agitated manic patient while waiting for the effects of other primary mood-stabilizing agents to become evident. The fact that lorazepam is well absorbed after intramuscular injection (unlike other benzodiazepines) has made it particularly useful for some very agitated patients.

Benzodiazepines are not effective antidepressants and may, in fact, exacerbate depressive symptoms in some patients. However, many depressed patients have anxiety and/or insomnia (either as a consequence of the depression or as a side effect of another medication) and may benefit from a benzodiazepine in addition to their specific antidepressant or mood-stabilizing medication.

Two studies have examined the prophylactic efficacy of benzodiazepines in bipolar disorder. One study demonstrated that clonazepam could successfully replace haloperidol in patients who required an adjunct to their maintenance lithium therapy (118). However, the other study demonstrated that patients who were relatively treatment refractory to the combination of neuroleptics and mood stabilizers could not successfully be treated with the combination of clonazepam and a mood stabilizer (119). Patients with anxiety and/or insomnia may benefit from the adjunctive use of a benzodiazepine. This is especially important for those patients who seem to be particularly vulnerable to the precipitation of an episode during periods of relative sleep deprivation. During these periods, the prompt institution of a benzodiazepine at bedtime may effectively decrease the risk of a relapse.

Although benzodiazepines may be helpful for many patients with bipolar disorder, two cautions are necessary. 1) Benzodiazepines have the potential to cause either dysphoria or disinhibition (with increased agitation) in some patients. 2) Benzodiazepines can produce dependency and in patients with comorbid substance use disorder can induce a relapse of another substance use disorder (120, 121). Patients with comorbid substance-related disorders who are taking benzodiazepines must be monitored particularly closely.

6. Antidepressants

Although antidepressant medications have been extensively studied in patients with unipolar depression (122) and in mixed groups of patients with unipolar and bipolar disorder, there are few sources of controlled data on their use in the depressive phase of bipolar disorder. In addition, all of these studies have methodologic limitations (41).

Zornberg and Pope reviewed seven controlled studies that examined the efficacy of tricyclic antidepressants in the treatment of bipolar depression (41). In general, the data indicate that tricyclic antidepressants are more effective than placebo for patients with bipolar depression. Their efficacy relative to lithium and other antidepressants is less certain. In addition, their utility when combined with lithium, or an alternative mood stabilizer, has not been systematically studied (although this is the manner in which they are frequently used).

Two controlled studies have tested monoamine oxidase inhibitors (MAOIs) in patients with bipolar depression. One study found moclobemide (a reversible MAOI) to be equivalent to imipramine among a heterogeneous group of depressed patients, including 33 bipolar patients (123). The other study showed that tranylcypromine was significantly superior to imipramine (without concomitant lithium) in the treatment of the anergic subtype of bipolar depression in patients with bipolar I and bipolar II disorder (124). It is unclear to what extent these findings would apply to bipolar patients without atypical features.

Selective serotonin reuptake inhibitors have not been well studied in the treatment of acute bipolar depression. One controlled study found that fluoxetine was superior to imipramine and placebo in the treatment of acute bipolar depression (125); some of the patients were receiving lithium and some were not (41). Conclusions about the efficacy and risks associated with these medications must await further systematic studies.

Case reports and two clinical trials suggest that bupropion is effective in the prevention and treatment of episodes of bipolar disorder, especially depressive episodes (126-130). Some investigators report that bupropion is less likely than other antidepressants to induce mania and hypomania, but the evidence supporting this is weak.

Virtually every available antidepressant agent has been associated with the emergence of mania in bipolar patients (41, 131, 132). The study of this issue is complicated, however, by the fact that patients with depression have a baseline risk of switching to mania. This risk has been difficult to characterize because of variations in patient groups and treatment regimens across studies. Of further concern is the fact that some investigators have reported an association between the use of antidepressants and the development of rapid cycling (133) and mixed affective states (134). It has therefore been hypothesized that antidepressants may worsen the overall course of bipolar disorder (133). Unfortunately, the phenomenon of antidepressants inducing the switch to mania, hypomania, rapid cycling, or mixed affective states has not been systematically evaluated in most studies of antidepressants and bipolar depression. It is therefore unknown whether different antidepressants are more or less likely to induce the switch process, although recent preliminary data suggest that bupropion may be less likely than tricyclic antidepressants to induce a switch (126).

In general, psychiatrists should be cautious in prescribing antidepressants for patients with bipolar disorder. However, as some bipolar patients continue to develop depression despite optimal use of mood stabilizers, antidepressants are often necessary for acute and/ or prophylactic treatment. Patients who require antidepressant treatment should receive the lowest effective dose for the shortest time necessary.

7. Novel and adjunctive pharmacologic treatments

A number of alternative treatments have been reported to be useful in the treatment of various phases of bipolar disorder (93, 135). These include calcium channel blockers, thyroid hormones, clozapine, psychostimulants, light therapy, and sleep manipulation. Some manic patients may respond to calcium channel blockers (136–146), although preliminary data suggest that these may be the same patients who respond to lithium, making these agents less useful in treatment-refractory patients.

Thyroid hormones thyroxine (T_4) and triiodothyronine (T_3), sometimes in "hyperthyroxinemic" (i.e., higher than physiologic) doses and regardless of baseline thyroid status, may have mood-stabilizing effects in patients with rapid-cycling bipolar disorder, usually when used adjunctively with other mood-stabilizing agents, such as lithium, carbamazepine, or valproate (50, 147, 148). Some investigative groups have recommended high initial doses of T_4 (150–400 µg/day), with an increase in dose to an end point of 50% above normal in the free thyroxine index (50, 147). The possibility of adverse cardiac effects, weight loss, depletion of bone mass, and anxiety must be considered (149–151); however, studies have not confirmed concerns about osteoporosis (152, and unpublished 1994 study of Gyulai et al.).

Retrospective and prospective open studies also suggest that the atypical antipsychotic agent clozapine may have mood-stabilizing as well as antipsychotic effects in bipolar patients with psychotic features, including those with rapid cycling and mixed episodes (62, 153, and unpublished 1992 study of Calabrese et al.). Although systematic studies in patients with bipolar disorder are lacking, clozapine appears to have a unique mechanism of action and side-effect profile compared with other neuroleptics. In particular, it does not appear to be associated with akathisia or acute extrapyramidal side effects or, more importantly, tardive dyskinesia. However, clozapine does cause serious side effects, such as seizures and potentially fatal leukopenia.

Psychostimulants, often in conjunction with an antidepressant medication, may be helpful in treatment-resistant depression, although the combination of psychostimulants and an MAOI may pose serious risks that require careful monitoring (122). Their use for the treatment of bipolar depression should be attempted very cautiously because they may precipitate mania.

Other drugs evaluated in the treatment of acute mania, including cholinergic drugs, β-blockers, serotonergic agents (such as fenfluramine, methysergide, and L-tryptophan), and the α-2 adrenergic agonist clonidine, have generally produced unpromising results.

Nonpharmacologic somatic treatments other than ECT, such as sleep deprivation and light therapy, have not yet been rigorously studied in patients with bipolar disorder. However, as noted in the Practice Guideline for Major Depressive Disorder in Adults (122), light therapy is effective for some patients with seasonal patterns of depressive episodes and may be useful in promoting regular sleep/wake cycles (154). The specific role of light therapy for patients with bipolar disorder, and its potential to induce mania, needs further clarification. Sleep deprivation may be useful for bipolar depression, although it may induce mania.

C.   Electroconvulsive Therapy

ECT is efficacious in the treatment of both phases of bipolar disorder. Since the treatment data are specific to the phase of the disorder, they will be discussed separately.

1.   Acute mania

ECT has been demonstrated to be rapidly effective as a treatment for acute mania (155). In a review of the studies in which ECT was used to treat acute manic episodes, 470 of 589 patients (80%) showed marked clinical improvement (155). Retrospective analyses of the efficacy and safety of ECT and lithium (with or without antipsychotic drugs) have found both to be roughly equivalent in efficacy (156–158). In controlled prospective studies, ECT was found to be equal to or more effective than pharmacotherapy (159–161).

Many manic patients will experience a relatively rapid response to ECT. For example, in one study with very strict clinical standards, complete remission occurred after six treatments (161). Recommended frequency is three treatments per week; no differences in response rate were found with more frequent treatments (161). The efficacy of frequent and/or prolonged ECT has not been supported by retrospective (156–158, 162) or prospective (160, 161) studies.

ECT is typically not considered a first-line treatment for manic episodes, given that a majority of patients will exhibit an acute response to a mood-stabilizing medication, which may then be continued for maintenance treatment. Consequently, the majority of manic patients treated with ECT are likely to be resistant to conventional antimanic pharmacological agents. One prospective study examined the efficacy of ECT in such medication-resistant patients and found that 13 of 24 (54%) responded to ECT (161). The role of ECT for patients who fail to respond to other mood stabilizers has not been systematically examined.

The rare syndrome of manic delirium that may be associated with severe hyperthermia represents a primary indication for the use of ECT, as ECT is rapidly effective and has a high margin of safety (163–166). ECT should also be considered as a first-line treatment in the presence of pregnancy, neuroleptic malignant syndrome, catatonia, and general medical conditions that preclude the use of standard pharmacological treatments.

2. Acute bipolar depression

ECT is generally considered the most effective antidepressant treatment available, although no study has focused exclusively on the use of ECT in bipolar depression (167–169).

The efficacy of ECT in the treatment of mixed groups of patients with unipolar and bipolar depression has been established in a series of double-blind studies comparing ECT with the administration of anesthesia alone and with antidepressant medications and in studies comparing different forms of ECT administration (170). Patients with psychotic depression may be particularly responsive to ECT. Several investigators have compared rates of response to ECT in patients with bipolar and unipolar depression (157, 171–173). In general, the unipolar/bipolar distinction does not have predictive value with regard to short-term ECT outcome. Consequently, ECT is considered an extremely effective treatment for the depressed phase of bipolar disorder. There is limited information on the efficacy of ECT in bipolar patients with established medication resistance. Recent studies suggest that approximately 50% of bipolar patients with acute depression who have failed at least one adequate trial of antidepressant medication show marked clinical improvement when treated with bilateral ECT (174).

ECT should be considered as a primary treatment in bipolar depression whenever a rapid response is necessary or when pharmacologic interventions are contraindicated (e.g., in pregnancy).

3. Implementing ECT treatment

ECT, like antidepressant medications, may provoke hypomania or mania. This phenomenon is relatively rare during the ECT course (175), and its management is uncertain. Some practitioners continue with ECT, while others discontinue ECT and start lithium treatment (169).

Patients receiving lithium during ECT may be at a higher risk for delirium and status epilepticus (176–182). However, adverse reactions to the combination of ECT and lithium are rare, and delirium associated with the combined treatment rapidly improves once lithium is discontinued. Benzodiazepines raise seizure threshold and reduce the duration of seizures and thus may impair the efficacy of ECT (177, 178, 183, 184). Antipsychotic drugs may be continued during the course of ECT for psychotic or highly agitated patients, but are generally discontinued after such symptoms remit. Like benzodiazepines, anticonvulsants may interfere with the production or duration of seizures and preferably should be discontinued. However, patients maintained on anticonvulsants to treat a concurrent seizure disorder may be safely treated with ECT, often with excellent clinical results.

ECT is extremely safe when administered using modern methods, which include current anesthesia practice, alterations in the delivery of the electrical stimulus, the selected use of unilateral treatment, and advanced cardiopulmonary monitoring. At this time no absolute contraindications to ECT are known. The reader is referred to the 1990 report of the APA Task Force on Electroconvulsive Therapy as the best available summary of indications, complications, side effects, and general implementation of ECT (169).

D.   Psychotherapeutic Treatments

Psychiatric management and pharmacologic therapy are essential components of treatment for acute episodes and for prevention of future episodes in patients with bipolar disorder. In addition, other specific psychotherapeutic treatments may be critical components of the treatment plan for some patients. Patients with bipolar disorder suffer from the psychosocial consequences of past episodes, the ongoing vulnerability to future episodes, and the burdens of adhering to a long-term treatment plan that may involve some unpleasant side effects. In addition, many patients have clinically significant mood instability between episodes. The goals of psychotherapeutic treatments (including psychiatric management) are to reduce distress and improve the patient's functioning between episodes and to decrease the frequency of future episodes (185). Most patients with bipolar disorder will struggle with some of the following issues: 1) emotional consequences of periods of major mood disorder and diagnosis of a chronic mental illness; 2) developmental deviations and delays caused by past episodes; 3) problems associated with stigmatization; 4) problems regulating self-esteem; 5) fears of recurrence and consequent inhibition of normal psychosocial functioning; 6) interpersonal difficulties; 7) marriage, family, childbearing, and parenting issues; 8) academic and occupational problems; and 9) other legal, social, and emotional problems that arise from reckless, violent, withdrawn, or bizarre behavior that may occur during episodes. For some patients, a specific psychotherapy (in addition to psychiatric management) will be needed to address these issues, although the form, intensity, and focus of psychotherapeutic treatment are likely to vary over time for each patient.

In addition to psychiatric management (see section II.A.), there are a range of specific psychotherapeutic interventions that may be helpful for some patients. In general, judgments regarding the efficacy of these treatments are based on strong clinical consensus regarding their beneficial effects for selected patients, rather than on formal controlled trials. The individual treatment approaches include psychodynamic, interpersonal, behavioral, and cognitive. In addition, couples therapy, family therapy, and group therapy may be indicated for some patients. Formal studies are currently being conducted for many of these treatments in patients with bipolar disorder.

The available psychotherapeutic treatments are discussed as separate entities, even though in practice psychiatrists commonly use a combination or synthesis of different approaches depending on the patient's needs and preferences.

1. Specific psychosocial interventions

Research on the application of specific psychosocial interventions for patients with bipolar disorder is sparse. The research summarized here involves formal psychotherapies that have as their goals many of the features of psychiatric management.

Inpatient family intervention (186) has been applied both in schizophrenia and bipolar disorder. Family treatment is brief (approximately six sessions) and includes a psychoeducational component. Goals include accepting the reality of the illness, identifying precipitating stresses and likely future stresses inside and outside the family, elucidating family interactions that produce stress on the patient, planning strategies for managing and/or minimizing future stresses, and bringing about the patient's family's acceptance of the need for continued treatment after hospital discharge. Systematic study of this approach in patients with bipolar disorder is limited, although there is some evidence that it is helpful for some patients (187).

Behavioral family management is a treatment for patients who have recently been hospitalized for an episode of mania. Behavioral family management is based on a home-centered psychosocial treatment for schizophrenia developed by Falloon (188). The treatment includes psychoeducation, communication skills training, and problem-solving skills training. A behavioral family treatment intervention has also been outlined (189). Although definitive trials of behavioral family treatment have not been completed, preliminary evidence suggests that behavioral family management/ behavioral family treatment in concert with adequate pharmacotherapy leads to a substantial decrease in relapse rates.

A pilot study of the impact of family therapy and psychoeducation (in addition to pharmacologic and milieu treatment) on patients with bipolar disorder has been reported (190). Patients who were randomly assigned to the family therapy group had lower rates of family separations, greater improvements in level of family functioning, higher rates of full recovery, and lower rates of rehospitalization for 2 years following family treatment.

A cognitive behavioral treatment package for patients with bipolar disorder has been developed by Basco and Rush (191). The goals of the program are to educate the patient regarding bipolar disorder and its treatment, teach cognitive behavioral skills for coping with psychosocial stressors and attendant problems, facilitate compliance with treatment, and monitor the occurrence and severity of symptoms.

The observation that many bipolar patients experience less mood lability when they maintain a regular pattern of daily activities (including sleeping, eating, physical activity, and emotional stimulation) has led to the development of a formalized psychotherapy called interpersonal and social rhythm therapy (192). This form of psychotherapy is currently being tested in combination with pharmacotherapy in a randomized clinical trial during the maintenance phase of bipolar disorder.

2. Specific psychotherapies for depressive episodes

There are a range of psychotherapeutic interventions that may be useful for patients with major depressive episodes. Some of these interventions have been studied in patients with bipolar depression as well as in those with unipolar depression. Others have only been studied in patients with unipolar depression. We did not identify any completed controlled studies of psychotherapeutic treatments in patients with bipolar (and not unipolar) depression, although some studies are underway. It is not clear to what extent patients with bipolar and unipolar depression are similar in their responsiveness to psychotherapy. However, it seems likely that the following treatments may benefit some patients with bipolar depressive disorders, especially when the depressive episodes seem to be precipitated or exacerbated by psychosocial issues or are the cause of significant psychosocial morbidity. This discussion is summarized from the APA Practice Guideline for Major Depressive Disorder in Adults (122).

Psychodynamic psychotherapy and psychoanalytic treatments are based on observed beneficial effects of clarifying intrapsychic processes that may precipitate and/or perpetuate affective dysregulation in vulnerable patients. Once these forces are made conscious, difficulties can be anticipated and mastered or conflicts neutralized through the process of insight. Mastery and insight, experienced in the supportive or interpretive relationship with the therapist, permit the patient not only to overcome ongoing negative or disorganizing effects of illness but to ward off recurrent dysregulation. In vulnerable individuals who are excessively sensitive to loss and who use reaction formation and aggression turned inward as defense mechanisms to control the aggressive impulse, the detection and alteration of these psychodynamic mechanisms are of central importance in the treatment of depression (193). The supportive psychodynamic approach seeks to alleviate ongoing symptoms and help the patient adapt to life circumstances.

Interpersonal therapy seeks to recognize and explore depressive precipitants that involve interpersonal losses, role disputes and transitions, social isolation, or deficits in social skills (194). There is some evidence in controlled studies that interpersonal therapy without pharmacotherapy is effective in reducing depressive symptoms in the acute phase of less severe unipolar depressive episodes (195, 196) and that it is especially effective in ameliorating occupational and social aspects of the patient's dysfunction (197). There is evidence that monthly interpersonal therapy also has a prophylactic effect during the maintenance phase of unipolar depression (198). The role of interpersonal therapy in the maintenance phase of bipolar disorder is not known.

Behavior therapy of depression is based on a functional analysis of behavior theory (199) and/or social learning theory (200). The techniques involve activity scheduling (201, 202), self-control therapy (203), social skills training (204), and problem solving (205). Behavior therapy has been reported to be effective in the acute treatment of patients with mild to moderately severe unipolar depression, especially when combined with pharmacotherapy (206–209). Studies of the prophylactic value of behavior therapy in the acute phase of depression, once therapy is discontinued, have been inconclusive (210, 211). The utility of behavior therapy in continuation- and maintenance-phase treatment of patients with bipolar depression has not been subjected to controlled studies.

Cognitive therapy maintains that irrational beliefs and distorted attitudes toward the self, the environment, and the future perpetuate depressive affects and that these beliefs may be reversed through cognitive behavior therapy (212). There is some evidence that cognitive therapy reduces depressive symptoms during the acute phase of less severe, non-melancholic forms of unipolar depression (196, 213). Studies of the prophylactic effect of acute-phase cognitive behavior therapy in unipolar patients, once therapy is discontinued, have had mixed results. No randomized, controlled studies are available on the role of cognitive therapy for bipolar patients in either the acute or maintenance phase of treatment (211, 214–217).

The effects of protracted depression can lead to severe strains in marital and family relationships. Comprehensive treatment includes an assessment of and efforts to address these problems. Marital and family problems may be a consequence of depression, but may also increase vulnerability to depression and in some instances retard recovery (218, 219). Techniques for using marital and family approaches for the treatment of depression include behavioral approaches (218), a psychoeducational approach, and a "strategic marital therapy" approach (220). In addition, family therapy in the inpatient treatment of depressed patients has been studied (221). Research suggests that marital and family therapy may reduce depressive symptoms and the risk of relapse in patients with unipolar depression who have marital and family problems (217, 222). The role of these treatments for patients with bipolar disorder has not been formally studied.

The role of group therapy in the treatment of patients with depression is based on clinical experience, rather than on systematic controlled studies. Group therapy may be particularly useful in the treatment of depression in the context of bereavement or such common stressors as chronic illness. Individuals in such circumstances may benefit from the example of others who have successfully dealt with the same or similar challenges. The role of group therapy in patients with bipolar depression has not been formally studied.

3. Specific psychotherapies for manic episodes

Management of severe manic episodes poses one of the greatest challenges in psychiatry. While it is generally not beneficial to implement a specific psychotherapy during a manic episode, there are important psychosocial and environmental approaches that may be applied. A plan that sets and enforces clear limits in a firm and unprovocative manner is generally recommended, but may be difficult to implement. Isolation of the patient from other individuals may sometimes be required to protect both the patient and others. Clinical consensus seems to indicate that reducing external stimulation may help calm the manic patient. Thus, a quiet room with few distractions may be desirable. A regular schedule of meetings with the patient may be helpful.

4. Specific psychotherapies for associated comorbidity and complications

Patients in remission from bipolar disorder suffer from the psychosocial consequences of past episodes and ongoing vulnerability to future episodes. In addition, patients with this disorder remain vulnerable to other psychiatric disorders, including, most commonly, substance use disorders (223) and personality disorders (224, 225). Each of these comorbid disorders has particular consequences and increases the overall psychosocial vulnerability of the bipolar patient. Psychosocial treatments should address comorbidities and complications that are present.

Clinical experience and preliminary research suggest that group psychotherapy, in conjunction with appropriate medication, may help certain patients to address such issues as adherence to a treatment plan, adaptation to a chronic illness, regulation of self-esteem, and management of marital as well as other psychosocial issues (226–232).

5. Support groups

Many support groups provide useful information about bipolar disorder and its treatment. Patients in these groups often benefit from hearing the experiences of others who are struggling with such issues as denial versus acceptance of the need for medication, problems with side effects, and how to shoulder other burdens associated with the illness and its treatment. Advocacy groups such as the National Depressive and Manic-Depressive Association and the National Alliance for the Mentally Ill have many local chapters that provide both support and educational material to patients and their families.

E. Formulation and Implementation of a Treatment Plan

The psychiatrist should use the information presented in this guideline to arrive at treatment recommendations. Treatment decisions will of course depend on cross-sectional and longitudinal features of the patient's illness. Considerations involved in these decisions are discussed in this section.

1. Choosing the site of treatment

One of the first decisions the psychiatrist must make is the overall level of care that the patient requires. Such a decision will, in part, be determined by the particular options of hospital, partial hospital, and outpatient services that are available in a given community. Many of the factors that underlie the choice of treatment setting discussed here are broadly applicable.

Acute episodes of bipolar disorder are frequently of such severity that patients will require treatment in either a full or partial hospital setting. The decision about the appropriate site of treatment should be based on the same considerations that guide the care of all patients with a severe mental disorder. In general, the least restrictive setting that is likely to allow for safe and effective treatment should be chosen.

Abnormal mood states (either manic or depressed) are characteristically accompanied by impaired judgment, and a substantial number of patients with a full mood episode will have psychotic symptoms (1). Patients may engage in risky behaviors that are explicitly designed to cause harm (e.g., suicidal or homicidal behavior) or have unanticipated consequences that are nonetheless harmful (e.g., promiscuous sexual activity, substance abuse, reckless driving). Some patients with a major mood disorder may not be judged to be at imminent risk, but nevertheless may require inpatient or partial hospital treatment to facilitate adequate treatment.

Unfortunately, the impaired judgment associated with acute episodes may interfere with the patient's ability to make reasonable treatment decisions. As a result, considerable effort should be put into working with patients and their families to help them appreciate the clinical situation and the reasons for the treatment recommendations. Anticipation of such situations during periods of mood stability, and the development of a treatment plan in case of a major mood episode, is frequently helpful. A long-term relationship between the psychiatrist and the patient (and family) can facilitate these discussions. Despite all efforts, however, some patients with acute episodes of bipolar disorder will need to be hospitalized involuntarily in order to receive necessary treatment. Guidelines for instituting such action are determined by specific state laws regarding involuntary commitment. Some patients during manic episodes seem to be capable of presenting different clinical pictures to different parties (e.g., judges, family members, treating psychiatrist), which may lead to profound disagreements among those involved over the best course of action. One of the psychiatrist's tasks in such a case is to educate the other concerned parties about the nature of mania and the risks to the patient despite the patient's apparent ability to appear relatively healthy at times.

a. The patient lacking the capacity to cooperate with treatment. Patients who, along with any available social supports, are unable to care for themselves adequately, cooperate with outpatient treatment of their mood disorder, or provide reliable feedback to their psychiatrist regarding their clinical status are candidates for full or partial hospitalization, even in the absence of a tendency toward intentional self-harm.

b. The patient at risk for suicide or homicide. Patients with suicidal or homicidal ideation, intention, or plan require close monitoring. Patients at particularly high risk may benefit from hospitalization, during which close observation, restricted access to violent means, and more intensive treatment are possible. Some patients with bipolar disorder are prone to rapid mood fluctuations, especially in the context of substance use, making the assessment of suicide risk particularly difficult and highlighting the need to attempt to understand, for each individual patient, the potential precipitants to suicidal thoughts and actions.

c. The patient lacking psychosocial supports. Recovery from acute bipolar episodes is aided by an environment that encourages safety, constructive activity, positive interpersonal interactions, and compliance with treatment. If the home environment lacks these features or exposes the patient to undesirable or dangerous activities, such as alcohol or drug abuse, admission to a hospital or an intensive day program may be necessary.

d. Other factors influencing the need for hospitalization. Hospitalization may be necessary for patients with complicating psychiatric or general medical conditions that make outpatient treatment unsafe. Detoxification or withdrawal from psychoactive substances may necessitate hospitalization. Patients with bipolar disorder, especially those with psychotic symptoms, may engage in bizarre or imprudent behavior that may endanger their important relationships, reputation, or assets; hospitalization may be necessary to protect the patient and others. The presence of severe psychotic features, catatonia, severe depression, or severe mixed states and the risk of ultrarapid cycling are often factors to be considered. Patients who have not responded to outpatient treatment may need to be hospitalized in order to receive the type or intensity of treatment deemed necessary. Hospitalization may also be necessary for patients who cannot receive the type or intensity of outpatient treatment required because of the local community lacks appropriate resources.

2.   Development of a treatment plan

Before starting treatment with a patient with bipolar disorder, a comprehensive general medical and psychiatric evaluation should be conducted. Examination of an acutely ill patient is sometimes impossible, in which case the psychiatrist must rely on his or her best judgment about the patient's safety. The psychiatrist should consider potential general medical and substance-induced causes of manic or depressive symptoms, especially when dealing with a patient's first episode. Laboratory and other diagnostic studies should be guided by the psychiatrist's evaluation of the patient's condition and by the choice of treatment, as outlined in section II.B. Attention should be given to the patient's psychosocial stressors, social supports, and general living situation.

Bipolar disorder is a chronic condition that has potentially devastating effects on many aspects of the patient's life and that carries with it a high risk of suicide. Care of the patient involves multiple efforts to reduce the frequency and severity of episodes and to reduce the overall morbidity and mortality of the disorder.

3.   Psychiatric management

Patients with bipolar disorder need different types and intensities of care at different times. The psychiatrist should have a relationship with the patient (and family, if appropriate) that allows him or her to monitor the patient's status and adjust the treatment recommendations accordingly. Psychiatric management (see section II.A.) is the foundation for all of the treatments for bipolar disorder. The specific nature and focus of psychiatric management will change as the patient's psychiatric status fluctuates and ability to respond adaptively to the demands of the illness expands.

4.   Choice of a mood-stabilizing medication and/or ECT

Lithium, valproate, carbamazepine, and ECT are all used as primary agents in the treatment of patients with bipolar disorder. ECT is generally reserved for those patients who are unable to safely wait until a medication becomes effective, who are unable to safely tolerate one of the effective medications, who have been unresponsive to the available medications, or who prefer ECT.

Although the pharmacologic treatment of patients with bipolar disorder varies with the phase of the illness, almost all patients will require the use of a mood stabilizer for individual episodes, and many will require a mood stabilizer for maintenance treatment as well. Therefore, one of the first decisions a psychiatrist must make is which mood stabilizer to use to initiate treatment (even though many patients will require additional pharmacologic treatments as well).

The choice of medication depends on an individualized assessment of the risks and benefits of, and preferences for, each of the three mood stabilizers. This decision may be informed by prior response to a given medication. In addition, the potential need for maintenance treatment is frequently relevant to the decision.

a. Benefits.   Four placebo-controlled trials of lithium have all demonstrated its efficacy in patients with acute mania (34–38). On the whole, about 50% to 80% of patients are expected to have some response to lithium, although the percentage varies with the study and the definition of "response." Fewer studies have been conducted using valproate, but in one recent double-blind trial in acute mania valproate was shown to be significantly more effective than placebo, with 48% of the patients having at least a 50% reduction in mania rating scale scores at 3 weeks (39). This study showed valproate and lithium to be similarly efficacious; other studies specifically designed to address the comparative efficacy of these two medications are needed. The effect of carbamazepine in acute mania is more difficult to evaluate because of the methodologic limitations of available studies. The available data, however, are supportive of the efficacy of carbamazepine in mania, though its efficacy relative to lithium and valproate is not known.

Studies of bipolar depression are generally difficult to interpret because of methodologic flaws involving the inclusion of patients with different diagnoses (i.e., bipolar I, bipolar II, unipolar depression), the use of concomitant medication, and other design problems. The data are strongest for lithium, which has been shown to be effective for depressed patients with bipolar I disorder. In addition, all three mood stabilizers have been used successfully in conjunction with antidepressants for these patients.

Only lithium has been proven to decrease the frequency and severity of episodes during maintenance treatment. Both valproate and carbamazepine have demonstrated prophylactic effect as well, although the evidence base is smaller than that for lithium and the available studies have significant methodologic flaws.

b. Risks.   All three mood stabilizers are associated with potentially unpleasant dose-related side effects, most of which can be better tolerated over time or ameliorated by alterations in preparation, dose, or schedule. All of the mood stabilizers can interact with other medications, and care should be taken to avoid certain drug combinations or adjust doses accordingly.

Lithium has been extensively studied in the short- and long-term treatment of bipolar disorder. Lithium induces dose-related side effects that can be effectively controlled by dosage adjustment. However, its relatively narrow therapeutic window means that for some patients lower rates of side effects will be traded off against slightly lower efficacy. Some patients may have toxic reactions to lithium after substantial shifts in total body fluid levels brought on by general medical illness, changes in medications, or alcohol binges; unreliable patients may attain toxic lithium levels after unauthorized dosage increases (e.g., "as needed" use of extra lithium for "nerves"). In addition, lithium is dangerous in overdose. Potentially serious side effects at therapeutic doses are rare, but include the induction of serious dermatologic conditions (that resolve with cessation of medication) and the possibility of long-term renal effects (manifested by rising creatinine levels) after 10 or more years of treatment.

During short-term treatment with valproate, dose-related side effects may occur, most of which are relieved over time or by dosage adjustment. Valproate can cause potentially life-threatening effects on bone marrow, liver, and pancreas. These rare reactions cannot be reliably predicted by routine laboratory monitoring. It is essential that patients taking valproate be made aware of the early symptoms of these conditions and instructed to report their occurrence promptly. The therapeutic window for valproate is wider than that for lithium, making the occurrence of unintentional toxic levels less likely.

Carbamazepine produces dose-related side effects, many of which can be relieved over time or by alterations in dosage. Potentially life-threatening reactions that are not dose related include blood dyscrasias, hepatic failure, exfoliative dermatitis, and pancreatitis. These rare reactions cannot be reliably predicted by routine laboratory monitoring. It is essential that patients taking carbamazepine be made aware of the early symptoms of these conditions and instructed to report their occurrence promptly.

c. Patient preferences.   In choosing a medication, informed patients should consider many factors in addition to evidence about efficacy, including the specific side-effect profile (which may be informed by prior use of a particular medication), other burdens of taking the medication, and costs. These considerations may be particularly important in the choice of a maintenance medication.

For the three mood stabilizers, these considerations may be summarized as follows. Lithium requires more frequent blood monitoring, but if recommendations are followed, does not carry a significant risk of life-threatening reactions. The specific side effects of valproate and carbamazepine may be preferable to some patients, but both carry a very small, though not negligible, risk of life-threatening reactions. The costs of the three medications may vary, depending, in part, on the availability of generic preparations. In most situations, lithium will likely be the least expensive agent.

5.   Manic episodes

In addition to intensified psychiatric management, the primary treatment of a manic episode involves the use of a mood-stabilizing medication or ECT. The choice of ECT is governed by the same factors discussed earlier (i.e., safety, efficacy, and patient preference). ECT would be appropriate in those situations in which a rapid response is necessary, medications are contraindicated or have not been effective in the past, or the patient is known to prefer ECT as a first-line treatment. If the patient refuses blood testing, treatment with a mood stabilizer may be initiated and laboratory tests obtained once the patient has begun to respond and is more cooperative. The choice of a medication should be determined by the factors discussed earlier. If a new medication is to be started or if the patient is already on a mood stabilizer, the first step is to ensure adequate serum levels, as defined previously. It must be kept in mind, however, that within the documented therapeutic ranges for each of these medications, there is likely to be a dose-response curve for each patient. Therefore, within the target range, the precise choice of serum level will need to be guided by the patient's beneficial and adverse responses to the medication. Simultaneously, the patient's general medical condition, including thyroid status, should be checked and any abnormalities treated. Any antidepressant medications should be discontinued unless the addition of a mood stabilizer brings prompt cessation of the manic symptoms and the patient is thought to require continued use of the antidepressant to control depressive symptoms (e.g., the patient has a prior history of positive response to antidepressants).

Since mood stabilizers may take up to 2 to 3 weeks to become fully effective, many patients will require adjunctive medication in the interim to control agitated, psychotic, or otherwise dangerous behavior. Both benzodiazepines and neuroleptics have been shown to be helpful and often necessary for extremely agitated or psychotic patients. Benzodiazepines are safer; however, neuroleptics have been more widely used and studied. Some patients will not be able to safely tolerate the side effects of the mood stabilizer, in which case the initial medication should be replaced by one of the other available agents.

If after 2 to 3 weeks on a mood stabilizer at therapeutic levels the patient has not substantially improved, a second mood stabilizer or ECT may be added to the treatment regimen. These interventions may need to be instituted earlier in patients with severe forms of mania. It is usually considered preferable to add another mood stabilizer rather than substitute a second agent for the first to avoid the possibility of exacerbating the patient's condition as a result of the cessation of the first medication.

If the decision is made to use carbamazepine and valproate simultaneously, the dose of carbamazepine may need to be decreased and the dose of valproate increased because of their pharmacokinetic interactions. In addition, there is some concern about increased neurotoxicity from this combination, so careful monitoring is essential.

Patients with manic episodes may require the use of adjunctive agents (e.g., benzodiazepines, neuroleptics) beyond the initial phase of treatment and/or other medications to treat side effects from the mood stabilizer(s) or to treat comorbid conditions.

6. Depressive episodes

The treatment options for bipolar patients with depressive episodes include psychiatric management, mood-stabilizing medication, specific psychotherapy, antidepressant medication, and ECT.

Psychiatric management may need to be intensified to allow for: assessment of the patient's condition, with particular attention to the use of (or adequate dosage of) mood-stabilizing medication; the possible role of psychosocial factors (e.g., the loss of an important relationship) or general medical factors (e.g., abnormal thyroid functioning) that may be contributing to the depression and initiation of any specific intervention designed to address these factors; assessment and monitoring of the patient's psychiatric status, with particular vigilance for suicidality, changes in severity of depression, or signs of a switch to mania; and efforts to reduce the psychosocial morbidity associated with the depressive episode.

For patients who are already taking an adequate dose of a mood stabilizer when they become depressed, the continued use of the mood stabilizer and intensified psychiatric management may be combined with one or more of the following interventions: 1) a specific psychotherapy, 2) an antidepressant medication, and 3) ECT (although this may require temporary discontinuation of the mood stabilizer).

For patients who are not taking a mood stabilizer when they become depressed (or are not taking an adequate dosage), a mood-stabilizing medication should be initiated (or an adequate dosage achieved). Data show lithium to be the most efficacious mood stabilizer for depression in bipolar patients, so this agent would most often be the logical initial choice. Since clinical experience suggests that the antidepressant efficacy of lithium may not be evident for 4 to 6 weeks after adequate serum levels have been achieved (with the full effect taking somewhat longer), other treatments noted above should also be considered.

The decision to initiate a specific psychotherapy, and the particular choice of psychotherapy, depends on the factors discussed earlier, including knowledge of the patient's response to treatment of earlier episodes, as well as an assessment of the factors that may play a role in the precipitation, exacerbation, perpetuation, or psychosocial consequences of the episode. Further considerations are discussed in the Practice Guideline for Major Depressive Disorder in Adults (122).

Decisions regarding the use of antidepressant medication require an assessment of the benefits (e.g., the likelihood of relatively rapid relief of symptoms) and burdens (e.g., potential side effects of the medication, increased risk of developing a manic episode). The decision will therefore depend on the patient's specific clinical features (e.g., severity of depression, previous course of depressive episodes) and preferences (e.g., concerns about side effects, availability of supports in the event of a manic episode).

For some patients with mild depression or a history of self-limited depressive episodes that are not unduly disruptive, the combination of psychiatric management, with or without a specific psychotherapy, and use of a mood stabilizer may be sufficient.

The addition of an antidepressant medication to the mood-stabilizing regimen is likely to be beneficial for the following groups of patients: patients who cannot safely tolerate or are unwilling to tolerate a 4- to 6-week delay before response to the initiation (or dosage adjustment) of a mood-stabilizing medication; patients who have a history of beneficial response to previous treatment with an antidepressant medication; or patients who have not responded to the combination of psychiatric management, a mood stabilizer, and, if indicated, a specific psychotherapy.

All antidepressant medications that have been shown to be effective for patients with major depressive disorder are also probably effective for patients in the depressed phase of bipolar disorder. However, these medications are likely to increase the bipolar patient's baseline risk of developing a manic episode. The simultaneous use of a mood-stabilizing medication is recommended to decrease this risk. Patients who take antidepressant medications should be informed of the risks of developing a manic episode and should be educated about the early warning signs of such a switch. A plan should be made for immediate intervention should a switch to mania occur; it is frequently helpful to involve the patient's family in such a plan. Patients who refuse treatment with a mood stabilizer and prefer treatment with an antidepressant alone may be at particular risk of switching to mania and should be so informed.

Available data indicate that the choice of antidepressant agents for bipolar patients is governed by the same factors that guide the choice in unipolar patients. Thus, the prior response of the patient, the side effect profile, the presence of atypical features (which would favor the use of an MAOI or a selective serotonin reuptake inhibitor), and patient preference are relevant to the decision. As in all depressed patients, the presence of suicidality should be continually assessed. Suicidal patients may be most safely treated with agents that are less toxic in overdose (e.g., selective serotonin reuptake inhibitors).

ECT is another alternative for depressed patients. The use of ECT is governed by the same factors discussed previously, including the need for a rapid response, the presence of contraindications to the use of medication, the history of nonresponse to medication, or patient preference.

Treatment decisions for psychotically depressed patients are similar to those for all severely depressed patients. Although some patients with psychotic depression may respond to the combination of a mood stabilizer and an antidepressant, others will require the additional use of a neuroleptic. ECT is also an appropriate first-line treatment for these patients.

Patients with a major depressive episode may at times require other adjunctive agents, which are discussed in the Practice Guideline for Major Depressive Disorder in Adults (122).

7. Mixed episodes and ultrarapid cycling

The treatment principles for patients with mixed episodes are the same as those for patients with pure mania. Antidepressants may exacerbate mixed states and should be avoided, if possible. Preliminary data from one controlled study suggests that valproate may be more effective than lithium for patients with mixed episodes (C Bowden, personal communication); however, this finding needs to be tested in further studies.

Patients who experience rapid changes in mood state between depression and mania share many features with patients who have mixed states. A general medical evaluation should be conducted, with particular attention to thyroid status. If there are indications of decreased thyroid function, thyroxine or T_3 should be added and the measures of thyroid function brought into the upper range of normal distribution. Other general medical conditions, as well as comorbid alcohol or substance abuse, could be exacerbating the ongoing mood abnormality and should be treated. Some investigators believe that the use of antidepressants should be discontinued or avoided, if possible, and the subsequent course of illness reevaluated.

If these interventions are not sufficient to halt the ultrarapid cycling, treatment with a second mood stabilizer should be initiated and response over time (preferably after at least two cycles) carefully evaluated. If hypomanic and manic symptoms are relieved but depression persists, thyroid hormone or an antidepressant may be added. Occasionally, a third mood stabilizer may be necessary.

A small series of studies suggest the utility of very high doses of thyroid hormone, used concomitantly with mood-stabilizing agents, in the treatment of rapid-cycling patients (50, 147, 148). This is discussed in more detail in section II.B.7.

8.   Maintenance phase

Bipolar disorder is a recurrent and sometimes chronic disorder. Therefore, the psychiatrist should address maintenance and other long-term issues with the patient and the family as early in treatment as is feasible. The decision to implement maintenance pharmacotherapy should involve the participation of the psychiatrist, the patient, and, at times, family members. A decision to initiate maintenance treatment depends on 1) the probability of a recurrence with or without a mood-stabilizing agent, 2) the likely consequences of a recurrence, and 3) the benefits and burdens of taking a mood-stabilizing agent (233). Information about past episodes is essential in making these judgments.

Many psychiatrists recommend maintenance medication following a single manic episode, particularly if there are no contraindications to the use of a mood-stabilizing medication. Although this option should be made available to all patients after their first manic episode, clearly different patients may rationally make different decisions regarding the initiation and continuation of maintenance treatment depending on their individual circumstances and attitudes. Decisions regarding maintenance treatment should be reassessed whenever the patient's clinical status changes, or approximately annually in stable patients. It is likely that after two manic episodes, the benefits of prophylaxis would outweigh the burdens for most patients.

The choice of a maintenance medication should be guided by the factors discussed earlier. Data are strongest for the efficacy and safety of lithium in this phase. However, patients who are nonresponsive or acutely intolerant to lithium may benefit from an alternative mood stabilizer for maintenance. Additionally, some patients achieve better prophylaxis with a combination of mood stabilizers.

The choice of a target serum level should also be guided by the factors discussed previously. The narrow therapeutic window for lithium means that some patients will need to determine their preferred balance between side effects and efficacy. Other patients will be able to tolerate the higher range of therapeutic levels with easily remediable or only insignificant side effects. Many psychiatrists and their patients find that lithium levels between 0.6 and 0.8 meq/liter are optimal; others will prefer higher or lower doses.

During this phase, patients must deal with the psychological consequences of past episodes, the ongoing vulnerability to future episodes, and, for some patients, a significant degree of mood lability that falls short of a full mood episode. In addition to psychiatric management, some patients appear likely to benefit from a specific psychotherapeutic treatment. The range of available treatments and the factors guiding treatment choice and implementation are discussed in section II.D.

Even with optimal serum levels of a mood stabilizer and the appropriate use of psychotherapy, many patients will have occasional episodes of mania or depression. A critical role of psychiatric management is to help patients identify precipitants to, or early manifestations of, such episodes, so that treatment can be initiated promptly. Patients can benefit from anticipating and planning for such an event, so that critical treatment and other decisions can be made while the patient is still relatively euthymic.

The first step in treating early symptoms of a major mood episode is to ensure that the serum level of the mood stabilizer is adequate. In addition, the presence of a general medical condition (e.g., alteration in thyroid status or addition of a medication that may alter the bioavailability of the mood stabilizer) or a psychological factor (e.g., loss of a valued relationship) that could be contributing to the episode should be determined and addressed. Insomnia may be a precipitant or an early indicator of mania. Education about the importance of regular sleep habits and the occasional use of a benzodiazepine to promote regular sleep patterns are felt to be important for some patients in the prevention of full-blown manic episodes (234). Other subtle or early signs of mania can sometimes be managed with short-term use of a benzodiazepine or a neuroleptic.

Some patients will require additional treatments for a major mood episode, as described in sections II. A, B, C, and D.

9. Discontinuation of maintenance medication

Discontinuation of effective lithium prophylaxis is associated with an increased risk of early relapse. Such risk may be minimized by gradual, rather than rapid, discontinuation. In addition, there have been reports of patients who seem to develop a more severe and relatively nonresponsive form of the illness following discontinuation of effective prophylactic lithium. The risks associated with the discontinuation of maintenance valproate or carbamazepine are not clear.

The development of an episode during maintenance treatment does not necessarily imply treatment failure. Rather, the efficacy of a maintenance medication regimen should be assessed by comparing the actual course of the illness with the predicted course without medication. Although in practice such determinations may be difficult, it is important that an effective treatment not be abandoned in search of a regimen that will confer 100% protection against all future episodes. Severe or repeated breakthrough episodes should trigger a reassessment of the treatment plan. The use of life charts before and after the institution of maintenance treatment may be helpful. It is possible for patients to show a gradual decrease in responsiveness to a previously effective mood stabilizer. In this instance, switching to a medication with a novel mechanism of action, providing ECT, or discontinuing the new medication for a period of time followed by a renewed trial may be successful, at least temporarily, in reinitiating a treatment response.

F. Clinical Features Influencing Treatment

This section summarizes considerations pertaining to clinical features influencing treatment. The reader is referred to pertinent sections of the guideline that cover in greater detail subjects touched upon here.

1. Psychiatric factors

a. Psychotic or catatonic features.   Patients may experience delusions and/or hallucinations during episodes of mania or depression. These symptoms can be treated with mood stabilizers alone or with the addition of an antipsychotic agent. In addition, ECT may be used.

Occasionally, catatonic features may develop in patients during a manic episode. A careful assessment is indicated to rule out a general medical etiology and to clarify the psychiatric diagnosis. If the diagnosis of mania is confirmed, treatment should be directed accordingly. ECT has been successfully used for patients with catatonic features and is probably the treatment of choice (235). Neuroleptics and benzodiazepines have also been used.

b. Risk of suicide, homicide, and violence.   Among patients with psychiatric disorders, bipolar patients are among those at highest risk for suicide (236, 237). While patients with bipolar disorder have a mortality rate that is two to three times higher than that of the general population, the mortality rate of patients in long-term lithium treatment does not appear to differ significantly from that of the general population (238). Lithium maintenance treatment is associated with lowering the frequency of suicide attempts and completions (3).

Numerous risk factors for suicide among bipolar patients have been determined. In addition to general risk factors for suicide (e.g., previous suicide attempt, suicidal ideation, substance use in conjunction with another psychiatric disorder), patients with bipolar disorder have been shown to have other risk factors, including mood cycling within an episode and depressive turmoil, or rapid shifting from one mood state to another (e.g., from euphoria to anger to depression) (237). In these patients, absence of general risk factors should not be taken as reassurance that the patient is not at high risk for suicide (237). In general, a detailed evaluation of the individual patient is necessary to assess suicidal risk. Decisions must be made with the understanding that judgments of suicidality cannot be perfect, and it is prudent to err on the side of caution.

The potential for violence in patients with bipolar disorder is less well studied than is risk for suicide. Clinical experience attests to the presence of violent behavior in some of these patients, and violence may be an indication for hospitalization. In some instances, the threat is explicit through the patient's verbalizations and expressed intent. In other instances, the risk can only be inferred from the patient's agitation and dysphoric mood states combined with paranoid delusional thinking. When these features are associated with very rapid mood cycling, the risk of violence may be high.

c. Substance-related disorders. The rate of comorbidity between bipolar disorder and substance-related disorders is high. Substance abuse and its associated behaviors may lead psychiatrists and family members to fail to diagnose bipolar disorder. Conversely, the diagnosis of substance-related disorders may be overlooked in patients with bipolar disorder. In addition, substance abuse may worsen the course of bipolar disorder, perhaps by decreasing compliance with the treatment regimen (1).

Treatment for the substance use disorder and mood disorder should proceed concurrently, to the extent possible. The treatment of one disorder may have effects on the treatment of the other. For example, increased thirst secondary to lithium treatment may lead to increased alcohol consumption, and dehydration associated with alcohol abuse may increase serum lithium levels. Also, lithium may decrease the psychological effects of alcohol, thus stimulating greater alcohol consumption. As suicide risk often increases during alcohol detoxification, inpatient hospitalization may be required.

d. Other psychiatric comorbidities. Patients with comorbid personality disorders pose complicated diagnostic pictures. They are clearly at greater risk for experiencing intrapsychic and psychosocial stress that can precipitate or exacerbate major mood episodes. In addition, these patients may have particular difficulty adhering to long-term treatment regimens. The choice of a psychotherapeutic treatment should be guided by patient needs and preferences, but should include as an important focus the psychiatric management tasks required for adequate treatment of bipolar disorder.

The presence of a comorbid anxiety disorder may complicate the assessment of mood states in patients with bipolar disorder. The anxiety disorder should be assessed and treated concurrently with bipolar disorder.

The presence of attention deficit hyperactivity disorder, especially in children and adolescents, complicates the assessment of changes in mood states in patients with bipolar disorder. Early manifestations of mania and hypomania can be particularly difficult to distinguish from the ongoing symptoms of attention deficit hyperactivity disorder. Careful tracking of symptoms and behaviors is helpful. In addition, psychiatrists should consider the implications of pharmacologic treatments for attention deficit hyperactivity disorder on the course of the bipolar disorder (e.g., the use of tricyclic antidepressants or psychostimulants may exacerbate the course of bipolar illness).

The presence of comorbid conduct disorder in children and adolescents with bipolar disorder is likely to interfere with the development of a treatment alliance, decrease the likelihood of adherence to a long-term treatment regimen, increase the risk of substance use and other forms of risk-taking behavior, and increase the exposure of the patient to psychosocial stress, which could precipitate or exacerbate major mood episodes. Such patients may require intensive approaches to maximize potential treatment benefit and minimize risks from imprudent behavior.

2. Concurrent general medical conditions

The presence of a general medical condition may affect the treatment of a patient with bipolar disorder by exacerbating the course or severity of the disorder or by complicating treatment.

For example, the course of bipolar disorder may be exacerbated any condition that requires intermittent or regular use of steroids (e.g., asthma, inflammatory bowel disease) or that leads to abnormal thyroid functioning. Psychiatrists who treat HIV-infected patients often find that lower doses of mood stabilizers are indicated because of the patient's increased sensitivity to side effects.

The treatment of patients with bipolar disorder may be complicated by conditions that affect renal or hepatic function, which may restrict the choice or dosage of mood-stabilizing agents; require the use of diuretics that affect lithium excretion (e.g., edema); or are associated with abnormal cardiac conduction or rhythm, which may limit the choice of mood-stabilizing medications.

The possibility of adverse drug–drug interactions should always be considered whenever patients are taking more than one medication. Patients should be educated about the importance of informing their psychiatrist and other physicians about their current medications whenever new medications are prescribed.

3. Family history

The treatment of patients with bipolar disorder is not dependent on family history, although a positive family history may increase the chance that a patient with a major depressive episode may develop bipolar disorder. Thus, a careful history for prior episodes of mania or hypomania and adequate patient education about the risk of developing mania while taking an antidepressant medication are recommended.

4. Demographic and psychosocial variables

a. Children and adolescents.   The treatment of bipolar disorder in children and adolescents, based on numerous case reports and open trials, is similar to that for adults. Lithium has traditionally been used as a first-line mood stabilizer (239). However, overall response to lithium may be lower in younger patients with bipolar disorder than adults because children, and especially adolescents, with mania often have either mixed episodes or a predominance of psychotic symptoms, both of which are generally more refractory to treatment.

Several studies have documented the effectiveness of lithium for adolescents with bipolar disorder (240–243). The prophylactic effectiveness of lithium in preventing and reducing the rate of relapses in children and adolescents was demonstrated by Strober et al. (14). In this study, 37.5% of patients who completed an 18-month trial of lithium experienced at least one relapse compared to 92.3% of those who did not complete the trial. Further, those patients who completed the trial and who had at least one relapse had a decreased frequency of episodes during lithium treatment compared to baseline.

While the spectrum of lithium side effects seen in children and adolescents is similar to that seen in adults, the long-term effects of lithium in children and adolescents have not been studied. In particular, potential interactions with the developmental maturation of a child (e.g., with skeletal growth given lithium's interaction with calcium metabolism) need further research.

Children generally excrete lithium more rapidly than do adults (1); this reduced half-life means that dosage can frequently be adjusted after shorter intervals (244). Therapeutic levels are the same as for adults, with dosage adjustment recommended according to individual response.

The frequency of lithium monitoring in children and adolescents may be determined by the same considerations that apply to adult patients. While either serum or saliva sampling may be used to monitor lithium levels, serum sampling is recommended. Saliva sampling should be used only in extreme situations because saliva lithium levels are more variable, and therefore less reliable, than serum levels and children would need to avoid eating or drinking for 12 hours prior to saliva samples being obtained (245).

As in adults, adjunctive agents such as benzodiazepines, neuroleptics, and antidepressants are often used in combination with lithium. The specific risks of each of these agents should be carefully considered (e.g., tardive dyskinesia with neuroleptics, cardiac effects of tricyclic antidepressants, development or exacerbation of a substance-related disorder with benzodiazepines). Carbamazepine and valproate are also used either as adjuncts to lithium or alone. The use of these agents is primarily based on studies of adults; the literature on their use with children and adolescents is quite limited.

Although there are case reports of ECT being used effectively in children and adolescents with bipolar disorder, systematic studies are not available (246).

Psychosocial treatments are necessary to address the morbidity and sequelae of bipolar disorder in children and adolescents (247). Psychiatric management of children and adolescents must be informed by an assessment of the individual's emotional, social, and academic capacities and skills, as chronic mood lability and major mood episodes may interfere with normal development in these areas. Comorbid conditions, such as substance-related disorders and learning problems, also need to be addressed.

Some children and adolescents will benefit from a specific, more intensive intervention. For example, individual and/or family psychotherapy may be indicated to address interpersonal, intrapsychic, and social conflicts; school consultation may be necessary to develop an appropriate educational environment for the child or adolescent.

b. The elderly. There are patients who have a first manic episode after age 60. The majority of these patients had previous depressive episodes in their 40s and 50s. Any patient who has an onset of mania after age 60 should be evaluated especially carefully for general medical (including neurological) causes. These patients more often have concurrent general medical conditions and thus need a thorough general medical as well as psychiatric evaluation.

Many elderly patients appear to be more sensitive to lithium, requiring lower serum levels than younger patients to achieve similar beneficial and adverse effects. For example, it is common for elderly patients to be intolerant of levels above 0.7 meq/liter and to have a beneficial response at even lower levels. In addition, certain side effects (e.g., lithium-induced tremor) may be more common in elderly patients.

c. Family history and current family functioning.   A family history of bipolar disorder is common in patients with bipolar disorder. A positive family history may increase the likelihood that a patient with a major depressive episode will eventually have a manic episode and be diagnosed with bipolar I disorder. In addition, individuals with bipolar disorder who are considering having children may benefit from genetic counseling (27). Children of individuals with bipolar disorder have genetic as well as psychosocial risk factors for developing a psychiatric disorder (1). Patients may need help anticipating, assessing, and addressing their children's needs both during and between parental episodes.

Recognizing distress or dysfunction in the family of a patient with bipolar disorder is important because such ongoing stress may exacerbate the patient's condition or interfere with treatment. In addition, poor family functioning will increase the psychosocial risks for the patient's children and other family members, including siblings of children and adolescents with bipolar disorder. Even if dysfunction is not apparent, it is important to educate the family about bipolar disorder and enlist their support and cooperation.

d. Gender and pregnancy.   A number of issues related to gender must be considered when treating patients with bipolar disorder. Hypothyroidism is more common in women, and women may be more susceptible to the antithyroid effects of lithium. Because of the increased risk of birth defects associated with many medications used to treat bipolar disorder, the psychiatrist should encourage careful contraceptive practices for all female patients of childbearing age who are receiving pharmacologic treatment (248). Further, the metabolism of birth control pills is increased by carbamazepine and dosages may need to be adjusted accordingly. This effect does not occur with other medications used to treat bipolar disorder.

Pregnancy and the postpartum state are major factors to be considered in the treatment of women with bipolar disorder. Women with bipolar disorder may exhibit significant affective symptoms while pregnant or during the postpartum period (249). However, first trimester exposure to any of the three mood stabilizers—lithium, carbamazepine, and valproate—is associated with increased risk of birth defects. The absolute risk of major congenital anomalies among children of women treated with lithium during early pregnancy is estimated at 4% to 12%, compared to 2% to 4% in untreated comparison groups (248). Carbamazepine may have teratogenic effects, especially with first trimester exposure, including neural tube defects (250, 251), craniofacial defects, fingernail hypoplasia, and developmental delay. Valproate has been associated with a 1% to 2% risk of neural tube defects (252). Exposure to fluoxetine and tricyclic antidepressants during the first trimester may increase the risk of miscarriage (253).

Because of the risks of pharmacologic treatment, psychotherapeutic treatment alone is an important alternative for female patients who are pregnant or trying to conceive. In pregnant women who are manic, depressed, or psychotically depressed, the safest and most effective treatment is usually ECT.

Decisions regarding treatment with mood stabilizers for women who are pregnant or trying to conceive require careful discussion of risks, benefits, and alternatives. In women with severe bipolar disorder for whom discontinuation of pharmacologic treatment poses a substantial risk of increased morbidity, treatment with mood stabilizers should be discontinued for a period coinciding as closely as possible with that of embryogenesis, and preferably throughout the first trimester. Nevertheless, for some women with severe bipolar disorder, brief discontinuation of mood stabilizers will pose an unacceptable risk of increased morbidity. Therefore, if mood stabilizers are to be taken during all or part of the first trimester, the patient should 1) receive reproductive risk counseling as early as possible during the pregnancy; and 2) be offered monitoring of fetal development, including a fetal echocardiography and high-resolution ultrasound examination at 16–18 weeks' gestation and tests of serum and amniotic fluid α-fetoprotein levels (248). Throughout pregnancy, dosages of mood stabilizers may need to be adjusted because of changes in renal clearance and increases in hepatic metabolism induced by maternal hormones. Accordingly, regular monitoring of serum concentrations of mood stabilizers is recommended throughout pregnancy.

It is advisable to discontinue mood stabilizers a few days before delivery to minimize toxic effects on the infant and to resume treatment a few days afterward to reduce the risk of a postpartum episode. If pharmacologic treatment is continued, however, it is important to be aware of the large changes in total body water expected at the time of delivery. Lithium levels need to be monitored very closely after delivery until a stable level is achieved to avoid the risks of toxicity with higher levels and untreated mania with lower levels (254). Because psychotropic medications are excreted in breast milk and their long-term effects on the developing child are unknown, most authorities recommend against breast feeding if psychotropic medications are being used.

e. Cross-cultural issues.   Culture can influence the experience and communication of symptoms of depression and mania. Underdiagnosis or misdiagnosis, as well as delayed detection of early signs of recurrence, can be reduced by being alert to specific ethnic and cultural differences in reporting complaints of a major mood episode. Ethnic groups may differ in their response to antidepressant agents (255, 256).

f. Environment.   During the manic phase of bipolar disorder, maintaining a routine and calm environment is optimal. Since the manic patient is stimulated by outside events, television, videos, music, animated conversations, and alcohol can heighten manic thought processes and activities. Manic patients may also need room to pace or exercise as a way to use energy and ensure sleep. Patients and their families should be advised that during manic episodes patients may engage in reckless driving and that, at times, steps should be taken to limit access to a car.

g. Stressors.   An association between psychosocial stressors and the precipitation of mania in the first four episodes has been reported (257), although many episodes of mania have no identifiable precipitants (258). As the illness progresses, more episodes may seem to occur spontaneously. There have been occasional reports of an association between bereavement and the onset of mania, which may be mediated through poor sleep. Patients and their families should work with the psychiatrist to develop an understanding of the unique association for each individual patient between stressful events and the onset of symptoms; they should be encouraged to contact the psychiatrist during such times.

III.   Summary of Recommendations

A.   Coding System

Each recommendation is identified as falling into one of three categories of endorsement, by a bracketed Roman numeral following the statement. The three categories represent varying levels of clinical confidence in the recommendation.

[I]   indicates recommended with substantial clinical confidence.
[II]   indicates recommended with moderate clinical confidence.
[III] indicates options that may be recommended on the basis of individual circumstances.

B.   General Considerations

Patients with bipolar disorder suffer from a severe long-term psychiatric illness. Without treatment, patients with bipolar disorder will face substantial and prolonged distress and impairment, as well as the risk of significant morbidity and mortality. While effective treatments exist, there is no cure and even with optimal treatment most patients need some level of longitudinal psychiatric care. A careful and thorough psychiatric and general medical evaluation is essential prior to initiating treatment and at times of significant clinical change throughout the illness [I]. The presence of a substance use disorder should be ascertained and treated [I]. A graphic display of the course of the patient's disorder (e.g., a life chart) is frequently helpful in detecting patterns in the development and amelioration of episodes and their sequelae. Such information may be helpful in guiding and assessing attempts to decrease the frequency, severity, and consequences of future episodes. Treatment decisions depend on both cross-sectional and longitudinal features of the patient's illness.

1.   Choosing the site of treatment

The psychiatrist must determine the overall level of care that a patient with bipolar disorder needs; such a decision will depend, in part, on the availability of inpatient, partial hospital, and outpatient services in the community. In general, the least restrictive setting that is likely to allow for safe and effective treatment should be chosen. Factors guiding the choice of a treatment setting include [I]: the patient's ability to cooperate with treatment, the patient's risk for suicidal or homicidal behavior, the availability of psychosocial supports, and other clinical factors that make outpatient treatment unsafe or unlikely to be effective. Involuntary hospitalization may be necessary to protect and adequately treat the patient.

2.   Development of a treatment plan

Treatment must be preceded by a careful general medical and psychiatric examination to determine precipitants of the episode, barriers to treatment, and the presence of other disorders or factors that may complicate treatment or that require specific interventions. Patients with full-blown manic episodes may require treatment prior to the completion of a full assessment. Laboratory and other diagnostic studies should be guided by the psychiatrist's evaluation of the patient's condition and by the choice of treatment, as outlined in section II.B.

3.   Psychiatric management

Psychiatric management is the foundation for all of the treatments for bipolar disorder [I]. The intensity and focus of treatment may change as the patient's psychiatric status fluctuates and as the patient expands his or her ability to respond adaptively to the demands of the illness. The goals of psychiatric management include: establishing and maintaining a therapeutic alliance, monitoring the patient's psychiatric status, providing education regarding bipolar disorder, enhancing treatment compliance, promoting regular patterns of activity and wakefulness, promoting understanding of and adaptation to the psychosocial effects of bipolar disorder, identifying new episodes early, and reducing the morbidity and sequelae of the disorder. The patient's family and other social supports may be critical components of a treatment plan.

4.   Choice of a mood-stabilizing medication and/or ECT

Lithium, valproate, carbamazepine, and ECT are all used as primary agents in the treatment of patients with bipolar disorder [I]. ECT is generally reserved for those patients who are unable to safely wait until a medication becomes effective, who are not responsive to or unable to safely tolerate one of the effective medications, or who prefer ECT [I]. Most patients will require the use of a mood-stabilizing medication for the treatment of acute episodes, and many will require a mood stabilizer for maintenance treatment as well [I].

The choice of medication depends on an individualized assessment of the benefits and risks of, and preferences for, each of the three mood stabilizers. A discussion of these issues is summarized in section II.E.4. The data regarding efficacy and safety, in both the acute and maintenance phases, are most favorable for lithium [I]. However, some patients and psychiatrists will choose either valproate or carbamazepine based on preferences for the specific side-effect profile or based on a history of nonresponse or intolerance to lithium [II]. The use of any of these medications requires laboratory monitoring both prior to and during treatment. In addition, all three agents have recommended therapeutic ranges that may serve as general guidelines, but the specific dosage must be individualized for each patient [II]. These issues are discussed in section II.B.

C. Manic Episodes

The primary treatment of a manic episode involves the use of a mood-stabilizing medication or ECT [I]. The first step is to ensure that the patient has an adequate serum level of the medication. The choice of a target serum level may involve a compromise between maximizing efficacy and minimizing side effects. Simultaneously, the patient's general medical condition, including thyroid function, should be checked and any abnormalities treated [I]. The use of antidepressant medications should be discontinued or avoided, unless continued use is necessary based on knowledge of the patient's prior course [II].

Adjunctive benzodiazepines or neuroleptics may be used to manage symptoms of agitation, psychosis, or other dangerous behavior while awaiting the full effects of a primary mood stabilizer, or to augment the effects of the mood stabilizer [I].

If the patient has not significantly improved within 2 to 3 weeks, a second mood stabilizer should be added to the treatment regimen [II]. Pharmacokinetic interactions among medications must be kept in mind to ensure safe and effective treatment. Alternatively, ECT may be considered based on judgments about safety, efficacy, and patient preference [I].

D. Depressive Episodes

The treatment of depressed bipolar patients who are on an adequate dose of a mood-stabilizing medication includes intensified psychiatric management and continued use of the mood-stabilizing medication [II]. In addition, some patients will need one or more of the following: specific psychotherapy, antidepressant medication, and ECT.

For patients who are not taking an adequate dose of a mood stabilizer when they become depressed, a mood-stabilizing medication should be initiated (or an adequate dosage achieved) [II]. The strongest efficacy data are for lithium, so this agent would most often be the logical initial choice of mood stabilizer. Other treatments noted above should also be considered.

The decision to initiate a specific psychotherapy, and the particular choice of psychotherapy, depends on the factors discussed earlier, including knowledge of the patient's response to earlier episodes of treatment, as well as an assessment of the factors that may play a role in the precipitation, exacerbation, perpetuation, or psychosocial consequences of the episode [II].

Decisions regarding the use of antidepressant medication require an assessment of the benefits (e.g., the likelihood of relatively rapid relief of symptoms) and burdens (e.g., potential side effects of the medication, increased risk of developing a manic episode). The decision will therefore depend on the patient's specific clinical features and preferences [II].

The choice of antidepressant medication for bipolar patients is governed by the prior response of the patient to antidepressants, the side-effect profile, the presence of atypical features, the risk of inducing a manic episode, and patient preference [II].

ECT is another alternative for depressed patients [I]; its use is governed by the same factors discussed previously.

Treatment decisions for psychotically depressed patients are similar to those for all severely depressed patients. Although some patients with psychotic depression may respond to the combination of a mood stabilizer and an antidepressant, others will require the additional use of a neuroleptic [II]. ECT is also a possible treatment for these patients.

Patients with a major depressive episode may, at times, require other adjunctive agents. Further considerations are discussed in the Practice Guideline for Major Depressive Disorder in Adults (122).

E. Mixed Episodes and Ultrarapid Cycling

The treatment of patients with mixed episodes is guided by the same principles underlying the treatment of manic patients [II]. The use of antidepressants should be avoided if possible [II]. Patients who switch rapidly between depressive and manic states share many features with patients who have mixed episodes. Treatment of general medical conditions, including optimization of thyroid functioning, may be effective. Some patients may respond to the elimination of antidepressants from their treatment regimen [III]. Preliminary data suggest that patients with mixed mania may be more likely to respond to valproate, and patients with classic mania may be more likely to respond to lithium (III). Augmentation with thyroid hormone has been suggested by some investigators [III].

F. Maintenance Phase

All patients with bipolar disorder should be informed of the option of maintenance medication [I]. A decision to initiate maintenance medication treatment depends on a judgment regarding the probability of a recurrence with and without medication, the likely consequences of a recurrence, and the risks and other burdens associated with taking a maintenance medication. Such decisions should be made by the patient in conjunction with the psychiatrist and, if appropriate, family members [I]. Decisions regarding maintenance treatment should be reviewed at times of clinical change and approximately annually in stable patients [I].

Data are strongest for the efficacy and safety of lithium in the maintenance phase [I]. However, patients who are nonresponsive or intolerant to lithium, or for other reasons prefer an alternative medication, may benefit from either valproate or carbamazepine maintenance treatment [II]. The choice of a target serum level for each of these medications should be guided by the factors discussed previously and may need to be individualized according to the patient's response and preference.

In addition to psychiatric management, some patients will benefit from a specific psychotherapeutic treatment [II]. The range of available treatments and the factors guiding their choice and implementation are discussed in section II.D.

A critical role of psychiatric management is to help patients to identify precipitants or early manifestations of breakthrough episodes, so that treatment can be initiated promptly [I]. Patients can benefit from anticipating and planning for such events, so that critical decisions can be made during periods of relative mood stability.

Early signs of breakthrough episodes should be treated according to the guidelines for the treatment of acute episodes [II]. Insomnia may be either a precipitant or an early indicator of mania or depression. Education about the importance of regular sleep habits and the occasional use of benzodiazepines to promote normal sleep patterns may be useful in preventing the development of a manic episode [III]. Other early or subtle signs of mania may be treated with the short-term use of benzodiazepines or neuroleptics [II].

G.   Discontinuation of Maintenance Medication

Discontinuation of maintenance lithium should be gradual to minimize the risk of early relapse [II]. While it is not known what risks are associated with the discontinuation of maintenance valproate or carbamazepine, most clinicians recommend gradual reduction in dosage.

IV.   Research Directions

The relative effectiveness of various possible treatment regimens, including all three primary mood stabilizers, needs to be clarified in the full range of bipolar patients. The magnitude of the risks and benefits of these treatments should be clarified to enable patients and their psychiatrists to optimize individual treatment regimens. In addition, more data regarding the optimal treatment(s) for patients who have not responded to first- and second-line treatments are needed. Clinical decisions would be improved by better quantitative data on the course of this disorder with and without available treatments. A better understanding of the spectrum of patients' preferences for different treatments and outcomes would facilitate the development of general recommendations for treatment.

The treatment of bipolar depression is vastly understudied and is of substantial clinical importance given the number of bipolar patients who initially present with depression. The efficacy and safety of antidepressants in the acute and maintenance treatment of bipolar depression need further elucidation.

Psychosocial and biological research to elucidate factors leading to the initiation and exacerbation of episodes would pave the way for improved maintenance treatments. For example, research designed to clarify the role of emotional stress and sleep deprivation in the induction of episodes, and the efficacy of treatments aimed at reducing these factors, could lead to important new treatments for patients with this disorder.

Psychotherapeutic treatments for patients with bipolar disorder must be formalized to allow for careful study of their essential features and effectiveness in patients with bipolar disorder at specific phases.

The diagnosis and optimal treatment of bipolar disorder in children and adolescents require further study. In addition, the development and testing of interventions to improve the outcome for children of parents with bipolar disorder are important.

Research into the genetic mechanisms of bipolar illness is a high priority. Ascertaining the gene(s) responsible for bipolar illness carries with it the probability of early and more accurate diagnosis, as well as the potential for more specific treatments derived from an understanding of the illness at its molecular level.

The treatment implications for bipolar II disorder or schizoaffective disorder—as opposed to bipolar I disorder—need to be clarified. The optimal treatment of patients with bipolar disorder and comorbid psychiatric disorders (e.g., substance use, personality disorders) needs further study. In addition, the need for modifications in the treatment plan based on such factors as age, gender, culture, ethnicity, family history, and other psychosocial factors must be assessed in order to better individualize treatment.

V. Bipolar Disorder Guideline Reviewers and Consultants

Hagop S. Akiskal, M.D.
Lori Altshuler, M.D.
James Ballenger, M.D.
Richard Balon, M.D.
Donald Banzhaf, M.D.
David J. Barry, M.D.
Monica Ramirez Basco, Ph.D.
Mark S. Bauer, M.D.
Lee H. Beecher, M.D.
Carl C. Bell, M.D.
Deborah Blacker, M.D., Sc.D.
Charles H. Blackinton, M.D.
Mary C. Blehar, Ph.D.

Carrie M. Borchardt, M.D.
Jonathan F. Borus, M.D.
Nashaat Boutros, M.D.
Charles L. Bowden, M.D.
R.C. Bowen, M.D., F.R.C.P.(C.)
Robert Paul Cabaj, M.D.
Joseph Calabrese, M.D.
Oliver G. Cameron, M.D., Ph.D.
James M. Campbell, M.D.
Gabrielle Carlson, Ph.D.
Brendan T. Carroll, M.D.
K. Himasiri De Silva, M.D.
Ronald J. Diamond, M.D.

David L. Dunner, M.D.
Jean Endicott, Ph.D.
Irl Extein, M.D.
Terry F. Fitzgerald, Ph.D.
Lois T. Flaherty, M.D.
David L. Fogelson, M.D.
Ellen Frank, Ph.D.
Alan J. Gelenberg, M.D.
Barbara Geller, M.D.
Samuel Gershon, M.D.
Mary Gillette, Ph.D.
Katharine Gillis, M.D.
Sheila Hafter Gray, M.D.
John Greden, M.D.
John Greist, M.D.
George T. Grossberg, M.D.
Ellen Haller, M.D.
Constance Hammen, Ph.D.
Sandra G. Hershberg, M.D.
Abram M. Hostetter, M.D.
Michael Hughes, M.D.
Steven Hyman, M.D.
William S. James, M.D.
Kay Jamison, Ph.D.
James W. Jefferson, M.D.
Kathleen Kannenberg, M.A.,
    OTRLH
Roger G. Kathol, M.D.
David L. Keegan, M.D.
Martin B. Keller, M.D.
Lawrence L. Kennedy, M.D.
Howard D. Kibel, M.D.
Donald F. Klein, M.D.
David J. Kupfer, M.D.
Henry Lahmeyer, M.D.
Barry J. Landau, M.D.
William B. Lawson, M.D., Ph.D.
Alan B. Levy, M.D.
Ellen Liebenluft, M.D.
Francis Lu, M.D.
Stephan C. Mann, M.D.
Velandy Manohar, M.D.
Ronald L. Martin, M.D.

Marlin Mattson, M.D.
Jon McClellan, M.D.
J. Stephen Meredith, M.D.
Arnold E. Merriam, M.D.
Jerome A. Motto, M.D.
J. Craig Nelson, M.D.
Charles Nemeroff, M.D., Ph.D.
Arthur M. Nezu, Ph.D.
Andrei Novac, M.D.
John I. Nurnberger, Jr., M.D., Ph.D.
Joseph Parks, M.D.
Eugene Patterson, M.D.
Teri Pearlstein, M.D.
Glen N. Peterson, M.D.
Herbert Peyser, M.D.
Robert Prien, Ph.D.
John C. Racy, M.D.
Shahzad Rahman, M.D.
Lynn Rehm, Ph.D., ABPP
William H. Reid, M.D., M.P.H.
Ronald A. Remick, M.D.,
    F.R.C.P.(C.)
Richard Ries, M.D.
A. John Rush, M.D.
Gary Sachs, M.D.
Harold A. Sackeim, Ph.D.
Alan Schatzberg, M.D.
Stephen Scheiber, M.D.
Jerome M. Schnitt, M.D.
Mogens Schou, M.D.
Aimee Schwartz, M.D.
Paul M. Schyve, M.D.
Steven S. Sharfstein, M.D.
Michael Silver, M.D.
Issac Slaughter, M.D.
Joyce G. Small, M.D.
David A. Solomon, M.D.
Harvey Sternbach, M.D.
Andrew L. Stoll, M.D.
Stephen M. Strakowski, M.D.
John Strauss, M.D.
Patricia Suppes, M.D.
Margery Sved, M.D.

Clifton R. Tennison, M.D.
Claudewell Thomas, M.D.
Mauricio Tohen, M.D., Dr.P.H.
Ming T. Tsuang, M.D., Ph.D.
Robert J. Ursano, M.D.

Richard Weiner, M.D.
Myrna Weissman, Ph.D.
Peter Whybrow, M.D.
Philip Woollcott, Jr., M.D.
Herbert F. Young, M.D.

VI. Organizations That Submitted Comments

Academy of Psychosomatic Medicine
American Academy of Child and Adolescent Psychiatry
American Academy of Family Physicians
American Academy of Neurology
American Academy of Psychiatrists in Alcoholism and Addiction
American Academy of Psychoanalysis
American Association of Community Psychiatrists
American Association of Psychiatric Administrators
American Association of Psychiatrists from India
American Association of Suicidology
American Board of Psychiatry and Neurology
American College of Neuropsychopharmacology
American College of Occupational and Environmental Medicine
American Geriatrics Society
American Group Psychotherapy Association
American Occupational Therapy Association
American Psychiatric Electrophysiology Association
American Psychoanalytic Association
American Psychological Association
American Psychosomatic Society
American Society for Adolescent Psychiatry
American Society of Addiction Medicine
Association for Academic Psychiatry
Association for the Advancement of Behavior Therapy
Association of Gay and Lesbian Psychiatrists
Association of Women in Psychology
Baltimore-Washington Society for Psychoanalysis
Black Psychiatrists of America
Joint Commission on Accreditation of Healthcare Organizations
National Alliance for the Mentally Ill

National Association of Psychiatric Health Systems
National Association of Social Workers
National Association of State Mental Health Program Directors
National Community Mental Healthcare Council
National Depressive and Manic Depressive Association
National Guild of Catholic Psychiatrists
National Institute of Mental Health
National Mental Health Association
Recovery, Inc.
Society of Biological Psychiatry

VII. References

The bracketed letter following each reference indicates the nature of the supporting evidence, as follows:

[A] *Randomized controlled clinical trial.*   A study of an intervention in which subjects are prospectively followed over time; subjects are randomly assigned to treatment and control groups; both the subjects and the investigators are blind to the assignments.

[B] *Clinical trial.*   A prospective study in which an intervention is made and the results of that intervention are tracked longitudinally; study does not meet standards for a randomized clinical trial.

[C] *Cohort or longitudinal study.*   A study in which subjects are prospectively followed over time without any specific intervention.

[D] *Case-control study.*   A study in which a group of patients is identified and information about them is pursued retrospectively.

[E] *Review with secondary data analysis.*   A structured analytic review of existing data, e.g., a metanalysis or a decision analysis.

[F] *Review.*   A qualitative review and discussion of previously published literature without a quantitative synthesis of the data.

[G] *Other.*   Expert opinion, case reports, and other reports not included above.

1. Goodwin FK, Jamison KR: Manic-Depressive Illness. New York, Oxford University Press, 1990 [F]
2. Coryell W, Scheftner W, Keller, Endicott J, Maser J, Klerman GL: The enduring psychosocial consequences of mania and depression. Am J Psychiatry 1993; 150:720–727 [C]
3. Müller-Oerlinghausen B, Muser-Causemann B, Volk J: Suicides and parasuicides in a high risk patient group on and off lithium long-term medication. J Affect Disord 1992; 25:261–269 [C]
4. Coppen A, Standish-Barry H, Bailey J, Houston G, Silcocks P, Hermon C: Does lithium reduce the mortality of recurrent mood disorders? J Affect Disord 1991; 23:1–7 [C]

5. Shulman KI, Tohen M, Satlin A, Mallya G, Kalunian D: Mania compared with unipolar depression in old age. Am J Psychiatry 1992; 149:341–345 [C]

6. Weissman MM, Bruce ML, Leaf PJ, Florio LP, Holzer III CE: Affective disorders, in Psychiatric Disorders in America. Edited by Robins L, Regier DA. New York, Free Press, 1990 [C]

7. Weissman MM, Leaf PJ, Tischler GL, Blazer DG, Karno M, Bruce ML, Florio EF: Affective disorders in five United States communities. Psychol Med 1988; 18:141–153 [C]

8. Weller BW, Weller RA: Mood disorders, in Child and Adolescent Psychiatry: A Comprehensive Textbook. Edited by Lewis M. Baltimore, Williams & Wilkins, 1991 [F]

9. Carlson GA, Strober M: Manic depressive-illness in early adolescence: a study of clinical and diagnostic characteristics in six cases. J Am Acad Child Adolesc Psychiatry 1978; 17:138–153 [G]

10. Strober M, Carlson G: Bipolar illness in adolescents with major depression: clinical, genetic, and psychopharmacologic predictors in a three- to four-year prospective follow-up investigation. Arch Gen Psychiatry 1982; 39:549–555 [C]

11. Weller RA, Weller EB, Tucker SG, Fristad MA: Mania in prepubertal children: has it been underdiagnosed? J Affect Disord 1986; 11:151–154 [F]

12. DeLong GR, Aldershof AL: Long-term experience with lithium treatment in childhood: correlation with clinical diagnosis. J Am Acad Child Adolesc Psychiatry 1987; 26:389–394 [B]

13. Varanka TM, Weller RA, Weller EB, Fristad MA: Lithium treatment of manic episodes with psychotic features in prepubertal children. Am J Psychiatry 1988; 145:1557–1559 [B]

14. Strober M, Morrell W, Lampert C, Burroughs J: Relapse following discontinuation of lithium maintenance therapy in adolescents with bipolar I illness: a naturalistic study. Am J Psychiatry 1990; 147:457–461 [C]

15. Werry JS, McClellan JM, Chard L: Childhood and adolescent schizophrenic, bipolar, and schizoaffective disorders: a clinical and outcome study. J Am Acad Child Adolesc Psychiatry 1991; 30:457–465 [D]

16. Tohen M, Shulman KT, Satlin A: First-episode mania in late life. Am J Psychiatry 1994; 151:130–132 [C]

17. Gershon ES, Berrettini W, Nurnberger J, Goldin LR: Genetics of affective illness, in Psychopharmacology: The Third Generation of Progress. Edited by Meltzer HL. New York, Raven Press, 1987 [F]

18. Nurnberger JI, Gershon E: Genetics, in Handbook of Affective Disorders, 2nd ed. Edited by Paykel ES. New York, Churchill Livingstone, 1992 [E]

19. Akiskal HS: The clinical management of affective disorders, in Psychiatry, vol 1. Edited by Michels R, Cooper AM, Guze SB, Judd LL, Klerman GL, Solnit AJ. Philadelphia, JB Lippincott, 1985 [G]

20. Schou M: Lithium Treatment of Manic-Depressive Illness: A Practical Guide, 5th ed. New York, S Karger, 1993 [F]

21. Bohn J, Jefferson JW: Lithium and Manic Depression: A Guide, 2nd ed. Madison, WI, Lithium Information Center, Dean Foundation, 1993 [G]

22. Jefferson JW, Greist JH: Valproate and Manic Depression: A Guide, 2nd ed. Madison, WI, Lithium Information Center, Dean Foundation, 1993 [G]

23. Medenwald JR, Greist JH, Jefferson JW: Carbamazepine and Manic Depression: A Guide, 2nd ed. Madison, WI, Lithium Information Center, Dean Foundation, 1993 [G]

24. Gutheil TG: The psychology of psychopharmacology. Bull Menninger Clin 1982; 46:321–330 [G]

25. Jamison KR: Manic-depressive illness: the overlooked need for psychotherapy, in Integrating Pharmacotherapy and Psychotherapy. Edited by Beitman BD, Klerman GL. Washington, DC, American Psychiatric Press, 1991 [F]

26. Jamison KR, Akiskal HS: Medication compliance in patients with bipolar disorder. Psychiatr Clin North Am 1983; 6:175–192 [F]

27. Pardes H, Kaufman CA, Pincus HA, West A: Genetics and psychiatry: past discoveries, current dilemmas, and future directions. Am J Psychiatry 1989; 146:435–443 [G]

28. Post RM, Roy-Byrne PP, Uhde TW: Graphic representation of the life course of illness in patients with affective disorder. Am J Psychiatry 1988; 145:844–848 [G]

29. Kraepelin E: Manic-Depressive Insanity and Paranoia (1921). Translated by Barclay RM; edited by Robertson GM. New York, Arno Press, 1976 [G]

30. Meyer A: The Collected Papers of Adolph Meyer. Edited by Winters EE. Baltimore, Johns Hopkins University Press, 1950–52 [G]

31. Cade JFJ: Lithium salts in the treatment of psychotic excitement. Med J Aust 1949; 36:349–352 [G]

32. Jefferson JW, Greist JH, Acherman DL, Carroll JA: Lithium Encyclopedia for Clinical Practice, 2nd ed. Washington, DC, American Psychiatric Press, 1987 [F]

33. Goodwin FK, Ebert M: Lithium in mania: clinical trials and controlled studies, in Lithium: Its Role in Psychiatric Research and Treatment. Edited by Gershon S, Shopsin B. New York, Plenum Press, 1973 [E]

34. Schou M, Juel-Nielson, Strömgren E, Voldby H: The treatment of manic psychoses by administration of lithium salts. J Neurol Neurosurg Psychiatry 1954; 17:250–260 [B]

35. Maggs R: Treatment of manic illness with lithium carbonate. Br J Psychiatry 1963; 109:56–65 [B]

36. Goodwin FK, Murphy DL, Bunney WF Jr: Lithium carbonate treatment in depression and mania: a longitudinal double-blind study. Arch Gen Psychiatry 1969; 21:486–496 [B]

37. Stokes PE, Shamoian CA, Stoll PM, Patton MJ: Efficacy of lithium as acute treatment of manic-depressive illness. Lancet 1971; 1:1319–1325 [B]

38. Goodwin FK, Zis AP: Lithium in the treatment of mania: comparisons with neuroleptics. Arch Gen Psychiatry 1979; 36:840–844 [F]

39. Bowden CL, Brugger AM, Swann AC, Calabrese JR, Janicak PG, Petty F, Dilsaver SC, Davis JM, Rush AJ, Small JG, Garza-Treviño ES, Risch SC, Goodnick PJ, Morris DD: Efficacy of divalproex vs lithium and placebo in the treatment of mania. The Depakote Mania Study Group. JAMA 1994; 271:918–924 [A]

40. Janicak PG, Davis JM, Preskorn SH, Ayd FJ: Principles and Practice of Psychopharmacotherapy. Baltimore, Williams & Wilkins, 1993 [F]

41. Zornberg GL, Pope HG Jr: Treatment of depression in bipolar disorder: new directions for research. J Clin Psychopharmacol 1993; 13:397–408 [E]

42. Baastrup PC, Schou M: Lithium as a prophylactic agent: its effect against recurrent depression and manic-depressive psychosis. Arch Gen Psychiatry 1967; 16:162–172 [B]

43. Faedda GL, Tondo L, Baldessarini RJ, Suppes T, Tohen M: Outcome after rapid vs. gradual discontinuation of lithium treatment in bipolar disorders. Arch Gen Psychiatry 1993; 50:448–455 [B]

44. Suppes T, Baldessarini RJ, Faedda GL, Tohen M: Risk of recurrence following discontinuation of lithium treatment in bipolar disorder. Arch Gen Psychiatry 1991; 48:1082–1088 [E]

45. Schou M: Is there a lithium withdrawal syndrome? an examination of the evidence. Br J Psychiatry 1993; 163:514–518 [F]

46. Post RM, Leverich GS, Altshuler L, Mikalauskas K: Lithium-discontinuation-induced refractoriness: preliminary observations. Am J Psychiatry 1992; 149:1727–1729 [G]

47. Pazzaglia PJ, Post RM: Contingent tolerance and reresponse to carbamazepine: a case study in a patient with trigeminal neuralgia and bipolar disorder. J Neuropsychiatry Clin Neurosci 1992; 4:76–81 [G]

48. Schou M: Lithium prophylaxis: myths and realities. Am J Psychiatry 1989; 146:573–576 [F]

49. Arana GW, Hyman SE: Handbook of Psychiatric Drug Therapy, 2nd ed. Boston, Little, Brown, 1991 [F]

50. Bauer MS, Whybrow PC: Rapid cycling bipolar affective disorder. II. Treatment of refractory rapid cycling with high-dose levothyroxine: a preliminary study. Arch Gen Psychiatry 1990; 47:435–440 [G]

51. Smigan L, Wahlin A, Jacobsson L, von Knorring L: Lithium therapy and thyroid function tests: a prospective study. Neuropsychobiology 1984; 17:39–43 [B]

52. Bocchetta A, Bernardi F, Burrai C, Pedditzi M, Loviselli A, Velluzzi F, Martino E, Del Zompo M: The course of thyroid abnormalities during lithium treatment: a two year follow-up study. Acta Psychiatr Scand 1992; 86:38–41 [C]

53. Vestergaard P, Schou M, Thomsen K: Monitoring of patients in prophylactic lithium treatment: an assessment based on recent kidney studies. Br J Psychiatry 1982; 140:185–187 [C]

54. Schou M: Effects of long-term lithium treatment on kidney function: an overview. J Psychiatry Res 1988; 22:287–296 [F]

55. Gitlin MJ: Lithium-induced renal insufficiency. J Clin Psychopharmacol 1993; 13:276–279 [C]

56. von Knorring L, Wahlin A, Nystrom K, Bohman SO: Uraemia induced by long-term lithium treatment. Lithium 1990; 1:251–253 [G]

57. Cooper TB, Bergner PE, Simpson GM: The 24-hour serum lithium level as a prognosticator of dosage requirements. Am J Psychiatry 1973; 130:601–603 [C]

58. Gelenberg AJ, Kane JM, Keller MB, Lavori P, Rosenbaum JF, Cole K, Lavelle J: Comparison of standard and low serum levels of lithium for maintenance treatment of bipolar disorder. N Engl J Med 1989; 321:1489–1493 [A]

59. Pope HG Jr, McElroy SL, Keck PE Jr, Hudson JI: Valproate in the treatment of acute mania: a placebo controlled study. Arch Gen Psychiatry 1991; 48:62–68 [A]

60. Keck PE Jr, McElroy SL, Tugrul KC, Bennett JA: Valproate oral loading in the treatment of acute mania. J Clin Psychiatry 1993; 54:305–308 [B]

61. McElroy SL, Keck PE, Jr: Treatment guidelines for valproate in bipolar and schizoaffective disorders. Can J Psychiatry 1993; 38(3 suppl 2):S62–S66 [F]

62. McElroy SL, Dessain EC, Pope HG Jr, Cole JO, Keck PE Jr, Frankenberg FR, Aizley HG, O'Brien S: Clozapine in the treatment of psychotic mood disorders, schizoaffective disorder, and schizophrenia. J Clin Psychiatry 1991; 52:411–414 [G]

63. Keck PE Jr, McElroy SL, Nemeroff CB: Anticonvulsants in the treatment of bipolar disorder. J Neuropsychiatry Clin Neurosci 1992; 4:395–405 [F]

64. Ketter TA, Pazzaglia PJ, Post RM: Synergy of carbamazepine and valproic acid in affective illness: case report and review of literature. J Clin Psychopharmacol 1992; 12;276–281 [F]

65. Puzynski S, Kosiewicz L: Valproic acid amide as a prophylactic agent in affective and schizoaffective disorders. Psychopharmacol Bull 1984; 20:151–159 [B]

66. Hayes SG: The long-term use of valproate in primary psychiatric disorders. J Clin Psychiatry 1989; 50(3 suppl):35–39 [D]

67. Calabrese JR, Delucchi GA: Spectrum of efficacy of valproate in 55 patients with rapid-cycling bipolar disorder. Am J Psychiatry 1990; 147:431–434 [B]

68. Calabrese JR, Markovitz PJ, Kimmel SE, Wagner SC: Spectrum of efficacy of valproate in 78 rapid-cycling bipolar patients. J Clin Psychopharmacol 1992; 12(1 suppl):53S–56S [B]

69. McElroy SL, Keck PE Jr, Pope HG Jr, Hudson JI: The use of valproate in psychiatric disorders: literature review and clinical guidelines. J Clin Psychiatry 1989; 50(Mar suppl):23–29 [F]

70. Jacobsen FM: Low-dose valproate: a new treatment for cyclothymia, mild rapid cycling disorders, and premenstrual syndrome. J Clin Psychiatry 1993; 54:229–234 [B]

71. Rall TW, Schleifer LS: Drugs effective in the therapy of the epilepsies, in Goodman and Gilman's: The Pharmacological Basis of Therapeutics, 8th ed. Edited by Gilman LS, Goodman AG, Rall TW. New York, Macmillan, 1991 [F]

72. Rimmer EM, Richens A: An update on sodium valproate. Pharmacotherapy 1985; 5:171–184 [F]

73. Penry JK, Dean JC: The scope and use of valproate in epilepsy. J Clin Psychiatry 1989; 50(Mar suppl):17–22 [F]

74. Wilder BJ, Karas BJ, Penry JK, Asconape J: Gastrointestinal tolerance of divalproex sodium. Neurology 1983; 33:808–811 [B]

75. Goodman AG, Zall TW, Nies AS, Taylor P: Goodman and Gilman's: The Pharmacological Basis of Therapeutics, 8th ed. New York, Macmillan, 1991 [G]

76. Sovner R, Davis JM: A potential drug interaction between fluoxetine and valproic acid (letter). J Clin Psychopharmacol 1991; 11: 389 [G]

77. Stoll AL, Vuckovic A, McElroy SL: Histamine-2-receptor antagonists for the treatment of valproate-induced gastrointestinal distress. Ann Clin Psychiatry 1991; 3:301–304 [G]

78. Isojarvi JI, Laatikainen TJ, Pakarinen AJ, Juntunen KT, Myllyla VV: Polycystic ovaries and hyperandrogenism in women taking valproate for epilepsy. N Engl J Med 1993; 329:1383–1388 [G]

79. Pellock JM, Willmore LJ: A rational guide to routine blood monitoring in patients receiving antiepileptic drugs. Neurology 1991; 41:961–964 [G]

80. McElroy SL, Keck PE Jr, Pope HG Jr, Hudson JI: Valproate in the treatment of bipolar disorder: literature review and clinical guidelines. J Clin Psychopharmacol 1992; 12(1 suppl):42S–52S [F]

81. McElroy SL, Keck PE Jr, Pope HG Jr, Hudson JI, Faedda GL, Swann AC: Clinical and research implications of the diagnosis of dysphoric or mixed mania or hypomania. Am J Psychiatry 1992; 149:1633–1644 [F]

82. Post RM, Leverich GS, Rosoff AS, Altshuler LL: Carbamazepine prophylaxis in refractory affective disorders: a focus on long-term follow-up. J Clin Psychopharmacol 1990; 10:318–327 [C]

83. Lipinski JF Jr, Pope HG Jr: Possible synergistic action between carbamazepine and lithium carbonate: a report of three cases. Am J Psychiatry 1982; 139:938–939 [B]

84. Keck PE Jr, McElroy SL, Vuckovic A, Friedman LM: Combined valproate and carbamazepine treatment of bipolar disorder. J Neuropsychiatry Clin Neurosci 1992; 4:319–322 [B]

85. Lerer B, Moore M, Meyendorff E, Cho SR, Gershon S: Carbamazepine versus lithium in mania: a double-blind study. J Clin Psychiatry 1987; 48:89–93 [A]

86. Small JG, Klapper MH, Milstein V, Kellams JJ, Miller MJ, Marhenke JD, Small IF: Carbamazepine compared with lithium in the treatment of mania. Arch Gen Psychiatry 1991; 48:915–921 [A]

87. Colgate R: The ranking of therapeutic and toxic side effects of lithium carbonate. Psychiatr Bull 1992; 16:473–475 [G]

88. Ayd FJ: Acute self-poisoning with lithium. Int Drug Therapy Newsletter 1988; 23:1–2 [G]

89. Ragheb M: The clinical significance of lithium-nonsteroidal anti-inflammatory drug interactions. J Clin Psychopharmacol 1990; 10:350–354 [G]

90. Ballenger JC, Post RM: Carbamazepine in manic-depressive illness: a new treatment. Am J Psychiatry 1980; 137:782–790 [A]

91. Post RM, Uhde TW, Ballenger JC, Squillace KM: Prophylactic efficacy of carbamazepine in manic-depressive illness. Am J Psychiatry 1983; 140:1602–1604 [G]

92. Kramlinger KG, Post RM: The addition of lithium to carbamazepine: antidepressant efficacy in treatment-resistant depression. Arch Gen Psychiatry 1989; 46:794–800 [B]

93. Prien RF, Gelenberg AJ: Alternatives to lithium for preventive treatment of bipolar disorder. Am J Psychiatry 1989; 146:840–848 [F]

94. Lusznat RM, Murphy DP, Nunn CMH: Carbamazepine vs lithium in the treatment and prophylaxis of mania. Br J Psychiatry 1988; 153:198–204 [A]

95. Okuma T, Inanaga K, Otsuki S, Sarai K, Takahashi R, Hazama H, Mori A, Watanabe S: A preliminary double-blind study on the efficacy of carbamazepine in prophylaxis of manic-depressive illness. Psychopharmacology (Berl) 1981; 73:95–96 [A]

96. Placidi GF, Lenzi A, Lazzerini F, Cassano GB, Akiskal HS: The comparative efficacy and safety of carbamazepine versus lithium: a randomized, double-blind, 3 year trial in 83 patients. J Clin Psychiatry 1986; 47:490–494 [A]

97. Watkins SE, Callender K, Thomas DR, Tidmarsh SF, Shaw DM: The effect of carbamazepine and lithium on remission from affective illness. Br J Psychiatry 1987; 150:180–182 [A]

98. Murphy DJ, Gannon MA, McGennis A: Carbamazepine in bipolar affective disorder (letter). Lancet 1989; 2:1151–1152 [G]

99. Ketter TA, Post RM, Worthington K: Principles of clinically important drug interactions with carbamazepine. Part I. J Clin Psychopharmacology 1991; 11:198–203 [F]

100. Ketter TA, Post RM, Worthington K: Principles of clinically important drug interactions with carbamazepine. Part II. J Clin Psychopharmacology 1991; 11:306–313 [F]

101. Smith MC, Bleck TP: Convulsive disorders: toxicity of anti-convulsants. Clin Neuropharmacol 1991; 14:97–115 [F]

102. Seetharam MN, Pellock JM: Risk-benefit assessment of carbamazepine in children. Drug Safety 1991; 6:148–158 [F]

103. Prien RF, Caffey EM, Klett CJ: Comparison of lithium carbonate and chlorpromazine in the treatment of mania. Report of the Veterans Administration and National Institute of Mental Health Collaborative Study Group. Arch Gen Psychiatry 1972; 26:146–153 [A]

104. Lenox RH, Newhouse PA, Creelman WL, Whitaker TM: Adjunctive treatment of manic agitation with lorazepam versus haloperidol: a double-blind study. J Clin Psychiatry 1992; 53: 47–52 [A]

105. Shopsin B, Gershon S, Thompson H, Collins P: Psychoactive drugs in mania. A controlled comparison of lithium carbonate, chlorpromazine, and haloperidol. Arch Gen Psychiatry 1975; 32:34–42 [A]

106. Davis JM: Overview: maintenance therapy in psychiatry: II. Affective disorders. Am J Psychiatry 1976; 133:1–13 [E]

107. Mukherjee S, Rosen AM, Caracci G, Shukla S: Persistent tardive dyskinesia in bipolar patients. Arch Gen Psychiatry 1986; 43: 342–346 [C]

108. Tardive Dyskinesia: A Task Force Report of the American Psychiatric Association. Washington, DC, APA, 1991 [F]

109. Parker G, Roy K, Hadzi-Pavlovic D, Pedic F: Psychotic (delusional) depression: a meta-analysis of physical treatments. J Affect Disord 1992; 24:17–24 [E]

110. Spiker DG, Weiss JC, Dealy RS, Griffin SJ, Hanin I, Neil JF, Perel JM, Rossi AJ, Soloff PH: The pharmacological treatment of delusional depression. Am J Psychiatry 1985; 142:430–436 [A]

111. Kukopulos A, Reginaldi D, Laddomada P, Floris G, Serra G, Tondo L: Course of the manic-depressive cycle and changes caused by treatment. Pharmakopsychiatrie-Neuropsychopharmakol 1980; 13:156–167 [C]

112. Sernyak MJ, Woods SW: Chronic neuroleptic use in manic-depressive illness. Psychopharmacol Bull 1993; 29:375–381 [B]

113. Edwards R, Stephenson U, Flewett T: Clonazepam in acute mania: a double-blind trial. Aust N Z J Psychiatry 1991; 25:238–242 [A]

114. Chouinard G, Young SN, Annable L: Antimanic effect of clonazepam. Biol Psychiatry 1983; 18:451–466 [F]

115. Chouinard G: Clonazepam in acute and maintenance treatment of bipolar disorder. J Clin Psychiatry 1987; 48(Oct suppl):29–37 [F]

116. Bradwejn J, Shriqui C, Koszycki D, Meterissian G: Double-blind comparison of the effects of clonazepam and lorazepam in acute mania. J Clin Psychopharmacol 1990; 10:403–408 [A]

117. Chouinard G, Annable L, Turnier L, Holobow N, Szkrumelak N: A double-blind randomized clinical trial of rapid tranquilization with I.M. clonazepam and I.M. haloperidol in agitated psychotic patients with manic symptoms. Can J Psychiatry 1993; 38(suppl 4):S114–S121 [A]

118. Sachs GS, Weilburg JB, Rosenbaum JF: Clonazepam vs neuroleptics as adjuncts to lithium maintenance. Psychopharmacol Bull 1990; 26:137–143 [F]

119. Aronson TA, Shukla S, Hirschowitz J: Clonazepam treatment of five lithium-refractory patients with bipolar disorder. Am J Psychiatry 1989; 146:77–80 [G]

120. Miller NS, Gold MS: Abuse, addiction, tolerance, and dependence to benzodiazepines in medical and nonmedical populations. Am J Drug Alcohol Abuse 1991; 17:27–37 [F]

121. Busto V, Sellers EM, Naranjo CA, Cappell HD, Sanchez-Craig M, Simpkins J: Patterns of benzodiazepine abuse and dependence. Br J Addiction 1986; 81:87–94 [C]

122. American Psychiatric Association: Practice Guideline for Major Depressive Disorder in Adults. Am J Psychiatry 1993; 150(Apr suppl) [F]

123. Baumhackl U, Biziere K, Fischbach R, Geretsegger CH, Hebenstreit G, Radmayr E, Stabl M: Efficacy and tolerability of moclobemide compared with imipramine in depressive disorder (DSM-III): an Austrian double-blind, multicentre study. Br J Psychiatry 1989; 155(Oct suppl):78–83 [A]

124. Himmelhoch JM, Thase ME, Mallinger AG, Houck P: Tranylcypromine versus imipramine in anergic bipolar depression. Am J Psychiatry 1991; 148:910–916 [A]

125. Cohn JB, Collins G, Ashbrook E, Wernicke JF: A comparison of fluoxetine imipramine and placebo in patients with bipolar depressive disorder. Int Clin Psychopharmacology 1989; 4:313–322 [A]

126. Sachs GS, Lafer B, Stoll AL, Banov M, Thibault AB, Tohen M, Rosenbaum JF: A double-blind trial of bupropion versus desipramine for bipolar depression. J Clin Psychiatry 1994; 55:391–393 [A]

127. Fogelson DL, Bystritsky A, Pasnau R: Bupropion in the treatment of bipolar disorders: the same old story? J Clin Psychiatry 1992; 53:443–446 [G]

128. Shopsin B. Bupropion's prophylactic efficacy in bipolar affective illness. J Clin Psychiatry 1983; 44(5, sec 2):163–169 [B]

129. Haykal RF, Akiskal HS: Bupropion as a promising approach to rapid cycling bipolar II patients. J Clin Psychiatry 1990; 51: 450–455 [G]

130. Wright G, Galloway L, Kim J, Dalton M, Miller L Stern W: Bupropion in the long-term treatment of cyclic mood disorders: mood stabilizing effects. J Clin Psychiatry 1985; 46:22–25 [F]

131. Wehr TA, Goodwin FK: Do antidepressants cause mania? Psychopharmacol Bull 1987; 23:61–65 [G]

132. Peet M: Induction of mania with selective serotonin re-uptake inhibitors and tricyclic antidepressants. Br J Psychiatry 1994; 164:549–550 [E]

133. Wehr TA, Goodwin FK: Rapid cycling in manic-depressives induced by tricyclic antidepressants. Arch Gen Psychiatry 1979; 36:555–559 [B]

134. Akiskal HS, Mallya G: Criteria for the "soft" bipolar spectrum: treatment implications. Psychopharmacol Bull 1987; 23:68–73 [G]

135. Prien RF, Potter WZ: NIMH workshop report on treatment of bipolar disorder. Psychopharmacol Bull 1990; 26:409–427 [F]

136. Dubovsky SL, Franks RD, Lifschitz M, Coen P: Effectiveness of verapamil in the treatment of a manic patient. Am J Psychiatry 1982; 139:502–504 [G]

137. Dubovsky S, Franks RD, Schrier D: Phenelzine-induced hypomania: effect of verapamil. Biol Psychiatry 1985; 20:1009–1014 [G]

138. Dubovsky SL, Franks RD, Allen S, Murphy J: Calcium antagonists in mania: a double-blind study of verapamil. Psychiatry Res 1986; 18:309–320 [A]

139. Dubovsky SL, Franks RD, Allen S: Verapamil: a new antimanic drug with potential interactions with lithium. J Clin Psychiatry 1987; 48:371–372 [G]

140. Dubovsky SL, Franks RD: Intracellular calcium ions in affective disorders: a review and an hypothesis. Biol Psychiatry 1983; 18:781–797 [F]

141. Hoschl C: Verapamil for depression? (letter). Am J Psychiatry 1983; 140:1100 [G]

142. Giannini AJ, Houser WL Jr, Loiselle RH, Giannini MC, Price WA: Antimanic effects of verapamil. Am J Psychiatry 1984; 141:1602–1603 [B]

143. Giannini AJ, Taraszewski R, Loiselle RH: Verapamil and lithium in maintenance therapy of manic patients. J Clin Pharmacol 1987; 27:980–982 [A]

144. Dose M, Emrich HM, Cording-Tommel C, Von Zerssen D: Use of calcium antagonists in mania. Psychoneuroendocrinology 1986; 11:241–243 [F]

145. Hoschl C, Kozeny J: Verapamil in affective disorders: a controlled, double-blind study. Biol Psychiatry 1989; 25:128–140 [B]

146. Garza-Treviño ES, Overall JE, Hollister LE: Verapamil versus lithium in acute mania. Am J Psychiatry 1992; 149:121–122 [A]

147. Stancer HC, Persad E: Treatment of intractable rapid-cycling manic-depressive disorder with levothyroxine: clinical observations. Arch Gen Psychiatry 1982; 39:311–312 [G]

148. Stein D, Avni J: Thyroid hormones in the treatment of affective disorders. Acta Psychiatr Scand 1988; 77:623–636 [F]

149. Banovac K, Papic M, Bilsker MS, Zakarija M, McKensie JM: Evidence of hyperthyroidism in apparently euthyroid patients treated with levothyroxine. Arch Intern Med 1989; 149:809–812 [C]

150. Stall GM, Harris S, Sokoll LJ, Dawson-Hughes B: Accelerated bone loss in hypothyroid patients overtreated with L-thyroxine. Ann Intern Med 1990; 113:265–269 [C]

151. Coindre JM, David JP, Riviere L, Goussot JF, Roger P, de Mascarel A, Meunier PJ: Bone loss in hypothyroidism with hormone replacement: a histomorphic study. Arch Intern Med 1986; 146: 48–53 [G]

152. Gyulai L, Lew PY, Bauer MS, Rubin L, Rounkin S, Jaggi J, Whybrow P: High dose thyroxine does not decrease bone density, in CME Syllabus and Scientific Proceedings in Summary Form, 146th Annual Meeting of the American Psychiatric Association. Washington, DC, APA, 1993 [F]

153. Suppes T, McElroy SL, Gilbert J, Dessain EC, Cole JO: Clozapine in the treatment of dysphoric mania. Biol Psychiatry 1992; 32:270–280 [B]

154. Deltito JA, Moline M, Pollak C, Martin LY, Maremmani I: Effects of phototherapy on non-season unipolar and bipolar depressive spectrum disorders. J Affect Disord 1991; 23:231–237 [B]

155. Mukherjee S, Sackeim HA, Schnurr DB: Electroconvulsive therapy of acute manic episodes: a review. Am J Psychiatry 1994; 151:169–176 [F]

156. Thomas J, Reddy B: The treatment of mania: a retrospective evaluation of the effects of ECT, chlorpromazine, and lithium. J Affect Disord 1982; 4:85–92 [D]

157. Black DW, Winokur G, Nasrallah A: Treatment of mania: a naturalistic study of electroconvulsive therapy versus lithium in 438 patients. J Clin Psychiatry 1987; 48:132–139 [C]

158. Alexander RC, Salomon M, Ionescu-Pioggia M, Cole JO: Convulsive therapy in the treatment of mania. Convulsive Therapy 1988; 4:115–125 [D]

159. Milstein V, Small JG, Klapper MH, Small IF, Miller MJ, Kellams JJ: Uni- versus bilateral ECT in the treatment of mania. Convulsive Therapy 1987; 3:1–9 [B]

160. Small JG, Klapper MH, Kellams JJ, Miller MJ, Milstein V, Sharpley PH, Small IF: Electroconvulsive treatment compared with lithium in the management of manic states. Arch Gen Psychiatry 1988; 45:727–732 [B]

161. Mukherjee S, Sackeim HA, Lee C: Unilateral ECT in the treatment of manic episodes. Convulsive Therapy 1988; 4:74–80 [B]

162. Strömgren LS: Electroconvulsive therapy in Aarhus, Denmark, in 1984: its application in nondepressive disorders. Convulsive Therapy 1988; 4:306–313 [D]

163. Heshe J, Roeder E: [Electroconvulsive therapy in Denmark. Review of the technique, employment, indications and complications.] Ugeskrift for Laeger 1975; 137:939–944 [G]

164. Kramp P, Bolwig TG: Electroconvulsive therapy in acute delirious states. Compr Psychiatry 1981; 22:368–371 [F]

165. Mann SC, Caroff SN, Bleier HR, Welz WK, Kling MA, Hayashida M: Lethal catatonia. Am J Psychiatry 1986; 143:1374–1381 [F]

166. Mann SC, Caroff SN, Bleier HR, Anttelo RE, Un H: Electroconvulsive therapy of the lethal catatonia syndrome. Convulsive Therapy 1990; 6:239–247 [F]

167. Janicak PG, Davis JM, Gibbons RD, Ericksen S, Chang S, Gallagher P: Efficacy of ECT: a meta-analysis. Am J Psychiatry 1985; 142:297–302 [E]

168. Hamilton M: Electroconvulsive therapy: indications and contraindications. Ann NY Acad Sci 1986; 462:5–11 [F]

169. The Practice of Electroconvulsive Therapy: Recommendations for Treatment, Training, and Privileging: A Task Force Report of the American Psychiatric Association. Washington, DC, American Psychiatric Press, 1990 [F]

170. Sackheim HA: The efficacy of electroconvulsive therapy in the treatment of major depressive disorder, in The Limits of Biological Treatments for Psychological Distress. Edited by Fisher S, Greenberg RP. Hillsdale, NJ, Erlbaum Publishing, 1989 [F]

171. Perris C, d'Elia G: A study of bipolar (manic-depressive) and unipolar recurrent depressive psychoses. IX. Therapy and prognosis. Acta Psychiatr Scand Suppl 1966; 194:153–171 [B]

172. Strömgren LS: Unilateral versus bilateral electroconvulsive therapy. Investigations into the therapeutic effect in endogenous depression. Acta Psychiatr Scand Suppl 1973; 240:8–65 [B]

173. Abrams R, Taylor MA: Unipolar and bipolar depressive illness. Phenomenology and response to electroconvulsive therapy. Arch Gen Psychiatry 1974; 30:320–321 [B]

174. Prudic J, Sackeim HA, Devanand DP: Medication resistance and clinical response to electroconvulsive therapy. Psychiatry Res 1990; 31:287–296 [B]

175. Devanand DP, Sackeim HA, Decina P, Prudic J: The development of mania and organic euphoria during ECT. J Clin Psychiatry 1988; 49:69–71 [G]

176. Small JG, Kellams JJ, Milstein V, Small IF: Complications with electroconvulsive treatment combined with lithium. Biol Psychiatry 1985; 20:125–134 [D]

177. Strömgren LS, Dahl J, Fjeldborg N, Thomsen A: Factors influencing seizure duration and number of seizures applied in unilateral electroconvulsive therapy: anaesthetics and benzodiazepines. Acta Psychiatr Scand 1980; 62:158–165 [A]

178. Standish-Barry HMAS, Bouras N, Hale AS, Bridges PK, Bartlett JR: Ventricular size and CSF transmitter metabolite concentrations in severe endogenous depression. Br J Psychiatry 1986; 148:386–392 [C]

179. Rudorfer MV, Linnoila M, Potter WZ: Combined lithium and electroconvulsive therapy: pharmacokinetic and pharmacodynamic interactions. Convulsive Therapy 1987; 3:40–45 [F]

180. El-Mallakh RS: Complications of concurrent lithium and electroconvulsive therapy: a review of clinical material and theoretical considerations. Psychopharmacol Bull 1987; 23:595–601 [F]

181. Ahmed SK, Stein GS: Negative interaction between lithium and ECT (letter). Br J Psychiatry 1987; 151:419–420 [G]

182. Small JG, Milstein V, Miller MJ, Sharpley PH, Small IF, Malloy FW, Klapper MH: Clinical, neuropsychological, and EEG evidence for mechanisms of action of ECT. Convulsive Therapy 1988; 4:280–291 [F]

183. Pettinati HM, Willis KW, Nilsen SM, Robin SE: Benzodiazepines reduce ECT's therapeutic effect, in New Research Program and Abstracts, 140th Annual Meeting of the American Psychiatric Association. Washington, DC, APA, 1987

184. Nettlebladt P: Factors influencing number of treatments and seizure duration in ECT: drug treatment, social class. Convulsive Therapy 1988; 4:160–168 [C]

185. Kahn DA: The use of psychodynamic psychotherapy in manic-depressive illness. J Am Acad Psychoanal 1993; 21:441–455 [F]

186. Haas GL, Glick ID, Clarkin JF, Spencer JH, Lewis AB, Peyser J, DeMane N, Good-Ellis M, Harris E, Lestelle V: Inpatient family intervention: a randomized clinical trial. II. Results at hospital discharge. Arch Gen Psychiatry 1988; 45:217–224 [B]

187. Clarkin JF, Glick ID, Haas GL, Spencer JH, Lewis AB, Peyser J, DeMane N, Good-Ellis M, Harris E, Lestelle V: A randomized clinical trial of inpatient family intervention. V. Results for affective disorders. J Affect Disord 1990; 18:17–28 [A]

188. Falloon IRH, Boyd JL, McGill CW: Family Care for Schizophrenia: A Problem-Solving Approach to Mental Illness. New York, Guilford Press, 1984 [G]

189. Miklowitz DJ, Goldstein MJ: Behavioral family treatment for patients with bipolar affective disorder. Behavior Modification 1990; 14:457–489 [G]

190. Miller IW, Keitner GI, Epstein NB, Bishop DS, Ryan CE: Families of bipolar patients: dysfunction, course of illness, and pilot treatment study, in Proceedings of the 22nd Meeting of the Society for Psychotherapy Research. Pittsburgh, Society for Psychotherapy Research, 1991 [B]

191. Basco MR, Rush AJ: Cognitive-behavioral therapy for bipolar disorder, in Cognitive Behavioral Treatment of Manic Depressive Disorder. New York, Guilford Press (in press) [F]

192. Frank E: Interpersonal and social rhythm therapy for bipolar disorder: integrating interpersonal and behavioral approaches. Behavior Therapist (in press) [F]

193. Karasu TB: Developmentalist metatheory of depression and psychotherapy. Am J Psychother 1992; 46:37–49 [G]

194. Klerman GL, Weissman MM, Rounsaville BJ, Chevron ES: Interpersonal Psychotherapy of Depression. New York, Basic Books, 1984 [G]

195. DiMascio A, Weissman MM, Prusoff BA, Neu C, Zwilling M, Klerman GL: Differential symptom reduction by drugs and psychotherapy in acute depression. Arch Gen Psychiatry 1979; 36: 1450–1456 [A]

196. Elkin I, Shea MT, Watkins JT, Imber SD, Sotsky SM, Collins JF, Glass DR, Pilkonis PA, Leber WR, Docherty JP, Fiester SJ, Parloff MB: National Institute of Mental Health Treatment of Depression Collaborative Research Program: general effectiveness of treatments. Arch Gen Psychiatry 1989; 46:971–982 [A]

197. Klerman GL, DiMascio A, Weissman M, Prusoff B, Paykel ES: Treatment of depression by drugs and psychotherapy. Am J Psychiatry 1974; 131:186–191 [A]

198. Frank E, Kupfer DJ, Perel JM, Cornes C, Jarrett DB, Mallinger AG, Thase ME, McEachran AB, Grochocinski VJ: Three-year outcomes for maintenance therapies in recurrent depression. Arch Gen Psychiatry 1990; 47:1093–1099 [B]

199. Ferster CB: A functional analysis of depression. Am Psychol 1973; 28:857–870 [F]

200. Bandura A: Social Learning Theory. Englewood Cliffs, NJ, Prentice-Hall, 1977 [F]

201. Lewinsohn PM, Antonuccio DA, Steinmetz-Breckinridge J, Teri L: The Coping with Depression Course: A Psychoeducational Intervention for Unipolar Depression. Eugene, OR, Castalia Publishing, 1984 [F]

202. Lewinsohn P, Clarke G: Group treatment of depressed individuals: the "Coping with Depression" course. Advances in Behaviour Research Therapy 1984; 6:99–114 [F]

203. Rehm LP: Behavior Therapy for Depression: Present Status and Future Directions. New York, Academic Press, 1980 [F]

204. Bellack AS, Hersen M, Himmelhoch JM: A comparison of social-skills training, pharmacotherapy and psychotherapy for depression. Behav Res Ther 1983; 21:101–107 [A]

205. Nezu AM: Efficacy of a social problem-solving therapy for unipolar depression. J Consult Clin Psychol 1986; 54:196–202 [B]

206. Thompson LW, Gallagher D, Breckenridge JS: Comparative effectiveness of psychotherapies for depressed elders. J Consult Clin Psychol 1987; 21:133–146 [A]

207. McLean PD, Hakstian AR: Clinical depression: comparative efficacy of outpatient treatments. J Consult Clin Psychol 1979; 47:818–836 [A]

208. Usaf SO, Kavanagh DJ: Mechanisms of improvement in treatment for depression: test of self-efficacy and performance model. J Cognitive Psychotherapy 1990; 4:51–70 [A]

209. Nezu AM, Perri MG: Social problem-solving therapy for unipolar depression: an initial dismantling investigation. J Consult Clin Psychol 1989; 57:408–413 [B]

210. Gallagher DE, Thompson LW: Treatment of major depressive disorder in older adult outpatients with brief psychotherapies. Psychotherapy: Theory, Research, and Practice 1982; 19:482–490 [A]

211. Gallagher-Thompson D, Hanley-Peterson P, Thompson LW: Maintenance of gains versus relapse following brief psychotherapy for depression. J Consult Clin Psychol 1990; 58:371–374 [A]

212. Beck TA, Rush AJ, Shaw BF, Emery G: Cognitive Therapy of Depression. New York, Guilford Press, 1979 [F]

213. Rush AJ, Hollon SD, Beck AT, Kovacs M: Depression: must pharmacotherapy fail for cognitive therapy to succeed? Cognitive Therapy and Research 1978; 2:199–206 [B]

214. Hollon SD, DeRubeis RJ, Seligman MEP: Cognitive therapy and the prevention of depression. Applied Preventive Psychol 1992; 1:89–95 [G]

215. Shea MT, Elkin I, Imber SD, Sotsky SM, Watkins JT, Collins JF, Pilkonis PA, Beckham E, Glass DR, Dolan RT, Parloff MB: Course of depressive symptoms over follow-up. Findings from the National Institute of Mental Health Treatment of Depression Collaborative Research Program. Arch Gen Psychiatry 1992; 49:782–787 [A]

216. Ross M, Scott M: An evaluation of the effectiveness of individual and group cognitive therapy in the treatment of depressed patients in an inner city health centre. J Royal College of General Practitioners 1985; 35:239–242 [A]

217. O'Leary KD, Beach SR: Marital therapy: a viable treatment for depression and marital discord. Am J Psychiatry 1990; 147: 183–186 [A]

218. Beach SRH, Sandeen EE, O'Leary KD: Depression in Marriage. New York, Guilford Press, 1990 [G]

219. Yager J: Patients with mood disorders and marital/family problems, in Annual Review of Psychiatry, vol 11. Edited by Tasman A. Washington, DC, American Psychiatric Press, 1992 [G]

220. Coyne JC: Inpatient family intervention, in Affective Disorders and the Family: Assessment and Treatment. Edited by Clarkin JF, Haas GL, Glick ID. New York, Guilford Press, 1988 [F]

221. Coyne JC, Kessler RC, Tal M, Turnbull J, Wortman CB, Greden JF: Living with a depressed person. J Consult Clin Psychol 1987; 55:347–352 [F]

222. Jacobson NS, Dobson K, Fruzzetti AE, Schmaling KB, Salusky S: Marital therapy as a treatment for depression. J Consult Clin Psychol 1991; 59:547–557 [A]

223. Regier DA, Farmer ME, Rae DS, Locke BZ, Keith SJ, Judd LL, Goodwin FK: Comorbidity of mental disorders with alcohol and other drug abuse. Results from the Epidemiologic Catchment Area (ECA) Study. JAMA 1990; 264:2511–2518 [C]

224. Blacker D, Tsuang MT: Contested boundaries of bipolar disorder and the limits of categorical diagnosis in psychiatry. Am J Psychiatry 1992; 149:1473–1483 [F]

225. Akiskal HS, Hirschfeld MA, Yerevanian BI: The relationship of personality to affective disorders. Arch Gen Psychiatry 1983; 40:801–810 [F]

226. van Gent EM, Vida SL, Zwart FM: Group therapy in addition to lithium therapy in patients with bipolar disorders. Acta Psychiatr Belg 1988; 88:405–418 [B]

227. Wulsin L, Bachop M, Hoffman D: Group therapy in manic-depressive illness. Am J Psychother 1988; 42:263–271 [F]

228. Graves JS: Living with mania: a study of outpatient group psychotherapy for bipolar patients. Am J Psychother 1993; 47:113–126 [B]

229. Shakir SA, Volkmar FR, Bacon S, Pfefferbaum A: Group psychotherapy as an adjunct to lithium maintenance. Am J Psychiatry 1979; 136:455–456 [B]

230. Volkmar FR, Bacon S, Shakir SA, Pfefferbaum A: Group therapy in the management of manic-depressive illness. Am J Psychother 1981; 35:226–234 [B]

231. Davenport YB, Ebert MH, Adland ML, Goodwin FK: Couples group therapy as an adjunct to lithium maintenance of the manic patient. Am J Orthopsychiatry 1977; 47:495–502 [G]

232. Ablon SL, Davenport YB, Gershon ES, Adland ML: The married manic. Am J Orthopsychiatry 1975; 45:854–866 [G]

233. Zarin DA, Pass TM: Lithium and the single episode: when to begin long-term prophylaxis for bipolar disorder. Med Care 1987; 25(12 suppl):S76–S84 [E]

234. Wehr TA: Sleep loss: a preventable cause of mania and other excited states. J Clin Psychiatry 1989; 50(Dec suppl):8–16 [F]

235. Gelenberg AJ: Catatonic syndrome. Lancet 1976; 1:1339–1341 [G]

236. Black DW, Winokur G, Nasrallah MA: Suicide in subtypes of major affective disorder: a comparison with general population suicide mortality. Arch Gen Psychiatry 1987; 44:878–880 [C]

237. Fawcett J, Scheftner W, Clark D, Hedeker D, Gibbons R, Coryell W: Clinical predictors of suicide in patients with major affective disorders: a controlled prospective study. Am J Psychiatry 1987; 144:35–40 [C]

238. Müller-Oerlinghausen B, Ahrens B, Grof E, Grof P, Lenz G, Schou M, Simhandl C, Thau K, Volk J, Wolf R, Wolf T: The effect of long-term lithium treatment on the mortality of patients with manic-depressive and schizoaffective illness. Acta Psychiatr Scand 1992; 86:218–222 [C]

239. Fetner HH, Geller B: Lithium and tricyclic antidepressants. Psychiatr Clin North Am 1992; 15:223–224 [F]

240. Hassanyeh F, Davison K: Bipolar affective psychosis with onset before age 16 years: report of 10 cases. Br J Psychiatry 1980; 137:530–539 [G]

241. Horowitz HA: Lithium and the treatment of adolescent manic depressive illness. Diseases of the Nervous System 1977; 38: 480–483 [G]

242. Hsu LK, Starzynski JM: Mania in adolescence. J Clin Psychiatry 1986; 47:596–599 [B]

243. Strober M, Morrell W, Burroughs J, Lampert C, Danforth H, Freeman R: A family study of bipolar I disorder in adolescence. Early onset of symptoms linked to increased familial loading and lithium resistance. J Affect Disord 1988; 15:255–268 [C]

244. Alessi N, Naylor MW, Ghaziuddin M, Zubieta JK: Update on lithium carbonate therapy in children and adolescents. J Am Acad Child Adolesc Psychiatry 1994; 33:291–304 [F]

245. Campbell M, Perry R, Green WH: Use of lithium in children and adolescents. Psychosomatics 1984; 25:95–106 [G]

246. Bertagnoli MW, Borchardt CM: A review of ECT for children and adolescents. J Am Acad Child Adolesc Psychiatry 1990; 29:302–307 [F]

247. Carlson GA: Bipolar disorder in children and adolescents, in Psychiatric Disorders in Children and Adolescents. Edited by Garfinkle BD, Carlson GA, Weller EB. Philadelphia, WB Saunders, 1990 [F]

248. Cohen LS, Friedman JM, Jefferson JW, Johnson EM, Weiner ML: A reevaluation of risk of in utero exposure to lithium. JAMA 1994; 271:146–150 [F]

249. Lier L, Kastrup M, Rafaelsen OJ: Psychiatric illness in relation to childbirth and pregnancy, II: diagnostic profiles, psychosocial and perinatal aspects. Nord Psykitr Tidsskr 1989; 43:535–542 [F]

250. Lindhout D, Meinardi H. Spina bifida and in-utero exposure to valproate (letter). Lancet 1984; 2:396 [G]

251. Rosa FW: Spina bifida in infants of women treated with carbamazepine during pregnancy. N Engl J Med 1991; 324:674–677 [D]

252. Centers for Disease Control: Valproate: a new cause of birth defects—report from Italy and follow-up from France. Morbidity and Mortality Weekly Report 1983; 32:438–439 [C]

253. Pastuszak A, Schick-Boschetto B, Zuber C, Feldkamp M, Pinelli M, Sihn S, Donnenfeld A, McCormack M, Leen-Mitchell M, Woodland C, Gardner A, Hom M, Koren G: Pregnancy outcome following first-trimester exposure to fluoxetine (Prozac). JAMA 1993; 269:2246–2248 [C]

254. Schou M, Amdisen A, Steenstrup OR: Lithium and pregnancy–II: hazards to women given lithium during pregnancy and delivery. Br Med J 1973; 2: 137–138 [G]

255. Marcos LR, Cancro R: Psychopharmacotherapy of Hispanic depressed patients: clinical observations. Am J Psychiatry 1982; 36:505–512 [G]

256. Escobar JI, Tuason VB: Antidepressant agents: a cross-cultural study. Psychopharmacol Bull 1980; 16:49–52 [B]

257. Ambelas A: Life events and mania: a special relationship? Br J Psychiatry 1987; 150:235–240 [G]

258. Swann AC, Secunda SK, Stokes PE, Croughan J, Davis JM, Koslow SH, Maas JW: Stress, depression, and mania: relationship between perceived role of stressful events and clinical and biochemical characteristics. Acta Psychiatr Scand 1990; 81:389–397 [C]

PRACTICE GUIDELINE

FOR

THE TREATMENT OF

PATIENTS WITH

SUBSTANCE USE

DISORDERS

Alcohol, Cocaine, Opioids

WORK GROUP ON SUBSTANCE USE DISORDERS

Steven M. Mirin, M.D., Chair

Steven L. Batki, M.D.
Oscar Bukstein, M.D.
Patricia Gonzales Isbell, M.D.
Herbert Kleber, M.D.
Richard S. Schottenfeld, M.D.
Roger D. Weiss, M.D.
Valery W. Yandow, M.D.

Contents

Treatment of Patients With Substance Use Disorders: Alcohol, Cocaine, Opioids

Introduction

This guideline seeks to provide guidance to psychiatrists who care for patients with substance use disorders. It summarizes somatic and psychosocial treatments that are used for such patients, as well as the data relevant to the choice of treatments, and is applicable to psychiatrists in any treatment setting who make treatment decisions with their patients. Psychiatrists care for such patients in a variety of practice settings and frequently work in collaboration with other professionals. The psychiatrist's precise role varies, depending on the specific clinical situation. The psychiatrist may provide all of the care or may work as part of a treatment team with other professionals: it is understood that in some situations the psychiatrist will not be directly providing all of the treatments recommended in this guideline.

The guideline is divided into four main sections. Section III provides an overview of the principles of treatment, and the evidence underlying them, that are broadly applicable to patients with all forms of substance use disorders. Sections IV, V, and VI discuss the treatment of patients with alcohol, cocaine, and opioid use disorders, respectively; these sections build on the general discussion in section III and are not intended to stand alone. Although some of the treatment principles discussed in each of these three sections may apply to a broader group of substances (e.g., there is an area of overlap between the treatment of patients with alcohol use disorders and treatment of patients with other sedative/hypnotic use disorders), the basis of the discussion and the resulting recommendations are based on data relevant to alcohol, cocaine, and opioids. These three substances were chosen because of their public health importance, the availability of a base of treatment research, and their utility in illustrating a variety of treatment modalities. A practice guideline on the treatment of patients with nicotine dependence is currently in development. The treatment of patients with other substance use disorders will be addressed in future guidelines.

The degree of specificity of recommendations in this guideline depends on the quality of available research and the degree of consensus among expert clinicians. By providing guidance in choosing among available treatment options and making specific recommendations whenever possible, the guideline reflects the variability in the availability of relevant research data and in the extent of clinical consensus. In section I, recommendations are summarized and coded according to their degree of clinical confidence.

The use of terminology in this guideline is consistent with DSM-IV. The term "substance-related disorders" encompasses substance use disorders and substance-induced disorders. The focus of this guideline is on the treatment of patients with substance use disorders, which include substance abuse and substance dependence. Many of these patients have coexisting conditions; psychiatrists should therefore consider, but not be limited to, the practice guidelines applicable to both substance use disorders and other comorbid disorders that may be present.

I. Summary of Recommendations

The following executive summary is intended to provide an overview of the organization and scope of recommendations in this practice guideline. The treatment of patients with substance use disorders requires the consideration of many factors and cannot adequately be reviewed in a brief summary. The reader is encouraged to consult the relevant portions of the guideline when specific treatment recommendations are sought. This summary is not intended to stand by itself. Unless otherwise noted, the principles and recommendations set forth under general substance use disorders (section III) apply to the treatment of patients with alcohol (section IV), cocaine (section V), and opioid (section VI) use disorders.

A. Coding System

Each recommendation is identified as falling into one of three categories of endorsement, indicated by a bracketed Roman numeral following the statement. The three categories represent varying levels of clinical confidence:

[I]   recommended with substantial clinical confidence.
[II] recommended with moderate clinical confidence.
[III] may be recommended on the basis of individual circumstances.

B. Substance Use Disorders:
General Treatment Principles and Alternatives

Substance use disorders constitute a major public health problem, costing our society in excess of $300 billion annually, including direct and indirect costs.

Individuals with substance use disorders are heterogeneous with regard to a number of clinically important features. Treatment for individuals with substance use disorders includes an assessment phase, the treatment of intoxication and withdrawal when necessary, and the development and implementation of an overall treatment strategy. Two general treatment strategies are used, depending on the clinical circumstances: drug free and substitution.

Substance use disorders may affect many domains of an individual's functioning and frequently require multimodal treatment. Goals of treatment include reduction in the use and effects of substances or achievement of abstinence, reduction in the frequency and severity of relapse, and improvement in psychological and social functioning.

1.   Assessment

A comprehensive psychiatric evaluation is essential to guide the treatment of a patient with a substance use disorder (I). The assessment includes a) a detailed history of the patient's past and present substance use and its effects on cognitive, psychological, behavioral, and physiologic functioning; b) a general medical and psychiatric history and examination; c) a history of prior psychiatric treatments and outcomes; d) a family and social history; e) screening of blood, breath, or urine for abused substances; and f) other laboratory tests to help confirm the presence or absence of comorbid conditions frequently associated with substance use disorders.

2.   Psychiatric management

Psychiatric management is the foundation of treatment for patients with substance use disorders (I). Psychiatric management has the following specific objectives: establishing and maintaining a therapeutic alliance, monitoring the patient's clinical status, managing intoxication and withdrawal states, developing and facilitating adherence to a treatment plan, preventing relapse, providing education about substance use disorders, and reducing the morbidity and sequelae of substance use disorders. Generally, psychiatric management is combined with specific treatments carried out in a collaborative fashion with professionals of various disciplines at a variety of sites, including community-based agencies, clinics, hospitals, detoxification programs, and residential treatment facilities.

3.   Specific treatments

The specific pharmacologic and psychosocial treatments for patients with substance use disorders are reviewed separately, although they are generally studied and applied in the context of treatment programs that combine a number of different treatment modalities. It is uncommon for a single treatment to be effective when used in isolation.

4.   Pharmacologic treatments

Pharmacologic treatments are beneficial for selected patients with substance use disorders (I). The categories of pharmacologic treatments are a) medications to treat intoxication and withdrawal states; b) medications to decrease the reinforcing effects of abused substances; c) medications that discourage the use of substances by inducing unpleasant consequences through a drug-drug interaction or by coupling substance use with an unpleasant, drug-induced condition; d) agonist substitution therapy; and e) medications to treat comorbid psychiatric conditions.

5.   Psychosocial treatments

Psychosocial treatments are essential components of a comprehensive treatment program (I). Although controlled studies are few in number and many have major design limitations, the available data, along with clinical experience, indicate that the following forms of treatment are effective for selected patients with substance use disorders: cognitive behavioral therapies, behavioral therapies, psychodynamic/interpersonal therapies, group and family therapies, and participation in self-help groups.

6. Formulation and implementation of a treatment plan

The goals of treatment and the specific choice of treatments needed to achieve these goals may vary among different patients and for the same patient at different phases of the illness. Since many substance use disorders are chronic, patients usually require long-term treatment, although the intensity and specific components may vary over time. A treatment plan is developed that includes the following components: a) psychiatric management; b) a strategy for achieving abstinence or reducing the effects or use of illicit substances; c) efforts to enhance ongoing compliance with the treatment program, prevent relapse, and improve functioning; and d) additional treatments necessary for patients with comorbid conditions.

7. Treatment settings

Treatment settings vary with regard to the availability of specific treatment modalities, the degree of restriction on access to substances that are likely to be abused, the availability of general medical and psychiatric care, and the overall milieu and treatment philosophy.

Patients should be treated in the least restrictive setting that is likely to be safe and effective (I). Decisions regarding the site of care should be based on patients' ability to cooperate with and benefit from the treatment offered, the need for structure and support, patients' ability to refrain from illicit use of substances, their ability to avoid high-risk behaviors, and the need for particular treatments that may be available only in certain settings (I). Patients move from one level of care to another on the basis of these factors and an assessment of their ability to safely benefit from a different level of care (I).

Commonly available treatment settings include hospitals, residential treatment facilities, partial hospital care, and outpatient programs. Hospitalization is appropriate for a) patients with a drug overdose that cannot be safely treated in an outpatient or emergency room setting; b) patients at risk for severe or medically complicated withdrawal syndromes; c) patients with comorbid general medical conditions that make ambulatory detoxification unsafe; d) patients with a documented history of not engaging in or benefiting from treatment in a less intensive setting (e.g., residential or outpatient); e) patients with a level of psychiatric comorbidity that would markedly impair their ability to participate in, comply with, or benefit from treatment or whose comorbid disorder would by itself require hospital-level care (e.g., depression with suicidal thoughts, acute psychosis); f) patients manifesting substance use or other behaviors that constitute an acute danger to themselves or others; or g) patients who have not responded to less intensive treatment efforts and whose substance use disorder(s) poses an ongoing threat to their physical and mental health (I).

Residential treatment is indicated for patients who do not meet the clinical criteria for hospitalization but whose lives and social interactions have come to focus predominantly on substance use, and who lack sufficient social and vocational skills and drug-free social supports to maintain abstinence in an outpatient setting (II). Residential treatment of 3 months or more is associated with better long-term outcome in such patients (II).

Partial hospital care should be considered for patients who require intensive care but have a reasonable probability of refraining from illicit use of substances outside a restricted setting (II). Partial hospital settings are frequently used for patients leaving hospitals or residential settings who remain at high risk for relapse. The latter include patients who are thought to lack sufficient motivation to continue in treatment, patients with severe psychiatric comorbidity and/or a history of relapse to substance use in the immediate posthospital or postresidential period, and those returning to high-risk environments who have limited psychosocial supports for remaining drug free. Partial hospital programs are also indicated for patients who are doing poorly in intensive outpatient treatment (II).

Outpatient treatment of substance use disorders is appropriate for patients whose clinical condition or environmental circumstances do not require a more intensive level of care (I). As in other treatment settings, a comprehensive approach using, where indicated, a variety of psychotherapeutic and pharmacologic interventions, along with behavioral monitoring, is optimal.

The duration of treatment should be tailored to individual needs and may vary from a few months to several years (I). Monitoring for substance use should be intensified during periods of high risk of relapse, including the early stages of treatment, times of transition to less intensive levels of care, and the first year following cessation of active treatment (I).

8.   Clinical features influencing treatment

Treatment planning and implementation should reflect consideration of comorbid psychiatric and general medical conditions, gender-related factors (including the possibility of pregnancy), age (e.g., for children, adolescents, and the elderly), social milieu and living environment, cultural factors, and family characteristics. The high prevalence of comorbid psychiatric disorders and the diagnostic distinction between substance use symptoms and other disorders should receive particular attention, and specific treatment for comorbid disorders should be provided (I).

C.   Alcohol Use Disorders: Treatment Principles and Alternatives

Psychiatric management (section III.C) forms the basis for the treatment of patients with alcohol use disorders.

1.   Treatment settings

Patients with alcohol withdrawal must be detoxified in a setting that provides for frequent clinical assessment and the provision of any necessary treatments (I). Some outpatient settings can accommodate these requirements and may be appropriate for patients deemed to be at low risk of a complicated withdrawal syndrome. However, those who have a prior history of delirium tremens, whose documented history of very heavy alcohol use and high tolerance places them at risk for a complicated withdrawal syndrome, who are concurrently abusing other drugs, who have a severe comorbid general medical or psychiatric disorder, or who repeatedly fail to cooperate with or benefit from outpatient detoxification are more likely to require a residential or hospital setting that can safely provide the necessary care (I). Patients in severe withdrawal (i.e., delirium tremens) require treatment in a hospital setting (I).

Most treatments for patients with alcohol dependence or abuse can be successfully conducted outside of the hospital (e.g., in outpatient, day hospital, or partial hospital settings) (II). However, patients who are unlikely to benefit from less intensive and less restrictive alternatives may need to be hospitalized at times during their treatment. The general criteria for hospitalization are summarized in sections III.G.1 and IV.B.

2. Pharmacologic treatments

The effectiveness of specific pharmacotherapies for alcohol-dependent patients is not well established. Naltrexone may attenuate some of the reinforcing effects of alcohol, but there are limited data regarding the long-term efficacy for patients with alcohol use disorders (II). Disulfiram is an effective adjunct to a comprehensive treatment program in reliable, motivated patients whose drinking may be triggered by events that suddenly increase alcohol craving (II). Patients with impulsive behavior, psychotic symptoms, or suicidal thoughts are poor candidates for disulfiram treatment (I).

In patients with clearly established comorbid psychiatric disorders, treatment specifically directed at these disorders is indicated (I). Such treatment must be coordinated with other treatments for the substance use disorder.

3. Psychosocial treatments

Psychosocial treatments found effective for selected patients with alcohol use disorders include cognitive behavioral therapies (II), behavioral therapies (I), psychodynamic/interpersonal therapy (III), brief interventions (II), marital and family therapy (II), and group therapies (II). Patient participation in self-help groups, such as Alcoholics Anonymous, is frequently helpful (II).

4. Management of alcohol intoxication and withdrawal

The acutely intoxicated patient should be monitored and maintained in a safe environment (II).

Symptoms of alcohol withdrawal typically begin within 4–12 hours after cessation or reduction of alcohol use, peak in intensity during the second day of abstinence, and generally resolve within 4–5 days. Serious complications include seizures, hallucinations, and delirium.

Clinical assessment of intoxicated patients and those manifesting signs and symptoms of withdrawal should include laboratory determination of the presence of other substances (I). The treatment of patients in moderate to severe withdrawal includes efforts to reduce central nervous system (CNS) irritability and restore physiologic homeostasis (I), and it requires the use of thiamine and fluids (I), benzodiazepines (II), and, in selected patients, other medications (II). Once clinical stability is achieved, the tapering of benzodiazepines and other medications should be carried out as necessary, and the patient should be observed for the re-emergence of withdrawal symptoms and the emergence of signs and symptoms suggestive of a comorbid psychiatric disorder (I).

5. Other clinical features influencing treatment

In addition to the considerations addressed in section III.H.3, the treatment of pregnant women with alcohol use disorders is complicated by the risk of fetal alcohol syndrome and the corresponding urgency of minimizing the intake of alcohol (I).

D.   Cocaine Use Disorders: Treatment Principles and Alternatives

Psychiatric management (section III.C) forms the basis for the treatment of patients with cocaine use disorders.

1.   Treatment settings

Clinical and research experience suggests that intensive (i.e., more than twice a week) outpatient treatment, in which a variety of treatment modalities are simultaneously used and in which the focus is the maintenance of abstinence, is effective for most patients with cocaine use disorders (II).

2.   Pharmacologic treatments

Pharmacologic treatment is not ordinarily indicated as an initial treatment for patients with cocaine dependence. However, patients with more severe dependence or individuals who fail to respond to psychosocial treatment should be considered for treatment with dopaminergic medications (III).

3.   Psychosocial treatments

Psychosocial treatments focusing on abstinence are effective for most patients with cocaine use disorders (II). The following specific types of psychotherapies have been evaluated and have been shown to have variable efficacy with different groups of patients: cognitive behavioral therapies (II), behavioral therapies (II), and psychodynamic psychotherapy (III). In addition, regular participation in self-help groups may improve the outcome for selected patients with cocaine use disorders (III).

4. Management of cocaine intoxication and withdrawal

Cocaine intoxication can produce hypertension, tachycardia, seizures, and paranoid delusions. The syndrome is usually self-limited and typically requires only supportive care (II). Acutely agitated patients may benefit from sedation with benzodiazepines (III).

Following cessation of cocaine use, anhedonia and craving are common. Most patients will not benefit from any currently available pharmacotherapy for withdrawal symptoms. The efficacy of dopamine agonists (e.g., amantadine, bromocriptine) in the treatment of acute cocaine withdrawal has not been clearly demonstrated (III).

5. Other clinical features influencing treatment

In addition to the considerations discussed in section III.H.3, the treatment of pregnant women with cocaine use disorders is complicated by the increased risk of prematurity, low birth weight, stillbirth, and sudden infant death syndrome and the corresponding urgency of minimizing the intake of cocaine (I).

E. Opioid Use Disorders: Treatment Principles and Alternatives

Psychiatric management (section III.C) forms the basis for the treatment of patients with opioid use disorders (I). Some opioid-dependent patients will be able to achieve abstinence from all opioid drugs; many others will require long-term maintenance with opioid agonists (e.g., methadone or LAAM [L-α-acetylmethadol or levomethadyl acetate]).

1. Treatment settings

In addition to the standard treatment settings described in section III.G, therapeutic communities have been found effective in the treatment of patients with opioid use disorders (II).

2. Pharmacologic treatments

Maintenance on methadone or LAAM is appropriate for patients with a prolonged history (>1 year) of opioid dependence and has been shown to reduce the morbidity associated with opioid dependence (I). The goals of treatment are to achieve a stable maintenance dose and to facilitate engagement in a comprehensive program of rehabilitation (I).

Maintenance on naltrexone is an alternative treatment strategy whose utility is often limited by lack of patient compliance and low treatment retention (II).

For some patients, abstinence can never be achieved, but important reductions in morbidity and mortality can be achieved through efforts to reduce the effects of opioid use.

3. Psychosocial treatments

Psychosocial treatments are effective components of a comprehensive treatment plan for patients with opioid use disorders (II). Cognitive behavioral therapies (II), behavioral therapies (II), psychodynamic psychotherapy (III), group and family therapies (III), and self-help groups (III) have been found effective for some patients with opioid use disorders. The choice of treatment should be made after consideration of the patient's preferences, the clinical issues to be addressed, associated comorbid psychopathology, and past response to various treatment modalities.

4. Management of opioid intoxication and withdrawal

Acute opioid intoxication of mild to moderate degree usually does not require specific treatment (II). However, severe opioid overdose, marked by respiratory depression, may be fatal and requires treatment in a hospital emergency room or inpatient setting (I). Naloxone will reverse respiratory depression and other manifestations of opioid overdose (I).

The treatment of opioid withdrawal is directed at safely ameliorating acute symptoms and facilitating entry into a long-term treatment program for opioid use disorders (I). Strategies found to be effective include methadone or LAAM substitution with gradual tapering (I); abrupt discontinuation of opioids, with the use of clonidine to suppress withdrawal symptoms (II); and clonidine-naltrexone detoxification (II). Buprenorphine substitution followed by abrupt discontinuation of buprenorphine (II) has also been found to be effective in laboratory settings but is not yet approved for use in clinical practice. Monitoring for the presence of other substances (particularly alcohol, benzodiazepines, or other anxiolytic or sedative agents) is essential because the concurrent use of or withdrawal from other substances can complicate the treatment of opioid withdrawal (I).

5. Other clinical features influencing treatment

A substantial number of opioid-dependent patients have comorbid psychiatric disorders that must be identified and treated concurrently with the patients' substance use disorders (I).

The use of opioids by injection is associated with high risk of general medical complications, such as bacterial endocarditis, hepatitis, HIV infection, and tuberculosis.

In addition to the considerations discussed in section III.H.3, the treatment of pregnant women with opioid use disorders is complicated by the increased risk of low birth weight, prematurity, neonatal abstinence syndrome, stillbirth, and sudden infant death syndrome and the corresponding urgency of minimizing the intake of opioids (I).

II. Disease Definition, Epidemiology, and Natural History

By any measure, substance use disorders constitute a major public health problem, costing our society in excess of $300 billion annually, including the costs of treatment, related health problems, absenteeism, lost productivity, drug-related crime and incarceration, and efforts in education and prevention (1). (The issues raised by nicotine use disorders are sufficiently different to warrant a separate guideline and are not included in this discussion unless specifically mentioned.)

The motivation for using any psychoactive substance is, in part, related to the acute and chronic effects of these agents on mood, cognition, and behavior. In some individuals the subjective changes (e.g., euphoria, tension relief) that accompany substance intoxication are experienced as highly pleasurable and lead to repetitive use. About 15% of regular users become psychologically dependent in that they come to believe that they are unable to function optimally in social, work, or other settings without experiencing some degree of substance intoxication. These individuals, in turn, are at high risk of developing one or more substance use disorders as defined in the DSM-IV criteria (2).

A. DSM-IV Criteria for Substance Dependence and Abuse

1. Criteria for substance dependence

A maladaptive pattern of substance use, leading to clinically significant impairment or distress, as manifested by three (or more) of the following, occurring at any time in the same 12-month period:

1) tolerance, as defined by either of the following:

   a) a need for markedly increased amounts of the substance to achieve intoxication or desired effect
   b) markedly diminished effect with continued use of the same amount of the substance

2) withdrawal, as manifested by either of the following:

   a) the characteristic withdrawal syndrome for the substance . . .
   b) the same (or a closely related) substance is taken to relieve or avoid withdrawal symptoms

3)   the substance is often taken in larger amounts or over a longer period than was intended

4)   there is a persistent desire or unsuccessful efforts to cut down or control substance use

5)   a great deal of time is spent in activities necessary to obtain the substance (e.g., visiting multiple doctors or driving long distances), use the substance (e.g., chain-smoking), or recover from its effects

6)   important social, occupational, or recreational activities are given up or reduced because of substance use

7)   the substance use is continued despite knowledge of having a persistent or recurrent physical or psychological problem that is likely to have been caused or exacerbated by the substance (e.g., current cocaine use despite recognition of cocaine-induced depression, or continued drinking despite recognition that an ulcer was made worse by alcohol consumption)

2. Criteria for substance abuse

A.   A maladaptive pattern of substance use leading to clinically significant impairment or distress, as manifested by one (or more) of the following, occurring within a 12-month period:

1)   recurrent substance use resulting in a failure to fulfill major role obligations at work, school, or home (e.g., repeated absences or poor work performance related to substance use; substance-related absences, suspensions, or expulsions from school; neglect of children or household)

2)   recurrent substance use in situations in which it is physically hazardous (e.g., driving an automobile or operating a machine when impaired by substance use)

3)   recurrent substance-related legal problems (e.g., arrests for substance-related disorderly conduct)

4)   continued substance use despite having persistent or recurrent social or interpersonal problems caused or exacerbated by the effects of the substance (e.g., arguments with spouse about consequences of intoxication, physical fights)

B.   The symptoms have never met the criteria for substance dependence for this class of substance.

In using the DSM-IV criteria, one should specify whether substance dependence is *with* physiologic dependence (i.e., there is evidence of tolerance or withdrawal) or *without* physiologic dependence (i.e., no evidence of tolerance or withdrawal). In addition, patients may be variously classified as currently manifesting a pattern of abuse or dependence or as in remission. Those in remission can be divided into four subtypes—full, early partial, sustained, and sustained partial—on the basis of whether any of the criteria for abuse or dependence have been met and over what time frame. The remission category can also be used for patients receiving agonist therapy (e.g., methadone maintenance) or for those living in a controlled drug-free environment.

B.   Disease Definition and Diagnostic Features

1.   Cross-sectional features

Patients presenting for treatment of a substance use disorder frequently manifest signs and symptoms of substance-induced intoxication or withdrawal. The clinical picture varies with the substance used, its dosage, the duration of action, the time elapsed since the last dose, the presence or absence of tolerance, and/or psychiatric or general medical comorbidity. The expectations of the patient, his or her style of responding to states of intoxication or physical discomfort, and the setting in which intoxication or withdrawal is taking place also play a role.

Patients experiencing substance-induced intoxication generally manifest changes in mood, cognition, and/or behavior. Mood-related changes may range from euphoria to depression, with considerable lability in response to, or independent of, external events. Cognitive changes may include shortened attention span, impaired concentration, and disturbances of thinking (e.g., delusions) and/or perception (e.g., hallucinations). Behavioral changes may include wakefulness or somnolence, lethargy or hyperactivity. Impairment in social and occupational functioning is also common in intoxicated individuals.

Other cross-sectional diagnostic features commonly found in patients with substance use disorders include those related to any comorbid psychiatric or general medical disorders that may be present. Psychiatric disorders commonly found in such patients include conduct disorder (particularly the aggressive subtype) in children and adolescents (3, 4), depression, bipolar disorder, schizophrenia, anxiety disorders, eating disorders, pathological gambling, antisocial personality disorder, and other personality disorders (5–13).

Examples of general medical problems that may be directly related to substance use include cardiac toxicity resulting from acute cocaine intoxication, respiratory depression and coma in severe opioid overdose, and hepatic cirrhosis after prolonged heavy drinking (14). Examples of general medical conditions frequently associated with opioid-dependent individuals who administer opioids by injection include subacute bacterial endocarditis, HIV infection, and hepatitis. Patients whose substance dependence is accompanied by diminished self-care and/or high levels of risk-taking behavior are at increased risk of experiencing malnutrition, physical trauma, and HIV infection (15).

2.   Longitudinal features

Patients with substance use disorders frequently present with a long history of repeated episodes of intoxication and withdrawal, interspersed with attempts to remain substance free. In patients who meet the DSM-IV criteria for substance abuse, episodes of intoxication may be sporadic and brief, rarely requiring general medical or psychiatric intervention.

Patients who meet the DSM-IV criteria for dependence often experience repeated episodes of intoxication that may last for weeks or months, interrupted by voluntary or involuntary periods of self-managed, or medically managed, withdrawal. Partial or complete withdrawal from abused substances may be followed by variable periods of self-imposed or involuntary (e.g., during periods of incarceration) abstinence, often ending in relapse to substance use and, eventually, resumption of dependence.

In some patients, dependence on a single substance may lead to use of, and ultimately dependence on, another substance (e.g., the development of alcohol dependence in patients already dependent on opioids or cocaine) (16). In such patients, replacement of one form of substance dependence by another may occur.

Although many individuals who abuse alcohol or illicit substances maintain their ability to function in interpersonal relationships and in the work setting, substance-dependent patients presenting for treatment often manifest profound psychological, social, general medical, legal, and financial problems. These may include disrupted interpersonal (particularly family) relationships, absenteeism, job loss, criminal behavior, poor academic or work performance, failure to develop adaptive coping skills, and a general constriction of normal life activities. Peer relationships often focus extensively on obtaining and using illicit drugs or alcohol. The risk of accidents, violence, and suicide is significantly greater than for the general population (17).

C. Natural History and Course

Not uncommonly, initial experiences with substance use take place before puberty. At the earliest stages of use, experimenters or casual users who go on to develop a substance use disorder are generally indistinguishable from their peers with respect to the type and frequency of substance use. However, early onset and/or regular use of "gateway" drugs, such as alcohol, marijuana, or nicotine, and early evidence of aggressive behavior, intrafamilial disturbances, and associating with substance-using peers contribute to, and predict, continued substance use and the subsequent development of abuse and dependence (18, 19).

In adolescents, growing preoccupation with substance use, frequent episodes of intoxication, use of drugs with greater dependence liability (e.g., opioids, cocaine), and a preference for routes of administration that result in quicker onset of drug effects (e.g., by injection, freebasing) and for more rapidly acting preparations (e.g., methamphetamine) presage the development of substance dependence. Although in most cases the onset of substance use disorders occurs in the late teens and early 20s, some individuals begin abusing substances in mid to late adulthood (20, 21).

Although experience with multiple substances often continues throughout adolescence, some individuals settle on a "drug of choice" early on. Drug preference is shaped by a variety of factors, including current fashion, availability, peer influences, and individual biological and psychological factors. Gender-specific differences in drug preference (e.g., heroin use in males, sedative/hypnotic and benzodiazepine use in females) have diminished somewhat over the last two decades. Although substance abuse and dependence appear to aggregate in families, some of this effect may be explained by the concurrent familial distribution of antisocial personality disorder, which may predispose individuals to the development of these disorders. On the other hand, genetic factors do affect the risk of developing alcoholism, particularly in males with biological male relatives who are also alcoholic (22, 23) and, to a lesser extent, in females with strong family histories of the disorder (24, 25). Finally, some clinicians have suggested, on the basis of retrospective reports from patients, that drug preference is also shaped by the "fit" between specific drug effects and the psychological needs of the user (26). However, there are no controlled studies to support this "self-medication" paradigm.

While there is considerable heterogeneity, for many patients substance dependence has a chronic course, often lasting for years. Periods of sustained use are interrupted by periods of partial or complete remission. Although some individuals are able to achieve prolonged periods of abstinence without formal treatment, abstinence or periods of greatly reduced substance use are more likely to be sustained by patients who are able to maintain active participation in formalized treatment and/or self-help groups (e.g., Alcoholics Anonymous) (27–30). Patients who experience a severe life crisis (e.g., loss of an important relationship, incarceration, or serious general medical sequelae of substance use) are generally more motivated to seek treatment, but most still require external support to maintain their motivation to continue in treatment beyond the initial stages (e.g., detoxification).

During the first several years of treatment, most substance-dependent patients continue to relapse, although with decreasing frequency. Risk of relapse is higher in the first 12 months after the onset of a remission. Many patients experience several cycles of remission and relapse before they conclude that a return to "controlled" substance use is not possible for them. Regardless of the treatment site or the modalities employed, the frequency, intensity, and duration of treatment participation are positively correlated with improved outcome (31).

The majority of patients treated for substance dependence (up to 70% in some studies) are eventually able to stop compulsive use and either abstain from abused substances entirely or experience only brief episodes of substance use that do not progress to abuse or dependence; only a minority of patients (15%–20%) exhibit a pattern of chronic relapse (i.e., over 10–20 years) requiring repetitive intervention. Of those who remain abstinent for 2 years, almost 90% are substance free at 10 years, and those who remain substance free for 10 years have a very high likelihood (i.e., >90%) of being substance free at 20 years (30, 32, 33). Prolonged abstinence, accompanied by improvement in social and occupational functioning, is more apt to occur in those who have lower levels of premorbid psychopathology, demonstrate the ability to develop new relationships, and consistently make use of self-help groups (e.g., Alcoholics Anonymous) (28, 34).

D. Epidemiology

Estimates developed by the Institute of Medicine (35) suggest that there are approximately 5.5 million individuals, or about 2.7% of the U.S. population over age 12, who clearly

(2.4 million) or probably (3.1 million) need treatment for drug use disorders and an additional 13 million who clearly or probably need treatment for alcohol use disorders. Of these, approximately two-thirds are men and approximately one-third concurrently have more than one substance use disorder (36).

Substance use disorders are associated with a significant increase in morbidity and mortality, particularly among men. Each year nonnicotine substance dependence is, directly or indirectly, responsible for at least 40% of all hospital admissions and approximately 25% of all deaths (500,000 per year) (37, 38). Approximately 100,000 deaths per year result directly from the use of illicit drugs or alcohol. Two-thirds of these deaths occur in individuals who are dependent on heroin or cocaine; nearly 40% occur in individuals between the ages of 30 and 39. Black men and women appear to be at much higher risk of drug-related mortality than their white counterparts. More than one-third of all new AIDS cases occur among users of intravenous drugs or individuals who have had sexual contact with such individuals, and AIDS-related illnesses account for about 8,000 deaths per year among intravenous drug users (39).

Substance use disorders also exert a profound impact on those who come in contact with these individuals. For example, approximately one-half of all highway fatalities involve either a driver or pedestrian who is intoxicated, and more than 50% of all cases of domestic violence occur under the influence of illicit drugs or alcohol (40). In addition, estimates based on urine testing in general populations suggest that between 7.5% and 15.0% of all pregnant women have had recent exposure to drugs of abuse (excluding alcohol) at the time they first seek prenatal care (41, 42).

Finally, substance use disorders are frequently associated with other forms of psychopathology. The lifetime prevalence of comorbid axis I psychiatric disorders in individuals with substance use disorders (including those with alcohol dependence or abuse) is between 20% and 90%, depending on the population screened and the rigor of the diagnostic criteria used, with treatment-seeking patients being at the higher end of the range (43–50). Approximately one-third of hospitalized psychiatric patients manifest comorbid nonnicotine substance use disorders (51, 52).

III. General Treatment Principles and Alternatives

Individuals with substance use disorders are heterogeneous with regard to a number of clinically important features:

- ❖ the number and type of substances used;
- ❖ the severity of the disorder and the degree of associated functional impairment;
- ❖ the associated general medical and psychiatric conditions;

❖ the patient's strengths (protective/resiliency factors) and vulnerabilities; and
❖ the social/environmental context in which the individual lives and will be treated.

Although the full spectrum of substance use disorders includes conditions that have a narrow impact on an individual's health and functioning, many patients have more severe conditions that broadly affect their health and functioning and that are long-term and/or relapsing in nature. Individuals with more severe conditions, which are less responsive to low-intensity treatments, are the focus of much of this guideline.

Treatment for individuals with substance use disorders may be thought of as occurring in phases:

❖ assessment phase, during which information on the aforementioned cross-sectional and longitudinal features, as well as other critical information, is obtained and integrated;
❖ treatment of intoxication/withdrawal, as necessary; and
❖ development and implementation of an overall treatment strategy.

Depending on the clinical circumstances, the treatment strategy may emphasize the individual's need to remain drug free or it may entail substitution of one presumably safer drug (e.g., methadone) for another (e.g., heroin). Substance use disorders may affect many domains of an individual's functioning, and they frequently require multimodal treatment. Some components of treatment may be focused directly on the substance use, and others may be focused on the associated conditions that have contributed to or resulted from the substance use disorder.

The specific pharmacologic and psychosocial treatments for patients with substance use disorders are reviewed separately, although they are generally studied and applied in the context of treatment programs that combine a number of different treatment modalities. It is uncommon for a single treatment to be effective when used in isolation.

A.   Goals of Treatment

Long-range goals of treatment for patients with substance use disorders include reduction in the use and effects of abused substances, the achievement of abstinence, reduction in the frequency of relapses, and rehabilitation. For some patients, abstinence can never be achieved or can be achieved only after many years of either continuous or episodic treatment. However, even in the absence of complete abstinence, important reductions in morbidity and mortality can be achieved through reduction in the frequency and intensity of substance use and its associated sequels.

1.   Abstinence or reduction in the use and effects of substances

The ideal outcome for patients with substance use disorders is total cessation of substance use. However, many patients are unable or unmotivated to reach this goal, particularly in the early phases of treatment. Such patients can still be helped to minimize the direct and indirect effects of substance use. Interventions discussed in this guideline may result in substantial reductions in the general medical, psychiatric, interpersonal, familial/parental, occupational, and other difficulties commonly associated with substance abuse or dependence. Reductions in the amount or frequency of substance use, substitution of a less risky substance, and reduction of high-risk behavior may also be achieved. Engagement of the patient in a long-term treatment that may eventually lead to further reductions in substance use and its associated morbidity is an important goal of early treatment.

Psychiatrists frequently encounter patients who wish to reduce their substance use to a "controlled" level. Some of these patients may be helped to reach a stable level of use (e.g., controlled drinking) that does not cause morbidity (53), while patients who cannot achieve this outcome (the majority) may subsequently be more motivated to accept a goal of total abstinence. For some patients, achieving sustained abstinence is a long-term goal, but the psychiatrist and patient may, for clinical reasons, decide that reduction in the use and/or the harmful consequences of substance use (without total abstinence) is a reasonable intermediate goal. On the other hand, a goal of "controlled" substance use may be unattainable for many patients, may dissuade some from working toward abstinence, and is inappropriate when the psychiatrist believes that any substance use carries a risk of acute or chronic risk (e.g., high-risk behaviors that could be harmful to the patient or others).

Patients who achieve total abstinence from abused substances have the best long-term prognosis, and many experienced psychiatrists feel that since substance use by these patients may be accompanied by disinhibition, increased craving for other drugs, poor judgment, and an increased risk of relapse, patients should be abstinent from all potential drugs of abuse, including alcohol (49, 54, 55).

Patients who agree to pursue a goal of achieving and maintaining abstinence should be advised about the possibility of relapse and participate in developing a treatment plan that includes methods for early detection of and intervention in episodes of relapse.

2. Reduction in the frequency and severity of relapse

Reduction in the frequency and severity of relapse is a critical goal of treatment (56). A major focus of relapse prevention is helping patients to identify situations that place them at high risk for relapse and to develop alternative responses other than substance use. High-risk situations may include craving, a complex phenomenon resulting from patients' acute or chronic physiologic responses to substance withdrawal or their classically conditioned responses to cues associated with substance availability or withdrawal (57–59). For some patients, interpersonal or social situations constitute risk factors for relapse.

It is important for psychiatrists and their patients to understand the chronic, relapsing nature of these disorders for many patients. A reduction in the frequency and severity of relapses may often be a more realistic goal than the complete prevention of any further episodes.

3. Improvement in psychological and social/adaptive functioning

Substance use disorders are associated with problems in psychological development and social adjustment, alienation from friends and family, impaired school or work performance, financial and legal problems, and deterioration of patients' general health (60). Substance dependence is associated with failure to develop age-appropriate interpersonal or coping skills or gradual atrophy of such skills (61). A substantial minority of substance-dependent individuals lack the educational, social, or vocational skills necessary to succeed in our society. Treatment specifically directed toward repairing disrupted relationships, reducing impulsivity, developing social and vocational skills, and obtaining and maintaining employment is important in itself, as well as in helping to maximize the patient's chances of remaining substance free.

B. Assessment

In evaluating a patient with a suspected or confirmed substance use disorder, a comprehensive psychiatric evaluation is essential. Information should be sought from the patient and, with the patient's consent, available family members and peers, current and past treaters, employers, and others as appropriate. The assessment may include the following:

1. A systematic inquiry into the degree of associated intoxication; the severity of associated withdrawal syndromes; most recent dose and time elapsed since most recent use; the mode of onset, quantity, frequency, and duration of use; and subjective effects of all substances used, including drugs other than the patient's "drug of choice."

2. A comprehensive general medical and psychiatric history, including a complete physical and mental status examination, to ascertain the presence or absence of comorbid general medical or psychiatric disorders, as well as signs and symptoms of intoxication or withdrawal. In some cases, psychological or neuropsychological testing may be indicated.

3. A history of any prior treatment for substance use disorders, including the following characteristics: setting, context (e.g., voluntary or involuntary), modalities used, compliance, duration, and short- (3-month), intermediate- (1-year), and longer-term outcome as measured by subsequent substance use, the level of social and occupational functioning achieved, and other outcome variables. Prior efforts to control or stop substance use outside of a formal treatment setting should be discussed, as well as the patient's attitudes toward his or her previous treatment and nontreatment experiences.

4. A complete family, social, and substance use history, including information on familial substance use disorders or other psychiatric disorders; familial factors contributing to the development or perpetuation of substance use disorders (e.g., enabling behav-

iors); school or vocational adjustment, peer relationships, and financial or legal problems; the impact of the patient's current living environment on his or her ability to
comply with treatment and remain abstinent in the community; and the specific
circumstances of the patient's substance use (where, with whom, how much, and by
what route of administration).

5. Qualitative and quantitative blood and urine screening for drugs of abuse and laboratory tests for abnormalities that may accompany acute or chronic substance use.
These tests may also be used during treatment to monitor for potential relapse.

6. Screening for infectious and other diseases often found in substance-dependent persons (e.g., HIV, tuberculosis, hepatitis). Such individuals, particularly those with evidence of compromised immune function, are felt to be at high risk for these disorders.
For example, patients exposed to social or environmental conditions conducive to
the spread of tuberculosis should be routinely screened for this disorder.

C. Psychiatric Management

Successful treatment of substance use disorders may involve the use of multiple specific
treatments, which may vary for any one individual, may change over time, and may involve
more than one clinician. Psychiatric management is crucial in the ongoing process of
choosing among various treatments, monitoring the patient's clinical status, and coordinating different treatment components. Psychiatric management has the following specific
objectives: establishing and maintaining a therapeutic alliance, monitoring the patient's
clinical status, managing intoxication and withdrawal states, developing and facilitating
adherence to a treatment plan, preventing relapse, providing education about substance
use disorders, and reducing the morbidity and sequelae of substance use disorders.

The frequency, intensity, and focus of psychiatric management must be tailored to
meet each patient's needs, and the type of management is likely to vary over time, depending
on the patient's clinical status. In each of these endeavors the psychiatrist should, when
appropriate, work collaboratively with members of other professional disciplines, community-based agencies, treatment programs, and lay organizations to coordinate and integrate the patient's care and to address his or her social, vocational, educational, and
rehabilitative needs.

1. Establishing and maintaining a therapeutic alliance

An essential feature of psychiatric management of patients with substance use disorders is
the establishment and maintenance of a therapeutic alliance wherein the psychiatrist empathically obtains necessary diagnostic and treatment-related information, gains the confidence of the patient and significant others, and is available in times of crisis. The frequency
and duration of treatment contacts should be sufficient to engage the patient and, where
appropriate, significant others in a sustained effort to participate in all relevant treatment

modalities and, where appropriate, self-help groups. Within the context of this alliance, learning, practicing, and internalizing changes in attitudes and behavior conducive to relapse prevention are the primary goal of treatment (62, 63). The strength of the therapeutic alliance has been found to be a significant predictor of psychotherapy outcome (64). For example, in a sample of persons with substance use disorders (65), a stronger alliance predicted less drug use and better psychological functioning during follow-up.

2. Monitoring the patient's clinical status

The ongoing evaluation of the patient's safety is critical, because the patient's clinical status may change over time. It is particularly important to monitor patients for the potential emergence of suicidal or homicidal thoughts or of treatment-emergent side effects.

The ongoing assessment of the patient's psychiatric status is also necessary, to ensure that the patient is receiving the appropriate treatment(s) and to monitor the patient's response to treatment (e.g., determining the optimal dose of a drug and evaluating its efficacy).

Because relapse is common and is inconsistently self-reported by patients (particularly when use is met with negative consequences or a judgmental response), laboratory monitoring through breath, blood, saliva, and urine testing for drugs of abuse may be helpful in the early detection of relapse. Such monitoring is often initially conducted on a frequent and random schedule, since many drugs and their metabolites may be detected for only a few days after use. Random urine screening for recent (i.e., within the last 1–3 days) substance use should be supplemented by nonrandom testing when recent substance use is suspected.

Methods of urine screening vary as to levels of sensitivity, specificity, and cost. The psychiatrist should be familiar with the applicability and sensitivity of the available analytic methods and collection procedures used in local laboratories, and he or she should specify the type of drug use suspected. Direct supervision of patient voiding and other "chain of custody" procedures will help to ensure the validity and reliability of the test results.

The decision whether to test a patient's breath, blood, or urine depends on the type of drug use suspected, the drug's duration of action, the sensitivity of the test employed, and the clinical setting in which care is being rendered. For example, serum testing is useful for assessing very recent substance use (since it reflects current serum levels). Alcohol can be detected for up to 24 hours in urine, but breath testing is frequently preferred because of the immediacy of the results, noninvasiveness of the procedure, and low cost. Finally, there is some evidence that elevation of certain state markers, such as mean corpuscular volume (MCV) or γ-glutamyl transpeptidase (GGT), may indicate that a patient has recently returned to drinking.

3. Managing intoxication and withdrawal states

In general, acutely intoxicated patients require reassurance and maintenance in a safe and monitored environment, with efforts to decrease external stimulation and provide orientation and reality testing. Clinical assessment is directed toward ascertaining which substances have been used, the route of administration, dose, time since the last dose, whether the level of intoxication is waxing or waning, and other diagnostic information as already described. Management of acute intoxication is also directed toward hastening the removal of substances from the body, which may be accomplished through gastric lavage, in the case of substances that have been recently ingested, or through techniques that increase the rate of excretion of drugs or their active metabolites. Drug effects may also be reversed by administering drugs that antagonize the effects of abused substances. Examples include the administration of naloxone to patients who have overdosed with heroin or other opioids.

Not all intoxicated individuals will develop withdrawal symptoms. Withdrawal syndromes usually occur in tolerant and/or physically dependent individuals who discontinue or reduce their substance use after a period of heavy and prolonged use. The specific signs and symptoms of withdrawal vary according to the substance used, the time elapsed since the last dose, the rate of elimination and duration of action of the substance in question, the concomitant use of other prescribed or nonprescribed drugs, the presence or absence of concurrent general medical or psychiatric disorders, and individual biological and psychosocial variables.

Many patients use multiple substances simultaneously to enhance, ameliorate, or otherwise modify the degree or nature of their intoxication or to relieve withdrawal symptoms. Intoxication with alcohol and cocaine, use of heroin and cocaine ("speedball"), and the combined use of alcohol, marijuana, and/or benzodiazepines by opioid-dependent patients are particularly frequent. Patients using multiple substances (including alcohol) are at risk for withdrawal from each of these.

4. Reducing the morbidity and sequelae of substance use disorders

The psychiatrist should engage the patient and significant others in developing a comprehensive treatment plan that addresses all areas of biological, psychological, and social functioning, the patient's vocational, educational, or recreational needs, and the treatment of any coexisting general medical or psychiatric disorders, including other substance use disorders, that may be present.

5. Facilitating adherence to a treatment plan and preventing relapse

Since substance-dependent patients are often highly ambivalent about giving up substance use, psychiatrists must monitor, throughout all phases of treatment, patient attitudes about participating in treatment and complying with specific recommendations. Barriers to treatment participation include denial of the problem by the patient and the patient's family or social network; patterns of behavior that facilitate substance use (e.g., criminal activity or continued contact with drug-using peers); the likely re-emergence of craving for abused substances; unproductive attitudes about the value of work, treatment, or interpersonal relationships; continued psychosocial or vocational dysfunction; and comorbid psychiatric or general medical problems. These barriers should be discussed at the beginning and throughout the course of treatment.

The psychiatrist may address these barriers by actively attempting to increase motivation through specific enhancing techniques (66), encouraging the patient to participate in self-help or professionally led groups that include recovering individuals; encouraging the development of a substance-free peer group and lifestyle; helping the patient develop techniques to improve interpersonal relationships in family, work, and social settings; encouraging the patient to seek new experiences and roles consistent with a substance-free existence (e.g., greater involvement in vocational, social, and religious activities); discouraging the patient from instituting major life changes that might increase the risk of relapse; and providing, or arranging for, treatment of comorbid psychiatric and general medical conditions (67, 68).

Relapse prevention efforts may include helping patients anticipate and avoid drug-related cues (e.g., instructing the patient to avoid drug-using peers), training patients in self-monitoring affective or cognitive states associated with increased craving and substance use, contingency contracting, teaching desensitization and relaxation techniques to reduce the potency of drug-related stimuli and modulate craving intensity, helping patients develop alternative, nonchemical coping responses to uncomfortable feelings and situations, and providing coping and social skills training to help patients become involved in satisfying drug-free alternative activities (69). Behavioral techniques to enhance the availability and perceived value of social reinforcement as an alternative to drug use or reward for remaining drug free have also been used (70).

A mutually acceptable therapeutic plan for intervening in situations in which there is a high likelihood of relapse to substance use should be developed in the early stages (e.g., first few weeks) of treatment and reviewed on a regular basis (e.g., monthly or more frequently) for patients for whom relapse is an immediate concern. It is frequently helpful to obtain the patient's agreement to 1) predetermined guidelines for obtaining information from family, friends, and employers with which to assess the patient's ability to remain substance free and 2) the clinical criteria for altering the type, intensity, or site of treatment.

6. Providing education about substance use disorders and their treatments

Patients with substance use disorders should receive some education and feedback in regard to their illness, prognosis, and treatment. The psychiatrist should educate patients and, where appropriate, significant others regarding the etiology and course of the disorder, the need for abstinence, the risk of switching addictions, the identification of relapse triggers, available treatments, and the role of family and friends in aiding or impeding recovery. Where appropriate, the psychiatrist should also provide education about associated general medical problems (e.g., HIV infection, the effects of alcohol and other drugs on the fetus), the advantages of using sterile needles, procedures for safer sex, birth control, and the availability of treatment services for drug-affected newborns. Educational efforts should be geared to the developmental and cognitive level of the patient.

7. Diagnosing and treating associated psychiatric disorders

An ongoing, longitudinal assessment of the patient may be critical to the accurate diagnosis of a comorbid condition (see section III.H.1). Comorbid psychiatric conditions may complicate the substance use treatment and may require the addition of specific treatments (e.g., an antidepressant medication for a patient with comorbid major depressive disorder).

D. Pharmacologic Treatments

Pharmacotherapy for patients with substance use disorders may be used 1) to ameliorate the signs and symptoms of drug intoxication or withdrawal; 2) to decrease the effect of an abused substance and, more specifically, to decrease its subjective reinforcing effects; 3) to make the use of an abused substance aversive by a) inducing unpleasant consequences through a drug-drug interaction or b) coupling substance use with an unpleasant drug-induced condition; 4) to use an agonist substitution strategy to promote abstinence from a more dangerous illicit substance (e.g., the use of methadone for individuals with opioid use disorders); and 5) to treat comorbid psychiatric or general medical conditions.

1. Medications to treat intoxication or withdrawal states

Patients who develop tolerance to a particular drug also develop cross-tolerance to other drugs in the same pharmacologic class. As a result, one can take advantage of cross-tolerance in the treatment of withdrawal states by replacing the abused drug with a drug in the same general class but with a longer duration of action and then slowly tapering the longer-acting drug in a way that allows time for the restoration of physiologic homeostasis. Examples include the use of methadone in the treatment of heroin withdrawal and benzodiazepines in the treatment of alcohol withdrawal (71–73). Clonidine is an example of an agent that ameliorates abstinence-related symptoms in patients withdrawing from opioids but is not a competitive agonist (74).

2. Medications to decrease the reinforcing effects of abused substances

A variety of medications have been used to block or otherwise counteract the physiologic and/or subjective reinforcing effects of abused substances. For example, the narcotic antagonist naltrexone blocks the subjective and physiologic effects of subsequently administered opioid drugs (e.g., heroin) (75, 76). Repetitive testing of antagonist-induced "blockade" of opioid effects theoretically leads to extinction of conditioned craving for opioids (77).

Because of their strong affinity for and binding to opioid receptor sites, the narcotic antagonists also displace opioid agonists from neuronal and other receptors and can, therefore, be used to treat acute opioid intoxication. Abstinence symptoms precipitated by narcotic antagonists have also been used as a provocative test for the presence of opioid dependence (71).

3. Medications that discourage the use of substances

The most prominent example within this category is disulfiram (Antabuse), a drug that inhibits the activity of aldehyde dehydrogenase, the enzyme that metabolizes acetaldehyde, the first metabolic breakdown product of alcohol. In the presence of disulfiram pretreatment, alcohol use results in the accumulation of toxic levels of acetaldehyde, accompanied by a host of unpleasant, potentially dangerous, and rarely lethal signs and symptoms (78–80).

Medications have also been used as part of a chemical aversion treatment in which conditioned stimuli signaling drug availability, or the abused substance itself, are coupled with drugs that produce highly unpleasant effects, such as succinylcholine, which interferes with respiratory function, or emetine, which induces vomiting. The use of aversive medications for this purpose has been tried with patients who have alcohol use disorders (81) and/or cocaine use disorders (82) with some success, but it is not recommended outside of specialized treatment settings.

4. Agonist substitution therapy

The use of agonist medications may help some patients to reduce illicit drug use by reducing or eliminating symptoms of withdrawal and by decreasing craving for that particular class of substances. An example is the use of methadone or LAAM in the treatment of opioid-dependent patients (section VI.C.1).

5. Medications to treat comorbid psychiatric conditions

Also refer to section III.B for important diagnostic considerations. The high prevalence of comorbid psychiatric disorders in substance-dependent patients implies that many such patients will require specific pharmacotherapy directed at their comorbid disorders. Examples include the use of lithium or other mood stabilizers for substance-dependent patients with bipolar disorder, the use of neuroleptics for patients with schizophrenia, and the use of antidepressants for patients with major or atypical depressive disorder.

Potential problems for substance-dependent patients receiving pharmacotherapy for comorbid psychiatric illnesses include potentiation of acute drug effects (e.g., in combining antidepressants and alcohol) and intentional or unintentional overdose. Certain drugs used to treat comorbid psychiatric illnesses may themselves be abused. For example, patients with comorbid alcohol dependence and panic disorder may abuse benzodiazepines, and patients with comorbid schizophrenia and neuroleptic-induced parkinsonism may abuse anticholinergics. Whenever possible, medications with low abuse potential and relative safety in overdose should be chosen, e.g., selective serotonin reuptake inhibitors for depression.

E. Psychosocial Treatments

The major psychotherapeutic orientations that have been studied in patients with substance use disorders are cognitive behavioral and psychodynamic/interpersonal therapies. Although controlled studies often have major design limitations, the available data, along with clinical experience, suggest that psychosocial interventions can be useful when adapted for the special needs of this patient population. In many cases, however, treatment effects may not be apparent until the patient has been consistently in treatment for 3 months or more (83). This section will review the treatment approaches, the principles underlying their use, and their application in the treatment of patients with substance use disorders. Studies of the efficacy of psychosocial treatments for alcohol, cocaine, and opioid disorders are discussed in sections IV.D, V.D, and VI.D. Two terms, "psychotherapy" and "drug counseling," are used by clinicians and in the literature to describe some of the treatments described in this section. In general, the term "drug counseling" is applied to treatment that is given by a nonprofessional and that narrowly focuses on specific strategies for avoiding drug use. "Drug counseling" in this sense may be accompanied by other specific treatments, including psychotherapy.

1. Cognitive behavioral therapies

Cognitive behavioral therapies focus on a) altering the cognitive processes that lead to maladaptive behaviors in substance users, b) intervening in the behavioral chain of events that lead to substance use, c) helping patients deal successfully with acute or chronic drug craving, and d) promoting and reinforcing the development of social skills and behaviors compatible with remaining drug free.

a. Cognitive therapy.　Cognitive therapy, initially developed by Beck et al. (84) for the treatment of depression and anxiety, has been modified by that group for the treatment of patients with substance use disorders (85). The foundation of cognitive therapy is the belief that by identifying and subsequently modifying maladaptive thinking patterns, patients can reduce or eliminate negative feelings and behavior (e.g., substance use).

b. Relapse prevention.　"Relapse prevention" is an approach to treatment in which cognitive behavioral techniques are used in an attempt to help patients develop greater self-control in order to avoid relapse (56, 86). Specific relapse prevention strategies include discussing ambivalence, identifying emotional and environmental triggers of craving and substance use, developing and reviewing specific coping strategies to deal with internal or external stressors, exploring the decision chain leading to resumption of substance use, and learning from brief episodes of relapse ("slips") about triggers leading to relapse and developing effective techniques for early intervention (56, 87).

In controlled studies, relapse prevention has generally been found over time to be as effective as other psychosocial treatments (53, 88), and it may be more effective than other psychosocial treatments for patients who are more severely dependent and those with concurrent sociopathy or high levels of psychiatric symptoms (89–91).

c. Motivational enhancement therapy. Motivational enhancement therapy, based on cognitive behavioral, client-centered, systems, and social-psychological persuasion techniques, was shown to have positive effects in eight of nine controlled studies (92–94). This brief treatment modality is characterized by an empathic approach in which the therapist helps to motivate the patient by asking about the pros and cons of specific behaviors, by exploring the patient's goals and associated ambivalence about reaching these goals, and by listening reflectively. Motivational enhancement therapy has demonstrated substantial efficacy in the treatment of substance-dependent patients (92).

2. Behavioral therapies

Operant behavioral therapy involves operant rewarding or punishing of patients for desirable (e.g., demonstrating treatment compliance) or undesirable (e.g., associated with relapse) behaviors (95–97). Rewards have included vouchers, awarded for producing drug-free urine samples, that can be exchanged for mutually agreed on items (e.g., movie tickets) or "community reinforcement," in which family members or peers reinforce behaviors that demonstrate or facilitate abstinence (e.g., participation in positive activities) (98).

Contingency management is a behavioral treatment based on the use of predetermined positive or negative consequences to reward abstinence or punish (and thus deter) drug-related behaviors. Negative consequences for returning to substance use may include notification of courts, employers, or family members. The effectiveness of contingency management depends heavily on the concurrent use of frequent, random, supervised urine monitoring for substance use. When negative contingencies are based on the anticipated response of others (e.g., spouses, employers), one should obtain the written informed consent of the patient at the time the contract is initiated (99).

Cue exposure treatment based on a Pavlovian extinction paradigm involves exposure of the patient to cues that induce drug craving while preventing actual drug use and, therefore, the experience of drug-related reinforcement (100). Cue exposure can also be paired with relaxation techniques and drug refusal training to facilitate extinction of classically conditioned craving (101, 102). Although two studies (103, 104) of cue exposure treatment showed encouraging results in laboratory settings, further studies are necessary before it can be recommended for general use.

Aversion therapy, which involves coupling drug or alcohol use with an unpleasant experience (e.g., mild electric shock or pharmacologically induced vomiting), is used in certain specialized facilities. Controlled trials of such treatment have had mixed results (105, 106).

3. Individual psychodynamic/interpersonal therapies

a. Individual psychodynamic psychotherapy.   Systematic investigations have examined the efficacy of specially adapted forms of psychotherapy when combined with other treatment modalities (e.g., pharmacotherapies and self-help groups). For example, Woody et al. found that psychodynamic psychotherapy facilitated continued abstinence in patients with a baseline period of sustained abstinence (i.e., 1 to 2 years) (107, 108). Patients with comorbid antisocial personality disorder and high levels of sociopathy have been found to be poor candidates for psychodynamic psychotherapy (107, 109). The efficacy of psychodynamic psychotherapy when used as the sole treatment modality has not been demonstrated by controlled studies.

A number of structured short-term psychodynamic treatments have recently been developed. Supportive-expressive therapy (110) is a modification of psychodynamically oriented treatment based on creating a safe and supportive therapeutic relationship in which patients are encouraged to deal with negative patterns in other relationships. The largest study of supportive-expressive therapy (107) was described in the preceding paragraph. When supportive-expressive therapy was compared to multimodal behavior therapy for alcohol use disorders, subjects in the former group had somewhat better outcomes (i.e., less drinking) than the latter group at 2-year follow-up but similar drinking outcomes at 3-year follow-up (111). However, because of the small number of subjects in the study and a higher follow-up rate among patients in the multimodal behavior therapy group, these results need to be replicated in carefully controlled trials. A multisite clinical trial of supportive-expressive therapy for cocaine dependence, funded by the National Institute on Drug Abuse (NIDA), is currently under way (section V.D.4).

The efficacy of psychodynamic psychotherapy and psychoanalysis has been suggested by case reports and other reports of clinical experience.

b. Individual interpersonal therapy.   Interpersonal therapy, described in detail by Klerman et al. (112), focuses on difficulties in current interpersonal functioning by using psychodynamic principles and techniques with some modifications, such as including limit setting and using advice and suggestions. Interpersonal therapy has been shown to be useful in the treatment of both opioid users and cocaine users with low levels of dependence (113). Neither interpersonal therapy nor psychodynamically oriented psychotherapy is indicated for patients with profound cognitive deficits resulting from heavy drinking or other causes.

4. Group therapies

Group therapies are regarded by some psychiatrists as the preferred mode of psychotherapeutic treatment for substance-dependent patients. Many types of group therapy have been used with this population, including modified psychodynamic, interpersonal, interactive, rational emotive, Gestalt, and psychodrama (114, 115). For patients able to tolerate the dynamics of group interaction, including group confrontation of their denial, dealing with issues of interpersonal conflict or closeness, and the sharing of painful experiences or affects, group therapy can be a supportive, therapeutic, and educational experience that can motivate and sustain patients struggling to cope with life stresses and drug craving while remaining drug free (116–118).

Group therapy offers patients opportunities to identify with others who are going through similar problems, to understand the impact of substance use on their lives, to learn more about their own and others' feelings and reactions, and to learn to communicate needs and feelings more adaptively. Group therapy can also be useful in providing a forum for discussing and updating the treatment plan and for developing and monitoring specific behavioral contracts that help prevent relapse (and re-establish abstinence when relapse occurs). Even when the patient is not in immediate danger with regard to substance use, attendance at a weekly therapy group and the opportunity to hear other people's concerns about abstinence underscore the need for constant vigilance. While for many patients regular attendance at 12-step meetings can serve a similar function, often patients slip away from Alcoholics Anonymous (AA) and Narcotics Anonymous when they are in the greatest difficulty. Participation in a therapy group increases accountability by providing opportunities for the therapist and other group members to note and respond to early warning signs of relapse.

5. Family therapies

Dysfunctional families, characterized by impaired communication among family members and an inability to set appropriate limits or maintain standards of behavior, are associated with poor short- and long-term treatment outcome for patients with substance use disorders (119). The goals of family therapy, in a formalized ongoing therapeutic relationship or through periodic contact, include encouraging family support for abstinence; providing information about the patient's current attitudes toward drug use, treatment compliance, social and vocational adjustment, level of contact with drug-using peers, and degree of abstinence; maintaining marital relationships; and improving treatment compliance and long-term outcome (120, 121). Controlled studies have shown family therapy to be effective for adolescents, patients on methadone maintenance, and patients with alcohol dependence.

Different theoretical orientations of family therapy include structural, strategic, psychodynamic, systems, and behavioral approaches. Family interventions include those focused on the nuclear family; on the patient and his or her spouse; on concurrent treatment for patients, spouses, and siblings; on multifamily groups; and on social networks (68, 122, 123).

Family interventions are indicated in circumstances in which a patient's abstinence upsets a previously well-established but maladaptive style of family interaction (121, 124) and in which other family members need help in adjusting to a new set of individual and familial goals, attitudes, and behaviors. Family therapy that addresses interpersonal and family interactions leading to conflict or enabling behaviors can reduce the risk of relapse for patients with high levels of family involvement. Structured family intervention techniques are often effective in breaking through denial and resistance to treatment and are appropriate when less confrontive measures fail. Similarly, coercion exerted by family members, employers, or courts is an effective and appropriate means of engaging otherwise noncompliant patients in treatment. The use of coercion per se does not adversely affect the long-term prognosis for such patients.

Couple and family therapy are also useful for promoting psychological differentiation of family members, providing a forum for the exchange of information and ideas about the treatment plan, developing behavioral management contracts and ground rules for continued family support, and reinforcing behaviors that help prevent relapse and enhance the prospects for recovery.

The duration of family therapy is determined by progress in addressing and altering patterns of family interaction that may have contributed to substance abuse in the index patient, as well as interpersonal or systemic difficulties that may arise as a consequence of the patient's remaining abstinent and that may increase the risk of relapse. Other important considerations include meeting with sufficient frequency so as to maintain open lines of communication and a therapeutic focus on family issues, the coordination of family therapy with other ongoing treatment interventions, referral of family members for individual or group treatment where necessary, defining the role of family members in monitoring compliance with medication regimens, and contingency contracts or participation in other treatment-related activities. In the case of adolescents or patients under guardianship, the roles of responsible family members in decisions about pharmacologic treatment, drug testing, hospitalization, financing of treatment, maintenance of confidentiality, requirements for living at home, and the sharing of parental responsibilities, particularly when the parents are separated or divorced, are among the important issues addressed by family therapy (125).

In many instances, formal termination of family treatment should be followed by renewed contact at times when the patient, the psychiatrist, or family members feel the need to reassess progress in treatment, intervene in behaviors that may ultimately lead to relapse, or reinforce familial interactions that enhance the patient's ability to remain substance free (126).

6. Self-help groups

Although there is little empirical evidence to support their efficacy, clinical experience suggests that participation in self-help groups can be an important adjunct to treatment for many patients with substance use disorders. Referral is appropriate at all stages in the treatment process, even for patients who may still be active substance users. These groups, which are generally based on the 12-step approach of AA and related groups, such as Narcotics Anonymous and Cocaine Anonymous, can provide critical support for patients in recovery. Patients who attend AA or Narcotics Anonymous regularly receive group support and repeated reminders of the disastrous consequences of alcohol or other drug use and the benefits of abstinence and sobriety. Straightforward advice and encouragement about avoiding relapse, the personalized support of a recovering sponsor, and opportunities for both structured and unstructured substance-free social events and interactions are important features of self-help groups. In addition, the process of working through the 12 steps with a sponsor provides a structured opportunity to re-assess the role of past life experiences and personal identity in the development and maintenance of substance use disorders.

Members of self-help groups can attend meetings on a self-determined or prescribed schedule, every day if necessary. Periods associated with high risk for relapse (e.g., weekends, holidays, and evenings) are particularly appropriate for attendance. A sponsor who is compatible with the patient can provide important guidance and support during the recovery process, particularly during periods of emotional distress and increased craving. Patients being treated with medication for comorbid psychiatric disorders should be referred to self-help groups in which such treatment is supported.

Self-help groups are useful for many, but not all, patients. The refusal to participate in self-help groups is not synonymous with resistance to treatment in general. Some self-help groups (e.g., Rational Recovery) do not follow the abstinence-oriented, 12-step approach of AA and related groups and are alternatives for patients who do not accept the philosophy and spiritual focus of AA. Young people generally do better in groups that include age-appropriate peers in addition to some older recovering members. Patients who require psychoactive medications (e.g., lithium, antidepressants) for comorbid psychiatric illness should be directed to groups in which this activity is recognized and supported as useful treatment, rather than another form of substance abuse. Self-help groups based on the 12-step model are also available for family members and friends (e.g., Al-Anon, Alateen, Nar-Anon). They provide group support and education about the illness, and they function to reduce maladaptive enabling behavior in family and friends.

F. Formulating and Implementing a Treatment Plan

The goals of treatment and the specific choice of treatments needed to achieve those goals (section III.A) vary among patients and, for the same patient, among different phases of the illness. Since many substance use disorders are chronic, patients may require long-term treatment, although the intensity and specific components may vary over time.

Decisions regarding the site and components of treatment depend on individual patient factors, with the least restrictive setting that is likely to be safe and effective generally being preferable (section III.G).

On the basis of the assessment (section III.B), a treatment plan is developed. The components of a treatment plan and the factors that go into their choice are summarized in the following list. It must be kept in mind, however, that the separation of components is done for heuristic reasons: in practice, the components, and the factors that underlie their potential utility, overlap considerably.

1. Psychiatric management (section III.C) is crucial to coordinating the use of multiple modalities applied in individual, group, family, and self-help settings. It includes the

following elements: establishment and maintenance of a therapeutic alliance, monitoring of the patient's clinical status, management of intoxication and withdrawal states, reduction in the morbidity and sequelae of substance use disorders, facilitation of adherence to a treatment plan and prevention of relapse, education about substance use disorders, and diagnosis and treatment of associated psychiatric disorders.

In addition to psychiatric management, a treatment plan must include specific interventions that address the objectives listed in items 2, 3, and 4. These interventions may include specific pharmacologic treatments, specific psychosocial treatments, or a combination of these.

2. A strategy for achieving abstinence or reducing the effects or use of illicit substances (or nonillicit substances that exacerbate the substance use disorder) must be developed and implemented. The range of available strategies depends, in part, on the severity of the disorder and the availability of an effective pharmacologic treatment (e.g., an antagonist to block the effects of the substance or an agonist to reduce craving).

3. Efforts to enhance ongoing compliance with the treatment program and prevent relapse (section III.C.5) and improve functioning (III.A.3) are critical. The likelihood of success in continued treatment compliance is improved by decreasing the patient's access to abusable substance(s); optimizing the use of any specific pharmacologic treatments; addressing factors that help precipitate and/or perpetuate substance use, including both external factors (e.g., living/social environment) and internal factors (e.g., other psychopathology); providing disincentives for substance use (e.g., through the use of monitoring or pharmacologic strategies); and helping the patient develop cognitive and behavioral strategies to support a substance-free lifestyle (97). Referral to self-help groups is frequently helpful during this phase of treatment. Specific rehabilitative interventions to improve functioning may be necessary for patients whose functional level is impaired to the extent that it interferes with their ability to comply with treatment or is not expected to improve satisfactorily with cessation of substance use.

4. Patients with comorbid conditions generally require additional treatments (e.g., a specific psychotherapy, an antidepressant medication) in order to achieve optimal outcomes.

A growing body of research has addressed the issue of "patient-treatment matching," especially for psychosocial treatments. Clinical features such as age at onset, severity of dependence, presence of polydrug use, level of social/occupational impairment, level and nature of additional psychopathology, the quality of relationships, spiritual experience or religious affiliation, and the presence of neuropsychological impairments have all been studied (31, 53, 86, 90, 91, 127–144). Although these studies have generated findings that may eventually have implications for clinical practice, most had relatively small numbers of subjects and many of the findings have not been replicated. In addition, many of these studies, particularly psychotherapy studies, employed highly trained, experienced therapists who were closely supervised and monitored throughout with regard to their adherence to the treatment model that they were using. It is also not known to what degree the findings from these studies will generalize to other settings and other clinicians. A large-scale, multisite patient-treatment matching study currently under way may help determine whether patient factors can be used to predict response to various psychosocial treatments and, if so, at what stage in the cycle of recovery and relapse (145). The choice of treatments for patients with substance use disorders depends on the patient's clinical status and preferences: patient preferences are particularly important since adherence to a treatment plan over time is a powerful predictor of its effectiveness. In general, clinical features that guide the choice of psychosocial treatment for non-substance-using populations are also helpful guides for patients with substance use disorders (e.g., patients with antisocial personality disorder tend to do better in structured behavioral or cognitive behavioral treatments) (91, 127).

A number of studies have shown that the amount and quality of treatment services received by individuals with substance use disorders are strong predictors of substance use outcome (146–150). There is also evidence that patients who receive more psychiatric services have better social adjustment outcomes (150), which might promote more abstinence over time.

G. Treatment Settings

Patients with substance use disorders may receive their care in a variety of settings. The choice of setting should be guided by the demands of the treatment plan (as described in section III.F and as determined by the patient's clinical status) and the characteristics of available settings. Treatment settings vary with regard to the availability of various treatment capacities (e.g., general medical care, psychotherapy), the relative restrictiveness with respect to access to substances or involvement in other high-risk behaviors, hours of operation, and overall milieu and treatment philosophy (e.g., the use of psychotropic medications for comorbid conditions).

1. Factors affecting choice of treatment setting

Patients should be treated in the least restrictive setting that is likely to prove safe and effective. Decisions regarding the site of care should be based on the patient's a) capacity and willingness to cooperate with treatment; b) capacity to care for himself or herself; c) need for structure, support, and supervision in order to remain safe and pursue treatment away from environments and activities that promote substance use; d) need for specific treatments for comorbid general medical or psychiatric conditions; e) need for particular treatments or an intensity of treatment that may be available only in certain settings; and f) preference for a particular treatment setting.

Patients should be moved from one level of care to another on the basis of these factors and the clinician's assessment of patients' readiness and ability to benefit from a less intensive level of care.

Studies comparing the short-, intermediate-, and long-term benefits of treatment in various settings (i.e., inpatient, residential, partial hospital, outpatient) suffer from a variety of methodologic problems, including heterogeneity of patient populations, high dropout rates, and reliance on patient self-reports uncorroborated by data from collateral sources. Stated treatment goals, program features, and outcome measures also vary across studies (151).

2. Commonly available treatment settings

The availability of different settings varies among communities. The settings described may be considered as points along a continuum of care. Key characteristics of settings that are not described in this section can be used to determine where, along this continuum, they would fit.

a. Hospitals. The range of services available in hospital-based programs typically includes detoxification; assessment and treatment of general medical and psychiatric conditions; group, individual, and family therapies; psychoeducation; and motivational counseling. Other important components of hospital-based treatment programs include the willingness and ability to introduce patients to self-help groups and to develop a plan for posthospital care that includes strategies for relapse prevention and, where appropriate, rehabilitation (152).

Hospital-based treatment settings may be secure (i.e., locked) or permit patients and visitors to come and go in a monitored but generally less restricted fashion. Secure hospital settings should be considered for patients with comorbid psychiatric conditions whose clinical state would ordinarily require such a unit (e.g., actively suicidal patients). Patients with poor impulse control and judgment who in the presence of an "open door" are likely to leave the program or obtain or receive drugs on the unit are also candidates for a secure unit. In some states patients can reside on a secure unit in "conditional voluntary" status, which requires written notice and a time delay (e.g., 3 days) before a patient-initiated request for discharge must be acted on or another disposition (e.g., commitment) is implemented. Such restrictions can provide a useful period of delay in which poorly motivated patients can reconsider their wish to leave the program prematurely.

Available data do not support the notion that hospitalization per se has specific benefits over other treatment settings beyond the ability to address treatment objectives that require a medically monitored environment (70, 153). Nonetheless, patients in one or more of the specific following groups may require hospital-level care:

1. Patients with drug overdoses that cannot be safely treated in an outpatient or emergency room setting (e.g., patients with severe respiratory depression or coma).
2. Patients in withdrawal who are either at risk for a severe or complicated withdrawal syndrome (e.g., patients dependent on multiple drugs, patients with a past history of delirium tremens) or who cannot receive the necessary assessment, monitoring, or treatment in an alternative setting.

3.   Patients with acute or chronic general medical conditions that make detoxification in a residential or ambulatory setting unsafe (e.g., patients with severe cardiac disease).
4.   Patients with a documented history of not engaging in, or benefiting from, treatment in a less intensive setting (i.e., residential or outpatient).
5.   Patients with marked psychiatric comorbidity who are an acute danger to themselves or others (e.g., patients who have depression with suicidal thoughts, acute psychosis).
6.   Patients manifesting substance use or other behaviors that constitute an acute danger to themselves or others.
7.   Patients who have not responded to less intensive treatment efforts and whose substance use disorder(s) poses an ongoing threat to their physical and mental health.

In general, the duration of hospital-based treatment should be dictated by the current need of the patient to receive treatment in a restrictive setting and by the patient's capacity to safely participate in, and benefit from, treatment in a less restrictive setting.

b. Residential treatment.   *Generic residential facilities.* Residential treatment is primarily indicated for patients whose lives and social interactions have come to focus exclusively on substance use and who currently lack sufficient motivation and/or drug-free social supports to remain abstinent in an ambulatory setting but who do not meet clinical criteria for hospitalization. For such patients, residential facilities provide a safe and drug-free environment in which residents learn individual and group living skills. As in the case of hospital-based programs, residential treatment programs should, at a minimum, also provide psychosocial, occupational, and family assessments; psychoeducation; an introduction to self-help groups; and referral for social or vocational rehabilitative services where necessary (154).

Many residential programs provide their own individual, group, and vocational counseling programs but rely on affiliated partial hospital or outpatient programs to supply the psychosocial and psychopharmacologic treatment components of their programs. Residential treatment settings should provide general medical and psychiatric care that is required to meet patient needs.

The duration of residential treatment should be dictated by the time necessary to achieve specific utilization criteria that would predict a successful transition to a less structured, less restrictive treatment setting (e.g., outpatient care); these may include demonstrated motivation to continue in outpatient treatment, the ability to remain abstinent even in situations where drugs are potentially available, the availability of a living situation and associated support system conducive to remaining drug free (e.g., family, drug-free peers), stabilization of any comorbid general medical or psychiatric disorder to the point where treatment can take place in an outpatient setting, and the availability of adequate follow-up care, including partial hospitalization and respite care if needed.

In some areas, residential treatment programs specifically designed for adolescents, pregnant or postpartum women, and women with young children are available, and such programs are preferred for these patient populations.

Therapeutic communities. Patients with opioid, cocaine, or polysubstance use disorders may benefit from referral to a long-term residential therapeutic community. These programs are generally reserved for patients with a low likelihood of benefiting from outpatient treatment (e.g., those with multiple prior treatment failures or profound characterologic problems that make treatment compliance unlikely) (155). The therapeutic community provides a secure, drug-free environment in which behavioral modeling and peer pressure are used to 1) shape residents' ability to modulate emotional distress without resorting to substance use and 2) resocialize them to pursue a drug-free lifestyle (156).

Characteristically, therapeutic communities are organized along strict hierarchies, with newcomers assigned to the most menial social status and work tasks. Residents achieve higher status and take on increasing responsibility as they demonstrate that they can remain drug free and conform to community rules. Confrontation, individually and in groups, is used to break through denial about the role of substance use in one's life, identify maladaptive behaviors and coping styles that lead to interpersonal conflict and vocational failure, suggest alternative ways of handling disturbing affects, and encourage the development of attitudes and beliefs that are incompatible with continued substance use.

Data regarding the effectiveness of therapeutic communities are confounded by the fact that only 15%–25% of patients admitted voluntarily complete the program, with maximum attrition occurring in the first 3 months (157). Follow-up studies of patients who continue in the treatment program suggest that a minimum of 3 months of treatment is necessary to demonstrate benefit and that the optimal length of stay may be considerably longer (i.e., 6 to 12 months). Therapeutic community program graduates have lower rates of relapse and better outcomes at 1-year follow-up than do patients entering outpatient treatment, although the clinical circumstances may have biased the findings (158, 159).

Reasonable candidates for treatment in a therapeutic community include 1) patients who need a highly structured setting in which to initiate treatment and 2) patients whose level of denial is such that interpersonal and group confrontation is deemed an important part of the initial approach to treatment. In choosing a therapeutic community, a program's ability to treat comorbid psychopathology should be carefully considered.

c. Partial hospitalization. Partial hospital care can provide an intensive and structured treatment experience for patients with substance dependence who require more services than those generally available in traditional outpatient settings. Randomized controlled trials have demonstrated that some patients who would ordinarily be referred for residential or hospital level care do just as well in partial hospital care (160).

Partial hospital programs should also be considered for patients leaving hospital or residential settings who are at high risk for relapse. The latter include patients in the early stages of treatment with questionable motivation to remain drug free, those with a history of past failure in the immediate posthospital or postresidential period, patients living in or returning to environments characterized by high drug availability or low levels of social support for remaining drug free, and those with severe psychiatric comorbidity.

The treatment components of partial hospital programs usually include individual, group, and family therapy; vocational and educational counseling; medically supervised use of adjunctive medications (e.g., narcotic antagonists, methadone); random urine screening for drugs of abuse; and treatment for any comorbid psychiatric disorders that may be present. As in other treatment settings, partial hospital programs should provide opportunities for patients to learn and practice coping strategies to reduce drug craving and avoid relapse. Patient and family education about substance use disorders and the opportunity to confront patient or family denial are also important program components. Partial hospital programs for adolescents should be affiliated or work closely with school-based counseling programs.

The duration of outpatient treatment should be tailored to individual patient needs and may vary from a few months to several years. Patients in partial hospital care typically begin by attending 4–12 hours per day, 3–7 days per week. The availability of evening and weekend care is particularly desirable. The duration or frequency of partial hospital visits should be tapered as patients demonstrate that they can remain substance free and make progress toward rehabilitation. The availability of community-based supports (e.g., non-drug-using friends or family), a job, and a living situation conducive to remaining abstinent are also important considerations in deciding when to decrease or discontinue partial hospital care.

d. Outpatient settings.   Outpatient treatment of substance use disorders is appropriate for those whose clinical condition or environmental circumstances do not require a more intensive level of care. As in other treatment settings, a comprehensive approach using, where indicated, a variety of psychotherapeutic and pharmacologic interventions, along with behavioral monitoring, is optimal. Treatment should encourage and be integrated with patient participation in self-help programs where appropriate (section III.E.6) (161).

As in the case of residential and partial hospital programs, high rates of attrition are a problem in outpatient settings, particularly in the early phase (i.e., first 6 months). Since intermediate- and long-term outcomes are highly correlated with retention in treatment, specific efforts should be directed toward motivating patients to remain in treatment (162); such efforts may include the use of legal, family, or employer-generated pressure where available (see sections III.H.6, III.H.8, and III.I.1).

H.   Clinical Features Influencing Treatment

Because of the chronic and relapsing nature of these conditions, the psychiatrist will often need to manage patients in intoxication and withdrawal states. These issues are discussed in sections III.D.1, IV.E.1, IV.E.2, V.E.1, V.E.2, VI.E.1, and VI.E.2.

1.   Psychiatric factors

a. Risk of suicide or homicide.   The frequency of both suicide attempts and completed suicides is substantially higher among patients with substance use disorders than in the general population (163–168). The incidence of completed suicide is approximately 3–4 times that found in the general population (167), with a lifetime mortality of approximately

15% (166). The presence of major depressive disorder substantially increases the suicide risk of these patients (169).

Substance use disorders are also associated with greater than average risk for other forms of violence, including homicide (170, 171). Anxiety, irritability, increased aggressivity, impaired impulse control, and impaired reality testing may be due either to the direct effects of the substance(s) or to a withdrawal syndrome. Substances whose use may be associated with aggression include cocaine, hallucinogens, phencyclidine (PCP), and alcohol (72, 172, 173). Substances that lead to withdrawal syndromes associated with a risk of violence include alcohol, opioids, and hypnotic sedatives (72). Patients intoxicated on marijuana or hallucinogens may inadvertently commit violent acts on the basis of their faulty perception of reality coupled with high levels of anxiety and paranoia (174–176).

An additional implication of these findings is the need to consider the diagnosis of substance use disorder in all individuals who present with a history of suicide or other form of violence.

b. Comorbid psychiatric disorders. The presence of psychiatric comorbidity affects the onset, clinical course, treatment compliance, and prognosis for patients with substance use disorders (29, 137, 148, 177, 178). Penick et al. (179) studied a Department of Veterans Affairs (VA) hospital outpatient population of patients with alcohol dependence or abuse; of these, 56% reported psychiatric comorbidity. High rates of personality disorders have been reported in patients with substance use disorders (12, 44, 180, 181). Patients with comorbid borderline or antisocial personality disorder appear to have a poorer response to treatment (182) and a greater risk of suicide (183).

All patients with substance use disorders should be carefully assessed for the presence of psychiatric comorbidity (184). In a study by McLellan et al. (31), patients with no comorbid psychiatric illness did well in all types of treatment settings, whereas patients with more severe psychiatric symptoms did poorly. Rounsaville et al. (185) found that patients with comorbidities benefit from specific treatment for their comorbid mental disorders.

Conversely, patients with identified psychiatric disorders should be routinely assessed for the presence of comorbid substance use disorders. In so doing, it is important to establish the chronology of symptom development (i.e., whether the signs and symptoms predate or follow the onset of repetitive substance use), whether symptoms were present during extended drug-free periods (e.g., of 3 months or more), and the impact of each disorder on the presentation, clinical course, and outcome of the other(s).

The probability that the patient has a comorbid psychiatric disorder is increased if 1) there is a clear history of similar signs and symptoms preceding the onset of the substance use disorder or evident during previous extended drug-free periods or 2) at least one first-degree biological relative has a documented history of similar illness (2).

In many cases, it is necessary to observe patients during a substance-free period before concluding that there is a comorbid psychiatric disorder and/or instituting specific treatment for that disorder. The length of the observation period is generally determined by balancing the following considerations: the degree of diagnostic certainty, the severity of the patient's condition, and the anticipated benefits and risks of the proposed treatment. For patients with a comorbid disorder, initial treatment efforts should be directed toward any substance-induced disorder (i.e., intoxication or withdrawal) that may be present. Once patients are stable, treatment for substance abuse or dependence, as well as any other disorder present, should proceed concurrently in the context of an integrated treatment program. However, a patient who is psychotic, suicidal, or homicidal may require intensive psychiatric treatment to stabilize the condition before he or she can be integrated into ongoing rehabilitative treatment for the substance use disorder(s).

Finally, it is incorrect to assume that treatment of a comorbid non-substance-related psychiatric disorder will by itself assure that the substance use disorder will also resolve. Even when a substance use disorder arises in the context of another psychiatric disorder, over time it often takes on a life of its own and usually requires specific treatment (186).

c. Use of multiple substances. A number of studies have shown that many patients entering treatment for a substance use disorder are abusing more than one substance. For some patients, there is a "drug of choice" and other substances serve as substitutes when the primary substance is unavailable. For others, multiple drugs are routinely used simultaneously. Concurrent use of two or more drugs may be motivated by the patient's wish to modify the effects of the primary drug of choice and/or to prevent or relieve withdrawal symptoms. In addition, many patients use multiple substances largely on the basis of their availability. Frequent drug combinations include cocaine and alcohol, cocaine and heroin, and heroin and benzodiazepines.

The assessment of patients with substance use disorder should routinely include questions about polydrug use. Treatment is most successful when it is directed toward establishing and maintaining abstinence or reduced use of all abused substances (including, for many patients, the use of nicotine) (187). Treatment may be complicated by 1) simultaneous intoxication or withdrawal from two or more drugs, 2) varying time frames for experiencing withdrawal symptoms in patients using multiple drugs, 3) the need to detoxify the patient from more than one drug, and 4) potential interactions between an abused substance and medications used to treat a comorbid substance use disorder (e.g., inadvertent precipitation of opioid withdrawal in patients treated with naltrexone for alcohol dependence).

2.   Comorbid general medical disorders

Concurrent general medical conditions frequently complicate the treatment of substance use disorders. Many patients with these disorders do not seek or receive adequate general medical care for a variety of reasons, including the chaotic and disorganized lifestyles often associated with substance abuse and lack of access to health care. Thus, the substance abuse treatment encounter may be the first opportunity to address the general medical care needs of these patients.

Because of their high prevalence, alcohol use disorders account for the majority of substance use problems encountered in general medical settings. Conversely, general medical problems related to alcohol dependence are frequently encountered in substance abuse treatment programs. Alcohol-related problems can affect almost all organ systems, most prominently the gastrointestinal and central nervous systems (188). Some of the more severe forms of alcohol-related injury to the CNS clearly have lasting effects on cognition, behavior, and the ability to comply with treatment. For example, the anterograde amnestic disorder found in patients with Korsakoff's syndrome dramatically limits the utility of treatment approaches that require the development of insight and/or the learning of new behaviors, such as maintaining abstinence. See also section V.E.3.

The following conditions contribute to an increased risk of death and disability in patients with substance use disorders: hepatitis, tuberculosis, motor vehicle accidents, falls, suicide, and homicide. Among injecting drug users, infectious diseases are the most common type of general medical comorbidity. From a public health standpoint, the most important of these are infection with HIV, tuberculosis, and sexually transmitted diseases. Approximately 30%–40% of inner-city intravenous drug users test positive for HIV (14, 189). The adoption of universal precautions against body contamination by infectious agents is a necessary part of protecting staff and patients against the spread of HIV (190). Sexually active patients should be specifically counseled in the use of safe sex practices. Needle exchange programs and effective treatment also reduce the spread of HIV infection (191).

The rise of treatment-resistant tuberculosis among patients with substance use disorders suggests the need to consider periodic tuberculosis screening for both patients and staff, along with efforts to reduce the spread of tuberculosis in treatment environments. Supervised on-site chemoprophylaxis or treatment for tuberculosis within substance abuse treatment programs is also strongly recommended (192, 193).

3. Pregnancy

Substance use during pregnancy has the following implications for both the mother and the developing fetus.

a. The health of the pregnant woman.   Pregnant women with substance use disorders are at high risk for sexually transmitted diseases (e.g., HIV infection), hepatitis, anemia, tuberculosis, hypertension, and preeclampsia. In addition, the presence of a substance use disorder may affect the woman's ability to maintain a healthy lifestyle, including proper nutrition, and obtain needed health care (e.g., prenatal care).

b. The course of the pregnancy.   Women with substance use disorders (depending on the substance) may be at greater than average risk for spontaneous abortions, preeclampsia, abruptio placentae, and early and prolonged labor, in addition to complications of other general medical conditions that may be due to the substance use (e.g., hypertension in cocaine users [194]).

c. Fetal development.   Some abused substances, including opiates, cocaine, and alcohol, are known to pass through the placenta and directly affect the fetus (195–197). This may happen at any stage of development but is particularly likely during the third trimester, when maternal fetal blood flow and rates of placental transport are increased. Fetal concentrations of abused substances average 50%–100% of maternal blood levels and in some instances are higher (196). The circulation of active drug metabolites is another source of fetal exposure to potentially toxic substances.

The fetus may be at higher than average risk of birth defects, cardiovascular problems, impaired growth and development, prematurity, low birth weight, and stillbirth (198–203). After delivery, the neonate may suffer from withdrawal of the substance, which may be difficult to recognize, particularly if the mother's diagnosis is not known by the pediatrician.

d. Child development.   Some substances (e.g., alcohol) are associated with long-term negative effects on physical and cognitive development (204).

e. Parenting behavior.   In addition to ongoing treatment for the substance use disorder, mothers with substance use disorders are frequently in need of education and training in parenting skills, social services, nutritional counseling, assistance in obtaining health and welfare entitlements, and other interventions aimed at reducing the likelihood of child abuse or neglect.

Goals of treatment of pregnant substance-using women include eliminating all alcohol and drug use, treating any comorbid general medical or psychiatric disorders, guiding the patient safely through the pregnancy, facilitating appropriate parenting behavior, and motivating the patient to remain in treatment after delivery to minimize the risk of relapse.

The optimal therapeutic approach is nonpunitive and maintains patient confidentiality. Education and counseling to help women make an informed decision about continuing or terminating a pregnancy should be made available to those who want it. Sexually active women and men likely to return to a drug-abusing subculture should be advised about reliable contraceptive techniques.

4.   Gender-related factors

Information on the natural history, clinical presentation, physiology, and treatment of substance use disorders in women is limited. Although women are estimated to comprise 34% of all persons with substance use disorders in the United States (205), psychosocial and financial barriers (e.g., lack of child care) prevent many women from seeking treatment. Other explanations for women's underuse of alcohol and drug treatment services may include women's perception of greater social stigma associated with their abuse of drugs and alcohol (206, 207). Once in treatment, women have been found to have a higher prevalence of primary comorbid depressive and anxiety disorders that require specific treatment, compared to men (207). Many women with substance use disorders have a history of physical and/or sexual abuse (both as children and as adults), which may also influence treatment planning, participation, and outcome (208). Female patients also tend to have more family responsibilities and may need more help with family-related problems. There is evidence that increasing the focus of treatment on concerns specific to women, such as adding treatment components that specifically address women's issues and increasing female staff, improves treatment outcomes for women (209, 210).

5. Age

a. Children and adolescents. Children and adolescents are generally more likely to have abuse rather than dependence disorders and are less likely to appreciate the need for entering and remaining in treatment. Assessment and treatment must take into account the cognitive, social, and psychological developmental levels of the patient and the possible role of substance use disorders in impeding the successful attainment of developmental milestones, including a sense of autonomy, the ability to form interpersonal relationships, and general integration into society. The assessment should also place particular emphasis on evaluating areas of the adolescent's adaptive functioning, such as academic progress, school behavior and attendance, and social functioning with peers and family members. Adolescents' typical position as dependent members of family systems, their desire to attain an independent identity, their general ambivalence about authority, their need to develop social skills and appropriate peer relationships, and their need for education or vocational training require specific treatment attention. Treatment should also address the ability of parents to communicate and set appropriate behavioral limits.

Some adolescents with substance use disorders also have comorbid psychiatric disorders, including conduct disorder, attention deficit hyperactivity disorder (ADHD), anxiety disorders (including social phobia and posttraumatic stress disorder), affective disorders, learning disabilities, and eating disorders (6). In addition, children reared in family environments in which other family members abuse or are dependent on alcohol or other substances are also at higher risk of physical or sexual abuse and may exhibit psychological and behavioral sequelae (including substance abuse) as a result (211, 212).

The clinical manifestations of comorbid psychiatric disorders in adolescents often vary from those noted in similarly diagnosed adults. Thus, assessment for and treatment of these disorders require professionals and staff who are familiar with their manifestations in children and adolescents and the use of specific psychosocial (i.e., individual, group, family) therapies, age-appropriate psychosocial treatments (including individual, group, and family psychotherapies), and medication when needed. Lack of attention to coexisting psychiatric disorders may impede progress in treatment and result in further impairment in adaptive functioning. Many adolescents with substance use disorders have preexisting and concurrent impulsive, oppositional, and conduct-disordered behaviors. Treatment should address these problems and the conduct-disordered behavior as well as focusing on the substance abuse itself. Treatment and assessment of adolescents may be further compromised by questions about whether diagnostic criteria developed for adults are appropriate for adolescents (6).

Generally, the range of treatment modalities used with adults can be used with adolescents as well. These modalities include cognitive behavioral approaches, psychodynamic/interpersonal approaches (individual, group, and family), self-help groups (213), and medications. Treatment is often delivered in a group therapy format. Although research data establishing the efficacy of specific treatment modalities for adolescent substance use disorders are sparse, program outcomes for adolescents appear to be enhanced by the availability of treatment that is developmentally appropriate, peer oriented, and setting specific; includes educational, vocational, and recreational services; and emphasizes family involvement in both treatment planning and the treatment itself (213).

b. The elderly.   Substance use disorders in elderly populations are an underrecognized and undertreated problem (214, 215). Abuse and dependence on prescribed medications, particularly benzodiazepines, hypnotic sedatives, and opioids, can contribute to excessive confusion and sedation in elderly patients, poor compliance with prescribed treatment regimens, and inadvertent overdose, particularly when these drugs are combined with alcohol (216). In addition, alcohol use disorders, as an extension of a longstanding disorder or of later onset, are a major problem among the elderly, particularly those living alone (217). Alcohol-related cognitive impairment, comorbid depressive disorder, dementia, poststroke syndromes, and other conditions common among the elderly may impair their ability to obtain or comply with treatment for substance abuse or for other general medical and psychiatric disorders (218).

6.   Social milieu or living environment

The patient's overall social milieu has an important impact on both the development of and recovery from substance dependence. The social milieu shapes attitudes about the appropriate context for substance use (e.g., the difference between social drinking on family occasions and recreational drinking to achieve intoxication). Role models among one's family or peers influence the social and psychological context for substance use, the choice of drug, and the degree of control exerted over substance-using behaviors.

Once a pattern of dependence or abuse has developed, motivation and ability to comply with treatment are influenced by the degree of support within the patient's immediate peer group and social environment for remaining abstinent. Continued involvement with a substance-abusing peer group or enabling family members and residence in an environment in which there is a high level of drug availability predict a poor outcome. Thus, addressing these issues is an important component of any treatment plan. Patients with high levels of psychosocial and environmental stressors need correspondingly high levels of community-based support or, in some cases, temporary relief from these stressors through treatment in a residential setting until the patient is able to develop specific relapse-prevention strategies that can be applied in a community setting. Sexually active individuals should be educated about the prevalence and prevention of HIV infection and other sexually transmitted diseases.

7.   Cultural factors

Current research suggests poorer prognoses for ethnic and racial minorities in conventional treatment programs, although this may be accounted for by social class differences (219–221). Although there is a paucity of research on the efficacy of culturally specific programming, treatment services that are culturally sensitive and address the special concerns of ethnic minority groups may improve acceptance of, compliance with, and, ultimately, the outcome of treatment. Training of staff and efforts to incorporate culture-specific beliefs about healing and recovery should be part of a comprehensive treatment program that serves different minority and ethnic groups (222).

8. Family characteristics

Substance use disorders exact an enormous toll on family members. High levels of interpersonal conflict, domestic violence, inadequate parenting, child abuse and neglect, separation and divorce, financial and legal difficulties, and drug-related general medical problems (e.g., AIDS, tuberculosis) all add to the family burden. In addition, children reared in family environments in which other family members abuse or are dependent on alcohol or other substances are also at increased risk of physical or sexual abuse (223).

Families with one or more members who have substance use disorders often display a multigenerational pattern of transmission of both substance abuse and other frequently associated psychiatric disorders (e.g., antisocial personality disorder, pathological gambling) (224). The impact of maternal substance use on both fetal development and childhood cognitive and emotional adjustment, coupled with the influence of genetically inherited risk factors (e.g., high genetic loading for alcoholism in males) and negative role models, all play a role in the development of substance use disorders across generational lines. In addition, pathological "enabling" behavior, the existence of psychiatric and general medical problems in parents and siblings, and high levels of social and/or transcultural stress also play a role in the development and perpetuation of substance use disorders.

The substantial burden imposed on families containing one or more members with substance use disorders, and the impact of family interactions in perpetuating or ameliorating these problems, affect the initiation of, perpetuation of, and recovery from the substance use disorders; the patient's motivation and ability to comply with treatment; and the patient's clinical course and outcome. These relationships, coupled with the high prevalence of substance use disorders, comorbid general medical and psychiatric disorders, psychosocial disability, and family burden, make family interventions extremely important in the treatment of these patients (120, 225).

I.   Legal and Confidentiality Issues

1.   Effect of legal pressure on treatment participation and outcome

Many patients with substance use disorders seek treatment in response to pressure from family members, employers, legal authorities, or other sources. While motivation for treatment is often regarded as a good prognostic sign, outcome studies of patients in therapeutic communities have shown that individuals who enter treatment under legal compulsion (e.g., a judge has made treatment a condition of probation or a mandatory alternative to incarceration) stay longer and do as well as comparable patients who enter treatment voluntarily (226, 227). Similarly, higher rates of compliance in treatment with the narcotic antagonist naltrexone have been reported for court-mandated patients and for physicians or other professionals who are at risk of losing their professional licenses should they fail to comply. Similar findings have been reported for professionals being treated for substance use problems by means of contingency contracting approaches in which the contingency for noncompliance with treatment is being reported to a professional board of registration (228).

2. Confidentiality and reporting of treatment information

To protect patients' privacy and encourage their entry into treatment, federal law and regulations mandate strict confidentiality for information about patients being treated for substance use disorders (i.e., 42 USC Section 290dd-3, ee-3; 42 C.F.R. Part 2). Disclosure of information from treatment records is prohibited unless the patient has given written consent, the disclosure is in response to a medical emergency, or there is a court order authorizing disclosure. Other instances in which patient confidentiality may be abrogated include disclosure in response to a crime committed at the treatment program or against program staff, and compliance with state laws addressing the psychiatrist's "duty to warn" third parties of a potential harm (by the patient); the initial reporting of child abuse or neglect may also abrogate confidentiality requirements. With regard to the last situation, psychiatrists should be familiar with reporting laws concerning the possible abuse and neglect of children and other dependents who may be at risk in the families of both male and female substance users.

Generally, federal law does not make specific reference to the confidentiality of information pertaining to the HIV/AIDS status of a patient in alcohol or drug treatment, but there are many different state laws restricting disclosure of such status.

3. Legal requirements for pharmacotherapy with opioids

Federal and state regulations govern the use of methadone and LAAM, the only two opioids approved by the Food and Drug Administration (FDA) for treating patients with opioid-related disorders. Federal law (P.L. 93-281) requires special registration of each physician using methadone or LAAM for maintenance or detoxification. The Drug Enforcement Administration will not register physicians without prior approval by the FDA and the state drug authority. FDA approval is contingent on practitioner willingness to comply with federal narcotic treatment regulations (229).

IV. Alcohol-Related Disorders: Treatment Principles and Alternatives

A. Overview

The focus of this section is on the treatment of patients with alcohol dependence or abuse. Treatment of these disorders may be complicated by episodes of intoxication and withdrawal, the treatment of which is discussed in sections IV.E.1 and IV.E.2.

The Epidemiologic Catchment Area (ECA) studies indicate that 13.8% of American adults have had either alcohol dependence or abuse sometime in their lives (230).

Alcohol use disorders have a variable course that is frequently characterized by periods of remission and relapse. The first episode of alcohol intoxication is likely to occur in the midteens, and the age at onset of alcohol dependence peaks in the 20s to 30s. The first evidence of withdrawal is not likely to appear until after many other aspects of dependence have developed. Although some individuals with alcohol dependence achieve long-term sobriety without active treatment, many need treatment to stop the cycles of remission and relapse.

The relationship between alcohol dependence and abuse is also variable. In one study (231), only 30% of male subjects with alcohol abuse at baseline met criteria for alcohol dependence 4 years later. The other 70% met criteria for either alcohol abuse or alcohol abuse in remission.

The long-term goals of treatment for patients with alcohol use disorders are identical to those for patients with any type of substance use disorder; these are discussed in section III.A and include abstinence (or reduction in use and effects), relapse prevention, and rehabilitation. There is some controversy in the literature, however, regarding the possible benefits of striving for a reduction in alcohol intake, as opposed to total abstinence, for those who are unlikely to achieve the latter. In a comprehensive review of the issue (232), Rosenberg concluded that a lower severity of pretreatment alcohol dependence and the belief that controlled drinking is possible were associated with the achievement of controlled drinking after treatment. Interventions aimed at achieving moderate drinking have also been used with patients in the early stages of alcohol abuse (see, e.g., references 233 and 234). Controlled drinking may be an acceptable outcome of treatment, for a select group of patients, when accompanied by substantial improvements in morbidity and psychosocial functioning. For most patients with alcohol dependence or abuse, however, abstinence is the optimal goal.

Numerous studies have documented the efficacy of alcoholism treatment; approximately 70% of all patients manifest a reduction in the number of days of drinking and improved health status within 6 months (151, 235).

The majority of patients who are treated for alcohol use disorders have at least one relapse episode during the first year following treatment. However, there is now considerable evidence that most individuals with alcohol use disorders drink less frequently and consume less alcohol after receiving alcoholism treatment, compared to their pretreatment drinking behavior (138, 236–238). For example, patients typically report drinking heavily on 75% of the days during a 3-month period before treatment. During posttreatment follow-ups patients are often abstinent on 70%–90% of the days, and they engage in heavy drinking on 5%–10% of the days (119).

Treatment also has been shown to bring about improvements in family functioning, marital satisfaction, and psychiatric impairments (137, 239, 240). Although improvements following alcoholism treatment are at least in part attributable to nontreatment factors, such as patient motivation (93), it is generally accepted that treatment does make a difference, at least in the short run.

Psychiatric management (section III.C) is the key component of a successful treatment plan.

B.   Choice of Treatment Setting

The range of available settings and the general criteria for choosing among them are described in section III.G. In general, the choice of a setting depends on the clinical characteristics of the patient, the preferences of the patient, the treatment needs, and the available alternatives. As in the treatment of all patients with substance-related disorders, the least restrictive setting that is likely to facilitate safe and effective treatment is preferred.

Most treatments for patients with alcohol dependence or abuse can be successfully conducted outside of the hospital (e.g., in outpatient, day hospital, or partial hospital settings) (138, 160). However, patients unlikely to benefit from less intensive and less restrictive alternatives may need to be hospitalized at times during their treatment. The general criteria for hospitalization are summarized in section III.G.2.a.

A large-scale epidemiologic study (241) showed that the mortality rates for male veterans with alcohol use disorders 3 years after discharge varied with the initial treatment setting. Veterans who completed inpatient rehabilitation had the lowest mortality rate, while the other groups, in order of increasing mortality rate, were 1) those who had at least 6 days of inpatient treatment (but did not complete the program), 2) those who were admitted for brief detoxification lasting less than 5 days, and 3) those who received no specific treatment for alcohol use disorders. Patients in this study were not randomly assigned to treatment conditions, so it is possible that self-selection influenced the results. However, the study provides preliminary evidence that more intensive treatment may lower the mortality associated with chronic alcohol use disorders.

With one exception (242), studies that have randomly assigned patients to different levels of treatment have generally not found an advantage for inpatient care over less restrictive settings (243–246). However, these studies have limited generalizability due to such problems as exclusion of patients who would ordinarily be considered to require inpatient treatment (140).

There is considerable evidence that longer treatment stays and treatment completion are associated with better outcomes (238, 247). This probably reflects the fact that better-motivated patients are more likely to stay in treatment and have better outcomes. However, patients randomly assigned to longer treatments typically do not have better outcomes than those randomly assigned to shorter treatments (138, 160).

Patients with alcohol withdrawal must be detoxified in a setting that provides for frequent clinical assessment and the provision of any necessary treatments. Some outpatient settings can accommodate these requirements and may be appropriate for patients deemed to be at low risk of a complicated withdrawal syndrome. However, those who have a prior history of delirium tremens, whose documented history of very heavy alcohol use and high tolerance places them at risk for a complicated withdrawal syndrome, who are concurrently abusing other drugs, who have a severe comorbid general medical or psychiatric disorder, or who repeatedly fail to cooperate with or benefit from outpatient detoxification are more likely to require a residential or hospital setting that can safely provide the necessary care. Patients in severe withdrawal (i.e., delirium tremens) require treatment in a hospital setting.

C. Pharmacologic Treatments for Dependence and Abuse

1. Naltrexone

Two independent double-blind, placebo-controlled studies (248, 249) have documented the efficacy of the narcotic antagonist naltrexone for the treatment of alcohol dependence. The study by O'Malley et al. (249) showed that naltrexone in doses of 50 mg/day was superior to placebo in terms of reduced drinking and the resolution of alcohol-related problems. Patients who received both naltrexone and coping skills training were the most successful at avoiding full relapse. These studies suggest the potential utility of this agent, particularly when combined with other therapeutic approaches, in preventing relapse. The mechanism by which naltrexone exerts its therapeutic effects is not adequately known but may involve blocking the primary subjective effects of a first drink. Animal studies suggest that part of alcohol's reinforcing effects relate to release of endogenous opioids, which are then blocked by naltrexone (250–252).

2. Disulfiram (Antabuse)

Pretreatment with disulfiram establishes conditions in which the subsequent use of alcohol results in a toxic and highly aversive reaction. Disulfiram inhibits the activity of aldehyde dehydrogenase, the enzyme that metabolizes acetaldehyde, a major metabolite of alcohol.

The usual therapeutic dose is 250 mg/day, although some patients achieve optimal benefit at either a higher or a lower dose (range, 125–500 mg/day). In the presence of disulfiram, alcohol consumption results in the accumulation of toxic levels of acetaldehyde, which in turn produce a host of unpleasant signs and symptoms, including a sensation of heat in the face and neck, headache, flushing, nausea, vomiting, hypotension, and anxiety. Chest pain, seizures, liver dysfunction, respiratory depression, cardiac arrhythmias, myocardial infarction, and death have also been reported. Understanding and explaining disulfiram's toxic, or lethal, effects to patients is a prerequisite for its use (253–255), so it should never be used without the patient's knowledge and consent.

Controlled trials have not demonstrated any advantage of disulfiram over placebo in achieving total abstinence, in delaying relapse, or in improving employment status or social stability (256, 257). However, some clinicians believe that this medication, when combined with other therapeutic interventions, has some benefit for selected individuals who remain employed and socially stable (80, 257–260). Treatment effectiveness is enhanced when compliance is encouraged through frequent behavioral monitoring (e.g., breath tests), group support for remaining abstinent (e.g., in group therapy or AA) (261), contingency contracting, or, where feasible, supervised administration of disulfiram. Patients who are intelligent, motivated, and not impulsive and whose drinking is often triggered by unanticipated internal or external cues that increase alcohol craving are the best candidates for disulfiram treatment. Poor candidates include patients who are impulsive, have poor judgment, or are suffering from a comorbid psychiatric illness (e.g., schizophrenia, major depression) whose severity makes them unreliable or self-destructive (79, 262).

Patients taking disulfiram must be advised to avoid all forms of ethanol (including, for example, that found in cough syrup). In addition, disulfiram interferes with the metabolism of many medications, including tricyclic antidepressants, so that care must be taken to avoid toxicity (263). Disulfiram can cause a variety of adverse effects; hepatotoxicity and neuropathies are rare but potentially severe. The medication should be avoided for patients with moderate to severe hepatic dysfunction, peripheral neuropathies, pregnancy, renal failure, or cardiac disease (257).

3. Lithium

The use of lithium to treat patients with alcohol use disorders not comorbid with bipolar disorder was supported by some early anecdotal reports and by a small double-blind, placebo-controlled study (264). However, a large VA collaborative study (265) showed no benefits of lithium over placebo for patients with or without depressive symptoms.

4. Antidepressants

Although past evidence regarding the efficacy of tricyclic antidepressants for depression associated with alcohol use disorders is equivocal (72), two studies showed improved mood and reduced alcohol consumption in open and double-blind placebo-controlled trials with desipramine (266, 267). Preliminary data indicate that selective serotonin reuptake inhibitors may significantly reduce problem drinking in nondepressed social drinkers (268) and in those with alcohol abuse or dependence (269, 270).

D.   Psychosocial Treatments

The psychotherapies described in section III.E have all been used in the treatment of alcohol use disorders (271). Several authors have reviewed the efficacy of various psychotherapies for alcohol use disorders (106, 135, 138). This section reviews the outcomes literature on cognitive behavioral therapies, behavioral therapies, psychodynamic/interpersonal therapies, brief interventions, marital and family therapy, group therapy, aftercare, and self-help groups.

1.   Cognitive behavioral therapies

There is abundant evidence that cognitive behavioral treatments aimed at improving self-control and social skills consistently lead to reduced drinking (106, 272, 273). Self-control strategies include goal setting, self-monitoring, functional analysis of drinking antecedents, and learning alternative coping skills. Social skills training focuses on learning skills for forming and maintaining interpersonal relationships, assertiveness, and drink refusal. Holder et al. (106) found that self-control training produced better outcomes than control treatments in 12 of 17 studies and that social skills training was more effective than the control condition in 10 of 10 studies. Two studies have demonstrated that patients with sociopathic features do better in cognitive behavioral treatment than in interactional treatment (91, 274). Longabaugh et al. found that patients with antisocial personality disorder who received cognitive behavioral treatment had better drinking outcomes at 18-month follow-up than those who received relationship-enhancing treatment.

Holder et al. (106) found that cognitive behavioral stress management interventions were effective in six of 10 studies reviewed. Monti et al. (103) found that inpatients who received cue exposure treatment paired with coping skills training had better outcomes than those who received only standard inpatient treatment. Cognitive therapy interventions that are focused on identifying and modifying maladaptive thoughts but do not include a behavioral component have not been as effective as cognitive behavioral treatments (106).

Behavioral self-control training consists of cognitive and behavioral strategies, including self-monitoring, goal setting, rewards for goal attainment, functional analysis of drinking situations, and the learning of alternative coping skills (275, 276). Although some studies of behavioral self-control training have included controlled drinking, as well as abstinence, as a goal for treatment, behavioral self-control techniques should be used with the explicit long-term goal of abstinence.

In several studies, increases in coping responses or "self-efficacy" (277) at the end of treatment predicted better drinking outcomes during follow-up (56, 134, 278). Individuals who report more frequent use of cognitive or behavioral strategies aimed at problem solving or mastery ("approach coping") typically have better drinking outcomes than those who rely on staying away from high-risk situations ("avoidant coping") (238, 279).

2. Behavioral therapies

Individual behavior therapy and behavioral marital therapy have been found to be effective treatments for patients with alcohol use disorders (95, 106, 138). The most well-studied behavioral approach to the treatment of patients with alcohol use disorders is the community reinforcement approach, which uses behavioral principles and usually includes conjoint therapy, training in job finding, counseling focused on alcohol-free social and recreational activities, monitoring of disulfiram, and an alcohol-free social club (280). Using random assignment to community reinforcement or standard hospital treatments, Azrin (98) found that patients in the community reinforcement group drank less, spent fewer days away from home, worked more days, and were institutionalized less over a 24-month follow-up. A second controlled study comparing a) the community reinforcement approach, b) disulfiram plus a behavioral compliance program, and c) regular outpatient treatment showed that patients treated with community reinforcement did substantially better on all outcome measures than those in the other treatment conditions (98).

3. Psychodynamic/interpersonal therapies

Holder et al. (106) concluded that there was little empirical evidence from controlled studies that either insight-oriented psychotherapy or counseling is an effective treatment for alcoholism. Individual psychotherapy produced better outcomes than a control condition in two of eight studies reviewed, and psychodynamically oriented group psychotherapy produced better outcomes in two of 11 studies. Generic counseling approaches (characterized as primarily directive and supportive) produced better outcomes than controls in one of eight studies reviewed. Existing studies of this modality may be limited by their short-term approaches.

4. Brief interventions

Brief interventions generally delivered over one to three sessions include an abbreviated assessment of drinking severity and related problems and the provision of motivational feedback and advice. In eight of nine controlled treatment trials reviewed by Holder et al. (106), brief interventions were found to be effective, although Chick et al. (281) reported negative results. Reviews by Babor (282) and Bien et al. (283) concluded that brief interventions a) are typically more effective (in terms of alcohol use, general health, or social functioning) than no intervention; b) often have efficacy comparable to that of traditional more intense, longer-term programs; and c) increase the effectiveness of later treatment. Even interventions that are very brief (i.e., a few hours) may have some positive effect

(284). Brief interventions are typically used (and are most successful) for less severely affected patients who have not received previous treatment for an alcohol disorder. Further research is needed to determine which patients are optimally served by receiving a brief intervention.

5. Marital and family therapy

The state of the patient's relationship with family members or significant others can be a critical factor in the posttreatment environment for patients who are married or living with family members (106, 285). O'Farrell et al. (240) contrasted behavioral marital therapy and interactional marital therapy with a no-treatment control group. Both treatment groups showed greater improvement in marital adjustment, and the behavioral marital therapy groups showed a greater degree of sobriety over a short-term follow-up period. Two other studies (244, 286) showed that patients who received behavioral marital therapy began to have better drinking outcomes than those who did not at 1-year follow-up. Studies also have indicated that spousal involvement in treatment leads to improved marital and alcohol use outcomes early in the posttreatment period (287), that patients in conjoint therapy are less likely to drop out of treatment (288), and that therapy aimed at improving the marriage as a whole seems to work better than couples therapy focused strictly on alcohol-related problems (e.g., therapy with minimal or only alcohol-focused spouse involvement) (239).

6. Group therapy

Outcome studies have typically supported the efficacy of behavioral and cognitive behavioral group treatments, including group marital therapy. While research data regarding the efficacy of dynamically oriented group psychotherapy are limited and there are no empirical data to support the effectiveness of group psychotherapy for all alcohol-dependent patients, there are considerable data suggesting effectiveness for some patients (106, 138). The results of patient-matching studies in which patients were randomly assigned to cognitive behaviorally oriented treatment groups or interactional therapy groups suggest that patients with less sociopathy and those with neurological impairment fare better in interactional therapy; those with higher levels of sociopathy and psychopathology fare better in cognitive behavioral groups (90, 91). Litt et al. (289), in a randomized controlled study, also found a patient-treatment matching effect.

7. Aftercare

Aftercare may be defined as the period following an intense treatment intervention (e.g., hospital or residential care) and may include partial hospital care, outpatient care, or involvement in self-help approaches, alone or in combination. Patients frequently report that aftercare is helpful in maintaining abstinence following primary treatment (290). Walker et al. (291) found that involvement in aftercare was a stronger predictor of outcome than length of hospitalization, neuropsychological functioning, or pretreatment drinking and social stability measures. McLatchie and Lomp (292) randomly assigned patients to mandatory, voluntary, or no aftercare for a 12-week period and found that aftercare completers had the lowest relapse rate, with no difference between the mandatory and voluntary groups. Gilbert (293) randomly assigned patients to one of three aftercare conditions that varied in the degree of therapists' efforts to maintain patients in aftercare over 30 appointments. Patients in the maximal effort group were the most likely to complete aftercare, and aftercare completers in all groups had better outcomes than noncompleters. Studies that did not include random assignment suggest that greater participation in aftercare is generally associated with lower severity (e.g., fewer drinks on drinking days) but not with diminished frequency of drinking (294). A controlled study by O'Farrell et al. (295) showed that a version of behavioral marital therapy that included relapse prevention techniques (56) and was delivered as an aftercare intervention led to better drinking outcomes. Cooney et al. (90) and Kadden et al. (91) compared 3-week inpatient aftercare programs consisting of a) cognitive behavioral therapy and coping skills training and b) insight-oriented, interactional group therapy, and they reported similar outcomes in the two groups.

8. Self-help groups

See also section III.E.6. "AA is a fellowship of men and women who share their experience, strength and hope with each other that they may solve their common problem and help others to recover from alcoholism. The only requirement for membership is a desire to stop drinking" (296). AA provides tools for its participants to maintain sobriety, including the Twelve Steps, group identification, and mutual help. It is a spiritual (not religious) program requiring belief in something beyond oneself (297). Al-Anon (spouses), Alateen (teenagers and children of alcoholics), and Adult Children of Alcoholics help family members and friends of alcoholics focus on the need to avoid enabling behaviors and care for oneself whether a loved one is drinking or not. Other mutual-help programs include Women for Sobriety, Rational Recovery, Double Trouble (for patients with alcohol dependence comorbid with other psychiatric disorders), and Mentally Ill Chemical/Substance Abusers.

While the effectiveness of AA has not been evaluated in randomized studies because of a host of ethical and practical problems associated with attempting to assign patients not to go to AA, several studies have suggested that AA can be an important support for promoting an alcohol-free lifestyle in patients who are willing to attend (138, 237, 238). A number of studies have examined the relationship between degree of participation in AA and drinking outcomes (29, 298, 299). There is some evidence that patients with greater severity of drinking problems, an affective rather than cognitive focus, a concern about purpose and meaning in life, better interpersonal skills, and a high need for affiliation are good candidates for AA (300, 301).

Patients are more likely to benefit from AA groups composed of individuals of similar age and cultural and occupational status. All patients should be encouraged to attend a minimum number of AA meetings (i.e., five to 10) to ascertain the appropriateness and utility of AA in helping them remain alcohol free.

E. Clinical Features Influencing Treatment

The treatment implications of various clinical features are summarized in section III.H. In addition to these considerations, specific patterns of comorbidities and sequelae need to be considered for patients with alcohol use disorders, including the management of intoxication and withdrawal states.

1. Management of intoxication

In general, the acutely intoxicated patient requires reassurance and maintenance in a safe and monitored environment, with efforts to decrease external stimulation and provide orientation and reality testing. Adequate hydration and nutrition are also essential. Clinical assessment should follow the guidelines previously described, with particular emphasis on the patient's general medical and mental status, substance use history, and any associated social problems. Patients presenting with signs of intoxication should also be assessed for the possibility of recent use of other substances that could complicate the clinical course. Patients with a history of prolonged or heavy drinking or a past history of withdrawal symptoms are at particular risk for medically complicated withdrawal syndromes, which may require hospitalization.

2. Management of withdrawal

The syndrome of mild to moderate alcohol withdrawal generally occurs within the first several hours after cessation or reduction of heavy, prolonged ingestion of alcohol; it includes such signs and symptoms as gastrointestinal distress, anxiety, irritability, elevated blood pressure, tachycardia, and autonomic hyperactivity (2). The syndrome of severe alcohol withdrawal especially occurs within the first several days after cessation or reduction of heavy, prolonged ingestion of alcohol; the syndrome includes such signs and symptoms as clouding of consciousness, difficulty in sustaining attention, disorientation, grand mal seizures, respiratory alkalosis, and fever (2).

Fewer than 5% of individuals with alcohol withdrawal develop severe symptoms, and fewer than 3% develop grand mal seizures (2, 204). In the past, the mortality rate for patients experiencing alcohol withdrawal delirium was as high as 20%, but currently it is closer to 1% because of improved diagnosis and medical treatment of such patients (204).

Thiamin should be given routinely to all patients receiving treatment for moderate to severe alcohol use disorders to treat or prevent common neurologic sequelae of chronic alcohol use (302–304) (see section IV.E.3).

Although pharmacotherapeutic agents are often used to ameliorate the signs and symptoms of alcohol withdrawal and to prevent a major abstinence syndrome, the relative importance of supportive and pharmacologic treatment for these patients is not well established (305, 306). Generalized support, reassurance, and frequent monitoring is sufficient treatment for approximately two-thirds of the patients with mild to moderate withdrawal symptoms (307). In one case-controlled study (305), 74% of hospitalized alcohol-dependent patients without serious comorbid general medical problems responded to supportive treatment for alcohol withdrawal. Patients in more severe withdrawal and those who developed hallucinations required pharmacologic treatment.

There are numerous reviews of the pharmacologic treatment of moderate to severe withdrawal (308–310). The pharmacotherapy is directed toward reducing CNS irritability and restoring physiologic homeostasis. This often requires use of fluids, benzodiazepines, and, in selected cases, other medications (72). Most patients should be monitored by using breath and/or urine testing to ensure that they have not resumed alcohol use.

Many authors (e.g., Ciraulo and Shader [204]) recommend use of benzodiazepines to control abstinence symptoms, which takes advantage of the cross-tolerance between alcohol and this class of drugs. A single oral loading dose of chlordiazepoxide, 200–400 mg, or diazepam, 20–40 mg or as needed, may be used. Orally administered chlordiazepoxide (50 mg every 2–4 hours), diazepam (10 mg every 2–4 hours), oxazepam (60 mg every 2 hours), and lorazepam (1 mg every 2 hours) are commonly used (306, 311). The total dose necessary to suppress CNS irritability and autonomic hyperactivity in the first 24 hours (i.e., the stabilization dose) is then given in four divided doses the following day, after which the dose can usually be tapered over 3–5 days, with monitoring for re-emergence of symptoms (312). For most patients, the equivalent of 600 mg/day of chlordiazepoxide is the maximum dose, and many patients require less; a few, however, may require substantially more (313). Patients in severe withdrawal and those with a history of withdrawal-related symptoms may require up to 10 days before benzodiazepines are completely withdrawn. Benzodiazepine administration should be discontinued once detoxification is completed.

For patients with severe hepatic disease, the elderly, and patients with delirium, dementia, or other cognitive disorders, short-acting benzodiazepines such as oxazepam or lorazepam are preferred by some clinicians. These agents have the advantage of being metabolized and excreted principally through the kidneys and may be more suitable for patients with poor hepatic function; they also do not have active intermediary metabolites that may accumulate. Unlike the longer-acting preparations, they can also be administered intramuscularly or intravenously. Because of their brief half-lives, the short-acting benzodiazepines need to be given more frequently (314–317).

Beta blockers (e.g., propranolol, 10 mg p.o. every 6 hours) have been used to reduce signs of autonomic nervous system hyperactivity (e.g., tremor, tachycardia, elevated blood pressure, diaphoresis) and, at higher doses, arrhythmias (318–320). Atenolol has been used for a similar purpose, usually combined with benzodiazepines (321), thus allowing use of lower doses of benzodiazepines and thereby reducing the sedation and cognitive impairment often associated with benzodiazepine use.

Clonidine, an α-adrenergic agonist (0.5 mg p.o. b.i.d. or t.i.d.) has been shown to reduce tremor, heart rate, and blood pressure (322, 323).

However, the use of either β blockers or clonidine alone for the treatment of alcohol withdrawal is not recommended, because of their lack of efficacy in preventing seizures.

Barbiturates (e.g., pentobarbital, phenobarbital, and secobarbital) may be useful in reducing withdrawal symptoms in patients refractory to benzodiazepines (324).

For patients manifesting delirium, delusions, or hallucinations, neuroleptics may be used, particularly haloperidol (0.5–2.0 mg i.m. every 2 hours as needed), in most cases less than 10 mg per 24 hours, although some patients may require considerably more. In such cases, neuroleptics are an adjunct to the benzodiazepines, since the former are not effective for treating the underlying withdrawal state.

The use of anticonvulsants to prevent seizures in patients with alcohol withdrawal syndromes is controversial (325, 326). For patients with a prior history of withdrawal-related seizures, benzodiazepines are generally effective for this purpose. For patients with a history of non-withdrawal-related seizures, their anticonvulsant medication should be continued or restarted. Patients currently taking phenytoin should have their dose increased to a minimum of 300 mg/day (327). Oral as well as intravenous loading doses of 10 mg/kg, not to exceed an administration rate of 50 mg/min, should be given to patients who have discontinued phenytoin during a drinking spree (328). The prophylactic use of phenytoin to prevent seizures during alcohol withdrawal is not indicated (329, 330). Carbamazepine (600–800 mg/day for the first 48 hours, then tapered by 200 mg/day) has also been demonstrated to be effective in preventing withdrawal-related seizures, although its tendency to lower white blood cell counts in some patients may pose an added risk of infection (331–335). Intramuscular magnesium sulfate has also been used for preventing withdrawal seizures (336).

3.   Comorbid psychiatric and general medical disorders

Many patients with alcohol dependence present with signs and symptoms suggestive of dysthymia, major depression, or anxiety disorder and, if a comorbid diagnosis is made, may require pharmacotherapy. Given the propensity of these patients to misuse prescribed medications, one should give preference to drugs that have low abuse potential. Patients with a high level of depression, impulsivity, poor judgment, or the potential for making a suicide attempt should receive drugs with low potential for lethality in overdose situations (e.g., selective serotonin reuptake inhibitors) (337, 338). Poor compliance with medication regimens coupled with high overdose risk also suggests the dispensing of limited amounts of medication and random blood or urine toxicology screening to verify the use of both prescribed and nonprescribed medications by such patients.

In the majority of patients, however, signs and symptoms of depression and anxiety are related to alcohol intoxication or withdrawal and remit in the first few weeks of abstinence (339). Consequently, most psychiatrists feel that observation over a 3- to 4-week drug-free period should occur before diagnosis of a comorbid affective or anxiety disorder and prescription of a disorder-specific drug. Others suggest that in selected cases earlier initiation of treatment is warranted. For example, depressed patients with a prior history of major depression unrelated to periods of alcohol use and/or a strong family history of affective disorder are more likely to have a comorbid primary depression that should be treated as soon as detoxification is completed (45, 47, 267, 340). Tricyclic antidepressants should be used with caution for alcohol-dependent patients with comorbid depression.

The risk of poor compliance, tricyclic-alcohol interactions, and the risk of overdose should be considered with such patients. In addition, tricyclic plasma levels may be lower than expected because of the alcohol-induced increase in liver microsomal oxidases (341, 342). Serotonin reuptake inhibitors may have less risk of morbidity and mortality in overdose situations and, therefore, are preferred (343). Lithium, valproate, or carbamazepine may be used with caution for patients with comorbid bipolar disorder.

The use of benzodiazepines for alcohol-dependent patients with comorbid anxiety or panic disorder is controversial. Benzodiazepines (and other CNS depressants) have high abuse potential in these patients. For patients with generalized or performance anxiety, β blockers (e.g., propranolol) and buspirone are preferable to benzodiazepines since they have no cross-tolerance with ethanol or other CNS depressants and minimal abuse potential. Buspirone has also been reported to reduce alcohol consumption in patients with high levels of comorbid anxiety (344, 345). In otherwise refractory cases of panic disorder, clonazepam or other long-acting benzodiazepines can be cautiously administered if the principles just outlined are observed.

Monoamine oxidase inhibitors (MAOIs) have been used to treat patients with atypical depressions, but the risk of poor compliance with dietary and drug restrictions (including those for alcohol) and subsequent adverse reactions (e.g., hypertension) is high (346).

Chronic high-dose alcohol use can affect several different organ systems, including the gastrointestinal tract, the cardiovascular system, and the central and peripheral nervous systems. Alcohol-induced gastrointestinal problems include gastritis, ulcers of the stomach or duodenum, and, in approximately 15% of heavy users, cirrhosis of the liver and pancreatitis (347–349). Alcohol-dependent patients also experience higher than average rates of cancer of the esophagus, stomach, and other parts of the gastrointestinal tract (350).

Common comorbid cardiovascular conditions include low-grade hypertension and increased levels of triglycerides and low-density lipoprotein cholesterol, which increase the risk of heart disease. Cardiomyopathy occurs primarily among very heavy drinkers.

Endocrine consequences of chronic alcohol use for men include decreases in serum testosterone, loss of facial hair, breast enlargement, decreased libido, and impotence (351); endocrine consequences for women include amenorrhea, luteal phase dysfunction, anovulation, early menopause, and hyperprolactinemia (350). Blunting of the thyroid-stimulating hormone response to thyrotropin-releasing hormone, hypoglycemia, ketosis, and hyperuricemia have also been reported (352).

Alcohol-induced peripheral myopathy with muscle weakness, atrophy, tenderness, and pain is accompanied by elevations in creatine phosphokinase levels and the presence of myoglobin in the urine. Severe cases can involve rapidly progressive muscle wasting.

Many patients seeking treatment of alcohol dependence manifest cognitive abnormalities. In chronically heavy drinkers, dementia with characteristic cognitive deficits can occur. More commonly, however, one sees a subtle cognitive dysfunction that still may hamper patients' ability to comprehend or comply with a treatment plan (353). For such patients active involvement of family members or other responsible parties should take place at the beginning of and throughout treatment. Initial placement in a more structured (e.g., residential) treatment setting may also be indicated to assess the impact of cognitive problems on the patient's ability to comply with short- and long-term treatment. In patients who remain abstinent, reversal of alcohol-induced cognitive disturbance is often observed over time (354).

Nervous system sequelae of chronic alcohol use are related to vitamin deficiencies, particularly deficiencies in thiamin and other B vitamins; they include peripheral neuropathies, cognitive deficits, severe memory impairment, and degenerative changes in the cerebellum (355).

Wernicke's encephalopathy is characterized by ophthalmoplegia, ataxia, and confusion (204, 356). Ocular abnormalities include nystagmus, eye muscle palsies, and pupillary abnormalities. The mortality rate for acute untreated Wernicke's encephalopathy is 15%–20% (357, 358). Recovery is incomplete in 40% of the cases.

The vast majority (approximately 80%) of patients with Wernicke's disease also develop Korsakoff's syndrome (alcohol amnestic disorder), characterized by anterograde and retrograde amnesia, disorientation, poor recall, and impairment of recent memory, coupled with confabulation. Lesions in the mammillary bodies and thalamic nuclei may be the result of vitamin deficiencies or the direct toxic effects of alcohol. Recovery is variable. In more than one-half of the patients, elements of Korsakoff's syndrome are permanent.

Ataxia in alcohol-dependent patients is most often due to cerebellar dysfunction. Central demyelinization of the paraventricular gray matter of the diencephalon of the brain stem and glial proliferation are the major pathologic findings.

These neurological complications should be treated vigorously with B complex vitamins (e.g., thiamin, 50–100 mg/day i.m. or i.v.). Some patients may require treatment over a prolonged period, and improvement may occur up to 1 year after treatment is begun (359).

Alcoholic hallucinosis during or after cessation of prolonged alcohol use may respond to antipsychotic medication. Unlike the visual hallucinations that may occur during alcohol withdrawal, these are primarily auditory and occur in conjunction with a clear sensorium (360).

Alcohol dementia, characterized by impairment in short- and long-term memory, abstract thinking, judgment, and other higher cortical functions and by personality change, is seen in chronically heavy drinkers. Usually the memory deficits are less severe than in Korsakoff's syndrome or Alzheimer's disease (361). Neuropathological abnormalities in the frontal lobes, in the area surrounding the third ventricle, or diffusely through the cortex have been reported.

4. Pregnancy

Also refer to section III.H.3. Alcohol-related disorders may have adverse effects on the health of the pregnant woman, the course of the pregnancy, fetal development, early child development, and parenting behavior. The most well-established effect of in utero substance exposure is fetal alcohol syndrome. Reported effects of fetal alcohol syndrome in children exposed to high doses of alcohol in utero include low birth weight, poor coordination, hypotonia, neonatal irritability, retarded growth and development, craniofacial abnormalities (including microcephaly), cardiovascular defects, mild to moderate retardation, childhood hyperactivity, and impaired school performance (204, 362, 363).

Goals of treatment of pregnant women with alcohol use disorders include eliminating the use of alcohol, treating any comorbid psychiatric or general medical disorders, guiding the patient safely through the pregnancy, facilitating appropriate parenting behavior, and motivating the patient to remain in treatment after delivery to minimize the risk of relapse.

5. Age: the elderly

Two studies suggest that the treatment needs of older adults with alcohol use disorders may be different from those of younger patients. Liskow et al. (364) found that patients aged 58–77 required higher benzodiazepine doses during a 5-day detoxification and may need longer detoxification than patients under 33. Kofoed et al. (365) reported that VA patients aged 54 or older who received specialized services for the elderly in a VA program remained in treatment longer and were four times as likely to complete the program than elderly patients who received conventional services, although posttreatment relapse rates were comparable in the two groups.

V. Cocaine-Related Disorders: Treatment Principles and Alternatives

A. Overview

The focus of this section is the treatment of patients with cocaine dependence or abuse. Treatment of these disorders may be complicated by episodes of intoxication and withdrawal, the treatment of which is discussed in sections V.E.1 and V.E.2, respectively.

Cocaine-related disorders are most commonly found in persons aged 18–30 and are almost equally distributed between males and females. In a 1991 study, 12% of the U.S. adult population reported using cocaine one or more times in their lifetimes. A community study conducted in the early 1980s indicated that about 0.2% of the adult population have had cocaine abuse at some time in their lives (2, p. 228). It is likely that the prevalence of abuse is now higher since the overall use of cocaine has increased since that time.

Cocaine smoking is associated with a more rapid progression from use to dependence or abuse than is intranasal use (366). Dependence is commonly associated with a progressive tolerance to the desirable effects of cocaine, leading to increasing doses. With continuing use there is a diminution of pleasurable effects due to tolerance and an increase in dysphoric effects. Few data are available on the long-term course of cocaine-related disorders (2).

The goals of treatment for patients with cocaine use disorders are identical to those for patients with other forms of substance use disorders; these are discussed in section III.A and include abstinence, relapse prevention, and rehabilitation.

Psychiatric management (section III.C) is an important component of a successful treatment plan.

B.   Choice of Treatment Setting

The range of available settings for substance-related disorders and the general criteria for choosing among them are described in section III.G. In general, the choice of a setting depends on the clinical characteristics of the patient, the preferences of the patient, the treatment needs, and the available alternatives. As in the treatment of all patients with substance-related disorders, the least restrictive setting that is likely to facilitate safe and effective treatment is preferred.

Several studies have indicated that most patients can be effectively treated for cocaine abuse in intensive outpatient programs (143, 367). Although in one nonrandomized study (368) a group of 149 inpatients fared better at 1-year follow-up than did patients treated in an outpatient setting, a randomized study (367) revealed no difference in outcome after 3 and 6 months between patients assigned to inpatient and partial hospital care.

C.   Pharmacologic Treatments for Dependence and Abuse

Although a number of studies have shown promising results with a variety of pharmacotherapeutic agents, no medication has been found to have clear-cut efficacy in the treatment of cocaine dependence (369–371). Consequently, pharmacologic treatment is not ordinarily indicated as an initial treatment for many patients with cocaine dependence. However, patients with more severe forms of cocaine dependence or individuals who do not respond to psychosocial treatment may be candidates for a trial of pharmacotherapy. Thus far, desipramine and amantadine appear to have had the most positive (although mixed) results, although other medications may prove to be more successful.

1.   Drugs to reduce symptoms of cocaine abstinence or craving

Over 20 different medications have been studied in the search for an effective pharmacologic treatment for cocaine dependence. Most of these studies have been hampered by methodological problems, including lack of adequate controls and consistent outcome measures (e.g., urine tests rather than self-reports), failure to standardize the type and "dose" of the accompanying psychosocial interventions, lack of clarity about the importance of craving in the maintenance of cocaine dependence, the role of craving in the natural course of untreated cocaine abstinence syndrome, and lack of agreement as to the exact meaning of the term "craving" (372, 373).

Gawin et al. (374) found desipramine to be more effective than either lithium or placebo in reducing cocaine use by outpatients without coexisting mood disorders. More recent reports (375–377) have failed to confirm these positive findings, possibly because of differences in patient population and route of cocaine administration.

Initial studies of carbamazepine in the treatment of cocaine dependence yielded some favorable results (378), but subsequent double-blind, placebo-controlled studies failed to establish the efficacy of carbamazepine for these patients (379, 380).

Other agents used in the treatment of cocaine dependence have included pergolide (381), L-dopa/carbidopa (382), fluoxetine (383, 384), flupentixol (385), bupropion (386), amantadine (387), and maprotiline (388). All have shown some promise, but in relatively small, uncontrolled trials. An uncontrolled study of phenelzine (389) also yielded moderate success, but this treatment carries a high risk of hypertensive crisis in individuals who relapse to cocaine use, and it is therefore not recommended.

The mixed opioid agonist/antagonist buprenorphine has shown some promise in open trials in the treatment of patients dually dependent on cocaine and opioids (390, 391), although a large-scale double-blind clinical trial comparing patients maintained on buprenorphine with those receiving methadone showed no decrease in cocaine use among the former group (392). Work by Schottenfeld et al. (393) suggests that higher doses of buprenorphine (12–16 mg/day) may be effective. Larger-scale clinical trials funded by NIDA are currently examining the effectiveness of buprenorphine in this population.

2. Drugs to block the subjective effects of cocaine

Attempts to find a drug that blocks or attenuates the subjective (e.g., euphorigenic) effects of cocaine have included trials of imipramine (394), desipramine (375), bromocriptine (395, 396), trazodone, neuroleptics (397), and mazindol (398). However, there is no convincing evidence that, at doses that can be tolerated by patients, any of these medications is effective in this regard.

D. Psychosocial Treatments

Although a wide variety of treatment approaches have shown promise in preliminary studies, no therapeutic modality has been shown to be consistently superior to others in the treatment of cocaine-dependent patients. To date, several approaches show promise, but they need further study in larger-scale studies involving a broader range of patients. Both clinical and research experience suggest that intensive (i.e., more than once a week) outpatient psychosocial treatment focusing on abstinence is the preferred approach (399). Kang et al. (400) found that once-a-week psychosocial treatment (e.g., family therapy, psychotherapy, or group therapy) was generally ineffective, while Weddington et al. (373) reported a high degree of success among patients assigned to twice-a-week psychotherapy with or without medication.

1. Cognitive behavioral therapies

Studies demonstrating the efficacy of cognitive behavioral treatment strategies for cocaine-dependent patients are few in number. However, cognitive behavioral relapse prevention has been shown to be somewhat more effective than interpersonal therapy for patients with severe cocaine problems, but for patients whose cocaine problems were less severe the two treatments were equally effective (89). Recent 1-year follow-up showed a positive emerging effect of the psychotherapy (83).

2. Behavioral therapies

Studies of contingency contracting have shown positive outcomes during the period when the contract is in effect, promoting treatment compliance and abstinence (228). However, in a controlled trial, Higgins et al. (97) demonstrated the efficacy of contingency contracting (i.e., vouchers) in the outpatient treatment of cocaine dependence, with positive effects maintained during the 3 months after the contingency voucher program ended. Higgins et al. (95–97) studied the efficacy of a community reinforcement approach and found better outcomes from community reinforcement counseling plus incentives than from 12-step counseling. Cue exposure therapy has also been used in the treatment of cocaine use disorders, with equivocal results (104).

3. Psychodynamic psychotherapy

Well-controlled trials of psychodynamically oriented treatments for cocaine abuse or dependence are limited. A case series of patients successfully treated with individual psychodynamically oriented psychotherapy was reported by Schiffer (401), and there is a preliminary report revealing a high rate of retention with modified psychodynamically oriented group psychotherapy (116). Spitz has also described the use of group therapy for this population (402).

4. Comparisons of specific psychotherapeutic interventions

Carroll et al. (89) compared relapse prevention treatment using behavioral and cognitive approaches with interpersonal psychotherapy in a 12-week study of 42 outpatients with cocaine use disorders and found no significant differences in overall treatment outcome between the two groups, although patients with more severe cocaine abuse problems fared slightly better with relapse prevention. In a second study of outpatient treatment, Carroll et al. (403) randomly assigned 139 subjects to one of four conditions: a) relapse prevention plus desipramine, b) clinical management plus desipramine, c) relapse prevention plus placebo, or d) clinical management plus placebo. By the end of the 12-week trial, all groups showed significant improvement, but there were no main effects for psychotherapy or medication. Patients with greater baseline severity of cocaine use had better outcomes with relapse prevention than with clinical management, whereas those with less severity did better with desipramine than placebo. Depressed subjects had better cocaine use outcomes than nondepressed subjects, and they did better in relapse prevention than in clinical management (403). At 6- and 12-month follow-up, Carroll et al. (83) found evidence that subjects who received relapse prevention had better cocaine use outcomes than those who received clinical management, but there were no differences in cocaine use between the desipramine and placebo subjects.

Higgins et al. (96) compared behavioral treatment, consisting of contingency management procedures and community reinforcement, with traditional 12-step drug counseling in a random-assignment study. Although the sample size was relatively small, the results indicated better treatment retention at 24 weeks (58% versus 11%) and greater abstinence at 16 weeks (42% versus 5%) in patients treated with behavioral therapy. In the Higgins et al. trial (97), all patients received community reinforcement counseling, but only one group received contingent vouchers. The group with vouchers was more likely to complete 24 weeks of treatment (75% versus 40%), had a longer average duration of continuous cocaine abstinence (mean=11.7 weeks, SE=2.0, versus mean=6.0 weeks, SE=1.5), and showed significant improvement on the drug and psychiatric scales of the Addiction Severity Index.

A large-scale, multisite study is currently under way to compare the efficacy of outpatient supportive-expressive psychodynamic therapy (110), cognitive therapy (85), and addiction counseling. The various psychosocial approaches for patients with cocaine and opioid use disorders have recently been reviewed (404).

5. Self-help groups

See also section III.E.6. Twelve-step approaches, such as Narcotics Anonymous and Cocaine Anonymous, are commonly used in the management of cocaine dependence (405, 406). In more traditional settings, peer-led counseling groups have reportedly been useful in reducing recidivism (407). In a study of day hospital rehabilitation for patients with cocaine use disorders (247), greater participation in self-help programs at 3 months posttreatment predicted less cocaine use at 6 months posttreatment, even after pretreatment patient characteristics and degree of success in the day hospital program were controlled. These findings suggest that participation in self-help programs may improve outcome, independent of other treatment-related factors.

E. Clinical Features Influencing Treatment

The treatment implications of various clinical features are summarized in section III.H. In addition to these considerations, specific patterns of comorbidities and sequelae need to be considered for patients with cocaine use disorders, including the management of intoxication and withdrawal states.

1. Management of intoxication

The treatment of acute cocaine intoxication has been the subject of relatively little systematic investigation. In general, since there is no specific cocaine antidote, treatment is typically symptomatic and supportive.

Cocaine intoxication can induce paranoid delusions. Although neuroleptic drugs have been reported to be effective, most individuals recover spontaneously within hours (372, 408) and thus require no treatment. Patients who become extremely agitated and/or potentially dangerous may require sedation (e.g., with a benzodiazepine). Acute cocaine use can also produce hypertension, tachycardia, and seizures. Animal data and some clinical experience suggest that all adrenergic blockers and dopaminergic antagonists should be avoided in treating acute cocaine intoxication. Labetalol has been cited in favorable case reports, but no clinical studies have been reported. Benzodiazepines are frequently used for acute cocaine intoxication, and favorable results have also been reported with ambient cooling (409). There is no evidence that anticonvulsants prevent cocaine-induced seizures, and they are not recommended for this purpose.

2. Management of withdrawal

Cessation of cocaine use does not always cause specific withdrawal symptoms, although anhedonia and drug craving are common (372). However, many people experience a characteristic withdrawal syndrome within a few hours to several days after the acute cessation of, or reduction in, heavy and prolonged cocaine use.

The clinical features and duration of the cocaine abstinence syndrome are still somewhat controversial and ill defined. An early uncontrolled outpatient study (372) characterized withdrawal as progressing through three phases: an acute "crash" phase, a period of more gradual withdrawal, and an extinction phase lasting 1 to 10 weeks. Acute withdrawal (crashing) is seen after periods of frequent high-dose use. Intense and unpleasant feelings of depression and fatigue, at times accompanied by suicidal ideation, have been described during this phase. More-recent inpatient studies (373, 410), however, have suggested that cessation of regular cocaine use is associated with relatively mild symptoms of depression, anxiety, anhedonia, sleep disturbance (i.e., insomnia or hypersomnia), increased appetite, and psychomotor retardation, which decrease steadily over several weeks.

Dopamine agonists, such as amantadine (200–400 mg/day), were initially thought to be effective in reducing symptoms of cocaine withdrawal, craving, and subsequent use (379, 411, 412), but two more-recent studies (373, 377) failed to confirm this finding. Similarly, initial studies of bromocriptine yielded promising results in the treatment of cocaine withdrawal (395, 413). Subsequently, Tennant and Sagherian (412) found a higher rate of cocaine-negative urine samples but a higher dropout rate among patients given bromocriptine than among patients given amantadine. Teller and Devenyi (414) found no reduction of cocaine craving in an inpatient study of bromocriptine, and Moscovitz et al. (415) found no significant difference between bromocriptine and placebo in reducing cocaine use in outpatients. There may be a subgroup of patients who will respond to some form of pharmacotherapy with reduced craving and, subsequently, reduced use (see section III.D). However, to date there are inadequate research data to help the psychiatrist identify such patients.

3. Comorbid psychiatric and general medical disorders

Several reports have addressed treatment of patients with comorbid psychiatric disorders who also have cocaine-related disorders (e.g., references 49, 55, 416–421). Specific treatments that have been reported effective in certain populations of patients with cocaine abuse include lithium for patients with comorbid bipolar disorder, desipramine for patients with comorbid depression, and bromocriptine for patients with comorbid ADHD (370, 416, 417, 422). In addition, Ziedonis and Kosten's double-blind trial (423) suggests that desipramine or amantadine treatment for depressed cocaine-abusing methadone maintenance patients may reduce cocaine use. Given the evidence to date, however, these treatments alone cannot be expected to reduce cocaine use in these patients and must therefore be accompanied by appropriate psychosocial treatment for cocaine use disorders (55, 416).

A range of general medical conditions are associated with the route of administration of cocaine. Intranasal use may cause sinusitis, irritation and bleeding of the nasal mucosa, a perforated nasal septum, or, when a Valsalva-like maneuver is performed to better absorb the drug, a pneumothorax. Smoking cocaine is associated with respiratory problems, such as coughing, bronchitis, and pneumonitis, resulting from irritation and inflammation of the tissues lining the respiratory tract. Puncture marks and "tracks," most commonly in the forearms, occur in persons who inject cocaine. HIV infection is associated with cocaine dependence as a result of frequent injections and increased promiscuous sexual behavior, while other sexually transmitted diseases, hepatitis, tuberculosis, and other lung infections are also seen (2).

General medical conditions independent of the route of administration of cocaine include a) weight loss and malnutrition due to appetite suppression, b) myocardial infarction, and c) stroke. Seizures, palpitations, and arrhythmias have also been observed. Among persons who sell cocaine, in particular, traumatic injuries due to violent behavior are common (2).

4. Pregnancy

Also refer to section III.H.3. Cocaine-related disorders may have adverse effects on the health of the pregnant woman, the course of the pregnancy, fetal development, early child development, and parenting behavior. Possible effects of cocaine use on the course of the pregnancy include irregularities in placental blood flow, abruptio placentae, and premature labor and delivery (2). Possible effects on fetal development include very low birth weight, congenital anomalies, malformations of the urogenital system, mild neurodysfunction, transient electroencephalogram abnormalities, cerebral infarction and seizures, vascular disruption syndrome, and smaller head circumference (2, 424–427). Cerebrovascular problems, including small brain hemorrhages, may be due to decreased placental blood flow and diminished fetal oxygen concentrations in cocaine-exposed fetuses (425).

Possible effects on early child development that have been reported in cocaine-exposed newborns include hypertonicity, spasticity and convulsions, hyperreflexia, irritability, and attention problems. However, the roles of exposure to cocaine or other substances, poor maternal nutrition, prematurity, low birth weight, and neonatal withdrawal in the development of these signs and symptoms remain unclear (428, 429). Signs of CNS irritability usually disappear within the first year of life, as do any differences in head circumference or retardation in brain growth. Studies in cocaine-exposed children reveal deficits in attention span at 7 months, and in utero exposure to amphetamines has been found to be associated with slightly lower IQs (albeit still in the normal range) in 4-year-olds (430). While no clear correlation between in utero drug exposure and subsequent intellectual or neurological development has been established, associated conditions, such as low birth weight, the complications of untreated (or undertreated) withdrawal, and congenital abnormalities, may have adverse effects on cognitive and psychosocial development.

For pregnant patients withdrawing from cocaine, consideration of the use of pharmacotherapies should take into account the risks and benefits to the mother and fetus. The possibility of concurrent heroin use should be considered.

VI. Opioid-Related Disorders: Treatment Principles and Alternatives

A. Overview

The focus of this section is on the treatment of patients with opioid dependence or abuse. Consistent with the DSM-IV criteria listed in section II.A, the ECA study indicated that 0.7% of the adult population have met DSM-III-R criteria for opioid dependence or abuse at some time in their lives and that the male-to-female ratio of those affected is 3:1 or 4:1 (431).

Treatment of opioid use disorders may be complicated by episodes of intoxication and withdrawal, the treatment of which is discussed in sections VI.E.1 and VI.E.2. Chronic opioid use typically leads to impairment in social, vocational, academic, and parental functioning. Comorbid general medical, psychiatric, and legal problems are also common. General medical conditions may be related to 1) the use of unsterile needles for intravenous drug self-administration (e.g., HIV infection, abscesses, "needle tracks"); 2) poor self-care and adverse living conditions (e.g., tuberculosis, malnutrition); and 3) the drug-using lifestyle (e.g., head trauma), as well as comorbid psychiatric disorders (see section VI.E.3). Finally, many opioid-dependent patients also abuse alcohol, cocaine, anxiolytics, sedatives, and/or other psychoactive substances and may become dependent on these as well.

Opioid dependence is associated with a high death rate—approximately 10 per 1,000 per year among untreated persons. Death most often results from overdose, accidents, injuries, or other general medical complications. Accidents and injuries due to violence associated with buying or selling drugs are also common and in some areas account for more opioid-related deaths than overdose or HIV infection.

The long-term course of opioid use is quite heterogeneous. Although many untreated individuals with an untreated opioid use disorder are able to maintain a pattern of abuse without ever meeting the DSM-IV diagnostic criteria for dependence, many do become dependent; among such patients, relapse following a long period of abstinence (e.g., after incarceration) is common. On the other hand, only about 10% of service personnel who became dependent on opioids in Vietnam continued use after their return home (although a substantial minority did become dependent on alcohol or amphetamines) (431). The latter finding suggests the importance of environmental and peer-related factors, along with drug availability, in the development and maintenance of this disorder.

The goals of treatment for patients with opioid use disorders are similar to those for patients with other substance use disorders (section III.A). Although some opioid-dependent patients are able to achieve abstinence from all opioid drugs, many require and benefit from opiate agonist maintenance (e.g., with methadone or LAAM).

Psychiatric management (section III.C) is an important component of a successful treatment plan. Denial and ambivalence about giving up opioid use often interfere with treatment compliance and should be addressed directly in both individual and group settings. Motivation for treatment is generally enhanced by the involvement of supportive family members, non-drug-using peers, and appropriate role models. Periodic monitoring of patients for the presence of opioids and other drugs in breath, blood, or urine is a necessary component of any treatment program. Maintenance of a therapeutic alliance is often difficult with opioid-dependent patients, particularly those with comorbid antisocial personality disorder. Many such patients require an initial period of treatment in a structured drug-free setting in which there is a high level of staff experience and expertise in confronting denial and setting limits. The use of coercive pressure to encourage the patient to remain in treatment (e.g., through the legal system) can also be a useful external support for patients with poor impulse control and high levels of ambivalence about abstaining from nonprescribed substances.

B. Choice of Treatment Setting

The range of available settings and the general criteria for choosing among them are described in section III.G. In general, the choice of a treatment setting depends on the clinical characteristics and preferences of the patient, the perceived treatment needs, and the available alternatives. As in the treatment of all patients, the least restrictive setting that is likely to facilitate safe and effective treatment is preferred.

Therapeutic communities have been shown to be effective in the treatment of patients with opioid dependence. Simpson and Sells (157) reported that in a large-scale study with a 12-year follow-up, individuals with opioid dependence treated in therapeutic communities had the most favorable outcomes, even after age and demographic variables were controlled for. However, these data are tempered by the fact that only 15%–25% of those admitted voluntarily completed the program (see section III.G.2.b).

Long-term treatment with methadone or LAAM is generally provided through specialized outpatient programs that are licensed to dispense these substances. Licensing requirements concerning these programs are discussed in section III.I.3.

C. Pharmacologic Treatments for Dependence and Abuse

1. Agonist substitution therapy

For many patients with chronic relapsing opioid dependence the treatment of choice is maintenance on long-acting opioids. Of these, methadone is the most thoroughly studied and widely used treatment for opioid dependence. LAAM is a longer-acting preparation that can be administered less frequently than methadone (discussed later in this section). Buprenorphine (section VI.E.2.d) is a partial opioid agonist that has shown promising results in the longer-term treatment of opioid dependence, but additional research is needed (392). The current formulation of buprenorphine for the treatment of opioid dependence is sublingual; an oral form remains to be developed. Experiments are being conducted on a combination of buprenorphine and low doses of naloxone to determine whether it reduces the chances for diversion and abuse.

The primary goals of methadone (or LAAM) maintenance are a) to achieve a stable maintenance dose that reduces opioid craving and illicit opioid use and b) to facilitate engagement of the patient in a comprehensive program designed to prevent dependence or abuse of other substances and promote rehabilitation.

Since maintenance on methadone leads to the development of physiologic dependence and perhaps other CNS adaptations, federal guidelines limit the use of this modality to patients with a prolonged (e.g., more than 1 year) history of opioid dependence including (with some carefully defined exceptions) demonstrated physiologic manifestations. For patients who meet these legal criteria, the choice of methadone maintenance treatment is a matter of patient preference, assessment of the patient's past response to treatment, the probability of achieving and maintaining abstinence with other treatment modalities, and the psychiatrist's assessment of the short- and long-term effects of continued use of illicit opioids on the patient's life adjustment and overall health status.

Methadone maintenance treatment has generally been shown to be effective in decreasing the psychosocial and general medical morbidity associated with opioid dependence, with overall improvements in health status, decreased mortality, decreased criminal activity, and improved social functioning. Several studies also support the usefulness of methadone maintenance in reducing the spread of HIV infection among patients who administer drugs by injection (191, 432).

No single dose of methadone is optimal for all patients. Some may benefit from maintenance on low doses (10–20 mg/day), while others require more than 100 mg/day to achieve maximum benefit. Although 40–60 mg/day of methadone is usually sufficient to block opioid withdrawal symptoms, higher doses (averaging 70–80 mg/day) are usually needed during maintenance treatment to block craving for opiates and associated drug use. In general, higher doses (i.e., >60 mg/day) are associated with better retention and outcome (146, 147). If higher doses are used, monitoring of plasma methadone concentrations may be helpful, with the aim of maintaining minimum levels of 150–200 ng/ml (433). Retention rates for patients in methadone maintenance programs exceed 60% at 6 months, with up to 90% reduction in illicit opioid use in the patients who remain in treatment (146, 434).

Key issues in methadone maintenance treatment include determining a dose sufficient to suppress opioid withdrawal and craving, deciding on the appropriate duration of treatment, and including this modality within a comprehensive rehabilitation program. Programs that stress rehabilitation and long-term methadone treatment have been associated with the availability of more general medical and psychiatric services (146–148) and higher overall program quality (146). A General Accounting Office study supported these findings and demonstrated that the majority of programs may fail to provide optimal treatment (435). In some studies, use of higher doses of methadone has been associated with better overall outcome (147); in others, high-dose methadone has been associated only with less heroin use (146). Behavioral monitoring, random urine testing to assess recent illicit drug use, and linking the results of urine tests to counseling and other contingencies also improve outcomes (148, 150).

LAAM is a long-acting preparation that also reduces craving for opioids. LAAM is usually prescribed in doses of 20–140 mg (average, 60 mg) (204). Some patients prefer LAAM to daily methadone since dosing can be as infrequent as three times per week (436), thus allowing for fewer clinic visits and expanded integration into work or other rehabilitative activities. While treatment with LAAM has been shown to be comparable to methadone treatment with respect to reduction of opioid use (436–438), retention rates are reportedly higher for patients treated with methadone at doses of 80–100 mg/day (204). In general, longer duration of LAAM treatment (i.e., >6 months) is associated with better outcome.

The criteria for withdrawing patients from long-term maintenance on methadone or LAAM include demonstrated progress toward a drug-free lifestyle, stability in personal and occupational adjustment, absence of other substance use disorders, and successful treatment and remission of any comorbid psychiatric disorder(s).

Precipitous discharge from maintenance programs and concurrent withdrawal of methadone are associated with a high rate of relapse to illicit opioid use (439, 440). Voluntary termination of methadone maintenance also carries a high risk of relapse, even for patients who have responded well to treatment. Patients who choose to voluntarily discontinue maintenance treatment should receive supportive treatment during detoxification and aftercare services to aid in maintaining abstinence (27). Patients who relapse repeatedly despite such support should be given the option of voluntary lifetime maintenance on methadone.

2.   Opioid antagonist treatment

Maintenance on the opiate antagonist naltrexone is an alternative to methadone maintenance. The goal of treatment is to block the effects of the usual street doses of heroin or other opioids, thereby discouraging opioid use and facilitating extinction of classically conditioned drug craving (57, 77). Because of its long duration of action (24 to 72 hours, depending on the dose), naltrexone can be administered three times per week (100 mg p.o. on Monday and Wednesday, 150 mg on Friday). Because it has no abuse potential, naltrexone can be an important adjunct in the treatment of patients with opioid use disorders (441).

Adverse effects of naltrexone may include dysphoria, anxiety, and gastrointestinal distress. Like other opioid antagonists, naltrexone can precipitate severe withdrawal symptoms when administered to patients who are physiologically dependent on opioids. In general, naltrexone should be administered only to patients who have been withdrawn from opioids under medical supervision and have remained opioid free for at least 5 days after the use of heroin or other short-acting opioids, or 7 days after the last dose of methadone or other longer-acting opioids. Before naltrexone treatment is begun, a test dose of naloxone, 0.8 mg i.m., should be used to assess the degree of opioid dependence. The interval between completion of opioid detoxification and initiation of naltrexone treatment is a period of high risk for relapse. For this reason rapid opioid withdrawal, with use of clonidine and naltrexone (see section VI.E.2.c), has been used to shorten the interval between detoxification and initiation of naltrexone maintenance (74, 442). Repeated naloxone doses have also been used with clonidine to shorten opioid detoxification.

Although naltrexone is extremely effective when taken as prescribed, its utility is often limited by lack of patient compliance and/or low treatment retention. Compliance is improved when drug administration is directly observed and supervised by a designated health care professional, responsible family member, or work supervisor (75). Treatment retention is facilitated by family involvement in treatment planning and by the use of behavioral contingencies (i.e., reinforcement or punishment) (443, 444). Higher rates of success with naltrexone have also been reported for court-mandated treatment and for physicians or other professionals who are at risk of losing their professional licenses if they do not comply with treatment (445).

D.   Psychosocial Treatments

Psychosocial interventions are a key component of a treatment plan that includes a strategy to facilitate abstinence from opioids (e.g., with the aid of an opioid antagonist) or that includes the use of an opiate agonist (e.g., methadone).

1. Cognitive behavioral therapies

Woody et al. (107, 109, 446, 447) randomly assigned methadone maintenance patients to one of three groups: a) drug counseling alone, b) drug counseling plus supportive-expressive psychotherapy, or c) drug counseling with cognitive behavioral therapy. Outcomes were determined at 7 and 12 months. In patients with moderate to high degrees of depression or other psychiatric symptoms, supportive-expressive or cognitive behavioral therapies were much more effective than drug counseling alone; for patients with low levels of psychiatric symptoms, all three treatment conditions were equally effective. These findings were essentially replicated in three community-based methadone maintenance clinics (448).

2. Behavioral therapies

A variety of behavioral techniques have been used in treating opioid-dependent patients. Cue exposure treatment has been demonstrated to be effective in reducing classically conditioned responses to drug-related cues in a small group of patients with opioid use disorders (104). The use of urine toxicology testing to monitor for illicit drug use and provision of rewards for abstinence or aversive consequences for illicit drug use have been shown to be effective in promoting treatment compliance and abstinence in both methadone maintenance and naltrexone programs during the period the contingencies are in effect (30, 75, 443, 449, 450). In one study (449), methadone take-home privileges contingent on two consecutive weeks of drug-free urine tests yielded a higher percentage of patients who were abstinent at 4 weeks than did control conditions.

McLellan et al. (148) evaluated whether the addition of contingency-based counseling, general medical care, and psychosocial services improved the efficacy of methadone maintenance treatment in a study of newly admitted opioid patients randomly assigned to three levels of care. Patients who received counseling and contingencies based on urine test results, in addition to methadone, had better drug use outcomes than those who received methadone only. Patients who, in addition, received on-site general medical and psychiatric care, employment services, and family therapy had the best outcomes of all three conditions. Methadone alone was effective treatment for only a small percentage of patients.

3. Psychodynamic psychotherapies

The utility of adding a psychodynamic therapy to a program of methadone maintenance has been investigated. Woody et al. (107, 448) found that supportive-expressive therapy was more effective than drug counseling alone for patients with high levels of other psychiatric symptoms (see section VI.D.1). Rounsaville et al. (113) attempted to compare the efficacy of a 6-month course of weekly individual interpersonal therapy with a low-contact comparison condition for individuals in a full-service methadone maintenance program (that included weekly group psychotherapy). Patients with opioid dependence who met the inclusion criteria (including the presence of an additional nonpsychotic psychiatric diagnosis) were randomly assigned to the two groups. However, only 5% of the eligible patients agreed to participate (compared to 60% in the Woody et al. study), and only about one-half completed the trial. The highly selective nature of the participants (i.e., 95% of eligible patients refused), the high attrition rate, and the lack of significant outcome differences between the two groups led to the conclusions that it is very difficult to engage opioid-dependent patients in individual interpersonal therapy and that the potential benefit of such treatment is unclear for those who participate.

4.   Group and family therapy

Psychodynamically oriented group therapy, modified for substance-dependent patients, appears to be effective in promoting abstinence when combined with behavioral monitoring and individual supportive psychotherapy (116). McAuliffe (451) reported that group relapse prevention based on a conditioning model of addiction, when combined with self-help groups, was more effective than no treatment in reducing opioid use, unemployment, and criminal activities in recently detoxified patients.

Family therapy has been demonstrated to enhance treatment compliance and facilitate implementation and monitoring of contingency contracting with opioid-dependent patients (see section III.E.5).

5.   Self-help groups

See also section III.E.6. Self-help groups, such as Narcotics Anonymous, are beneficial for some individuals in providing peer support for continued participation in treatment, avoiding drug-using peers and high-risk environments, confronting denial, and intervening early in patterns of thinking and behavior that often lead to relapse.

E.   Clinical Features Influencing Treatment

The treatment implications of various clinical features are summarized in section III.H. In addition to these considerations, specific patterns of comorbidities and sequelae need to be considered for patients with opioid use disorders, including the management of intoxication and withdrawal states.

1.   Management of intoxication

The care of patients with opioid use disorders is frequently complicated by episodes of relapse. Consequently, recognition and treatment of intoxication with opioids or other substances is an important aspect of ongoing treatment.

Acute opioid intoxication of mild to moderate degree usually does not require treatment. However, severe opioid overdose, marked by respiratory depression, may be fatal and requires treatment in a hospital emergency room or inpatient setting. The length of hospitalization depends on the severity of respiratory depression and associated general medical complications, the dose and half-life of the opioid used, the presence of other drugs of abuse, and the reason for the overdose. Uncomplicated overdose with an opioid that has a relatively short half-life (e.g., 3–4 hours for heroin) may be treated in an emergency room, with release after a few hours. Overdose with methadone or LAAM, however, requires closer observation for a minimum of 24–48 hours. Deliberate overdose as part of a suicide attempt requires thorough psychiatric evaluation in a hospital setting.

Patients with signs of respiratory depression, stupor, or coma need ventilatory assistance. An adequate airway should be established. Aspiration can be prevented by placing the patient on his or her side or by using a cuffed endotracheal tube. In cases where oral intake of opioids or other drugs within the previous 6 hours is suspected, gastric lavage should be carried out. In hypoglycemic patients, intravenous 50% glucose in water should be administered slowly. Pulmonary edema, where present, can be treated with positive-pressure ventilation.

Naloxone (Narcan), a pure narcotic antagonist, will reverse respiratory depression and other manifestations of opioid overdose. The usual dose is 0.4 mg (1 ml) i.v. A positive response, characterized by increases in respiratory rate and volume, a rise in systolic blood pressure, and pupillary dilation, should occur within 2 minutes. If there is no response, the same or a higher dose (e.g., 0.8 mg) of naloxone can be given twice more at 5-minute intervals. Failure to respond to naloxone suggests a concurrent, or completely different, etiology for the problem (e.g., barbiturate overdose, head injury). In patients who are physically dependent on opioids, naloxone may precipitate signs and symptoms of opioid withdrawal. These may appear within minutes and last several hours (74).

2. Management of withdrawal

The treatment of opioid withdrawal is directed at safely ameliorating acute symptoms of withdrawal and facilitating entry into recovery and/or rehabilitation programs. Four pharmacologic strategies are in general use: a) methadone substitution, with gradual methadone tapering; b) abrupt discontinuation of opioids, with use of clonidine to suppress withdrawal symptoms; c) clonidine-naltrexone detoxification, where withdrawal symptoms are precipitated by naltrexone and then suppressed by clonidine; and d) buprenorphine substitution, followed by discontinuation (abrupt or gradual) of buprenorphine.

a. Methadone substitution.   Methadone hydrochloride is highly effective in ameliorating the signs and symptoms of opioid withdrawal. While the use of narcotics to detoxify or maintain patients with opioid dependence requires special licensing (see section III.I.3), this regulation is waived for inpatients with life-threatening general medical or psychiatric conditions.

The procedure for opioid detoxification with methadone involves stabilizing the patient on a daily dose of methadone that is determined by the patient's response (based on objective signs of withdrawal) to a dose of 10 mg every 2–4 hours as needed (444, 452).

During the first 24 hours, 10–40 mg will stabilize most patients and control abstinence symptoms. Once the stabilization dose is determined, the drug can be slowly tapered (e.g., by 5 mg/day). In inpatient settings, detoxification from heroin or other short-acting opioids can usually be completed within 7 days, but a more gradual tapering will result in a smoother clinical course. The detoxification of patients from longer-acting opioids (e.g., methadone) generally is done over a much longer period (federal regulations allow methadone detoxification in licensed facilities to last as long as 180 days). The benefits of slow tapering include greater patient comfort and more time in which to strengthen other therapeutic interventions. When the methadone dose drops below 20–30 mg/day, many patients begin to complain of renewed (but milder) abstinence symptoms. These may be ameliorated by the addition of clonidine (see the following section). Unless patients can be sufficiently motivated to complete the course of treatment, the dropout and relapse rates during this stage of methadone-assisted withdrawal are very high (452).

b. Clonidine-assisted detoxification.   Clonidine is a nonopioid antihypertensive drug that has been used successfully to reduce symptoms of opioid withdrawal. It acts by stimulating midbrain α_2-adrenergic receptors, thereby reducing the noradrenergic hyperactivity that accounts for many of the symptoms of opioid withdrawal. Clonidine suppresses nausea, vomiting, diarrhea, cramps, and sweating but does little to reduce the muscle aches, insomnia, and drug craving that often accompany opioid withdrawal. Some patients are extremely sensitive to clonidine and experience profound hypotension, even at low doses.

Protocols for clonidine detoxification have been described by Kleber (74). On the first day of treatment, clonidine-aided detoxification involves 0.1 to 0.3 mg in three divided doses, which is usually sufficient to suppress signs of opioid withdrawal; inpatients can generally receive higher doses because of the greater availability of staff monitoring for hypotension and sedation. The dose is adjusted until withdrawal symptoms are reduced. If the patient's blood pressure falls below 90/60 mm Hg, the next dose should be withheld, after which tapering can be resumed while the patient is monitored for signs of withdrawal. In the case of short-acting opioids, such as heroin, clonidine-aided withdrawal usually takes 4–6 days, whereas withdrawal from methadone usually takes 10–14 days.

Although clonidine does not yet have FDA approval for the treatment of opioid withdrawal, it has some advantages over methadone in that it does not produce opioid-like tolerance or physical dependence, it avoids the postmethadone rebound in withdrawal symptoms, and patients completing a course of clonidine-assisted withdrawal can be immediately given an opioid antagonist (e.g., naltrexone) if indicated. The disadvantages of clonidine include insomnia, sedation, and hypotension as side effects. In addition, clonidine will not ameliorate some symptoms of opioid withdrawal, such as insomnia and muscle pain, which may require additional treatments. Contraindications to the use of clonidine include acute or chronic cardiac disorders, renal or metabolic disease, and moderate to severe hypotension (453).

In general, clonidine-assisted detoxification is easier to carry out in inpatient settings, where it is possible to use higher doses to block withdrawal symptoms while monitoring side effects (e.g., hypotension). Clonidine-induced sedation is also less of a problem for inpatients. However, with experienced staff, outpatient detoxification with clonidine is a reasonable approach. Outpatients should not be given more than a 3-day supply of clonidine for unsupervised use, since treatment requires careful dose titration and clonidine overdoses can be life threatening (454, 455).

While clonidine can be an effective alternative to methadone for treating opiate withdrawal, it does not substantially shorten the time required for withdrawal. In addition, the completion rate for clonidine-treated outpatients is relatively low and roughly comparable to that with methadone (454, 456).

c. Clonidine-naltrexone ultrarapid withdrawal. The combined use of clonidine and naltrexone has been demonstrated as safe and effective for rapidly withdrawing patients from heroin or methadone. Essentially, naltrexone-precipitated withdrawal is avoided by pretreating the patient with clonidine (456, 457). The technique is most useful for opioid-dependent patients who are in transition to narcotic antagonist treatment.

O'Connor et al. (458) reported that 95% of patients successfully completed detoxification with clonidine and naltrexone on an outpatient basis. However, the limitations of this method of detoxification include the need to monitor patients for 8 hours on day 1 (because of the potential severity of naltrexone-induced withdrawal) and the need for careful blood pressure monitoring during the entire detoxification procedure.

d. Buprenorphine. Buprenorphine is a partial opioid agonist. At low doses (2–4 mg/day sublingually), the drug blocks the signs and symptoms of opioid withdrawal. Because it is only a partial agonist, high doses (i.e., >8 mg/day) do not produce as much respiratory depression or other agonist effects as do comparably high doses of pure agonists (e.g., morphine). Patients treated with low doses may be able to stop taking the drug abruptly and experience milder symptoms of opiate withdrawal than after taking heroin or methadone. In experimental studies (459) buprenorphine has been shown to suppress heroin use in both inpatient and outpatient settings.

e. Other medications. There is considerable controversy, and few factual data, about the use of sedative-hypnotics or anxiolytics to treat the insomnia, anxiety, or muscle cramps associated with opioid withdrawal. Some psychiatrists maintain that the abuse potential of CNS depressants for these patients is too great and may also precipitate craving for opioids and relapse. Others feel that for carefully selected patients and with appropriate monitoring, use of benzodiazepines over a relatively brief period (i.e., 1–2 weeks) may be helpful in ameliorating the often-debilitating insomnia that can accompany opioid withdrawal (458). Diphenhydramine, hydroxyzine, and sedating antidepressants (e.g., doxepin, amitriptyline, and trazodone) have also been used for this purpose. It should be noted that these medications may also be abused, although much less often than the benzodiazepines (74).

f. Acupuncture. Studies on the efficacy of acupuncture or electrostimulation in the treatment of opioid withdrawal have yielded conflicting findings (460–465). Wen and Cheung (466) reported favorable results with 40 patients who received acupuncture combined with electrical stimulation, although the study was subsequently thought to have inadequate controls (467). Experts remain divided on the effectiveness of acupuncture in the treatment of withdrawal (463).

3. Comorbid psychiatric disorders

a. Comorbid symptoms. The reduction of opioid use in patients with preexisting comorbid psychiatric disorders may precipitate the reemergence of previously controlled symptoms (e.g., depression, mania, psychosis), which may in turn increase the risk of relapse to substance use (433).

In prescribing medications for comorbid non-substance-related psychiatric disorders, psychiatrists should be alert to the dangers of medications with high abuse potential and to possible drug-drug interactions between opioids and other psychoactive substances (e.g., benzodiazepines) (444, 446, 468). For example, use of MAOIs should be avoided because of potential drug-drug interactions with cocaine, opioids, or alcohol. In general, benzodiazepines having a rapid onset, such as diazepam and alprazolam, should be avoided because of their abuse potential (469). However, benzodiazepines having a slow onset and substantially lower abuse potential (e.g., oxazepam or clorazepate) can probably be used safely for selected patients provided that appropriate controls are applied (470). All other psychotherapeutic drugs should be prescribed cautiously, with random blood or urine monitoring to ascertain compliance.

b. Other substance use disorders. Dependence on alcohol, cocaine, or other drugs of abuse is a frequent problem for opioid-dependent patients. Cocaine abuse was found to be a problem for about 60% of patients entering methadone programs (146). In studies of opioid-dependent patients in active treatment, rates of cocaine use as high as 40% or more have been reported (471–474). Similarly, heavy drinking is a problem for an estimated 15%–30% of methadone-maintained patients, and benzodiazepine abuse may be just as common in this population (475, 476). Comparable data regarding rates of comorbid substance use disorders in patients treated in naltrexone programs are not generally available.

Comorbid substance use disorders require special attention, since treatment directed at opioid dependence alone is unlikely to lead to cessation of other substance use. Treatment is generally similar to that described for individual substances elsewhere in this guideline. Increased frequency of behavioral monitoring (e.g., daily breath or twice-weekly urine toxicology testing), intensified counseling, contingency contracting, referral to specific self-help groups (e.g., AA), and specialized pharmacologic treatments (e.g., disulfiram) have all been used with varying degrees of success. Two studies suggest that higher methadone doses coupled with intensive outpatient treatment may decrease cocaine use by methadone-maintained patients (252).

Opioid-dependent patients who are also dependent on other substances, particularly CNS depressants, should be stabilized with methadone and then gradually withdrawn from other drugs. Efforts to abruptly eliminate all drugs of abuse will not be successful with all patients. In such cases, elimination of the drugs one at a time may be warranted.

Use of aversive contingencies, such as methadone dose reduction or even withdrawal, for continued abuse of cocaine (or sedatives or alcohol) by patients in methadone maintenance treatment is controversial. Some psychiatrists believe that requiring methadone withdrawal for persistent drug abuse causes many patients to cease or greatly limit use, while failure to enforce such limits implicitly gives patients license to continue use. Others believe that methadone withdrawal is never justified for patients abusing alcohol or other drugs because of the proven efficacy of methadone in reducing intravenous heroin use, improving social and occupational functioning, and providing the opportunity to continue to motivate patients to reduce other drug use.

4. Comorbid general medical disorders

The injection of opioids may result in the sclerosing of veins, cellulitis, abscesses, or, more rarely, tetanus infection. Other life-threatening infections associated with opioid use by injection include bacterial endocarditis, hepatitis, and HIV. HIV infection rates have been reported to be as high as 60% among persons dependent on heroin in some areas of the United States (2). Counseling on how to reduce HIV risk should be a routine part of treatment for intravenous opioid users (14).

Tuberculosis is a particularly serious problem among individuals who inject drugs, especially those dependent on heroin. Infection with the tubercle bacillus occurs in approximately 10% of these individuals. For non-HIV-infected patients who test positive for the purified protein derivative of tuberculin (PPD), the lifetime risk of developing active tuberculosis is approximately 10%, and the 1-year risk is 7%–10% (477). Guidelines regarding prophylactic treatment for patients with a positive skin test have been published (478).

In addition to the presence of life-threatening infections, opioid dependence is associated with a very high rate of death from overdose, accidents, injuries, or other general medical complications (2, p. 253).

5. Pregnancy

Also refer to section III.H.3. Opioid use disorders may have adverse effects on the health of the pregnant woman, the course of the pregnancy, fetal development, early child development, and parenting behavior. In pregnant women these effects include a) poor nourishment, with accompanying vitamin deficiencies or iron and folic acid deficiency anemias; b) general medical complications from frequent use of contaminated needles (abscesses, ulcers, thrombophlebitis, bacterial endocarditis, hepatitis, urinary tract infections, and HIV infection); c) sexually transmitted diseases (gonorrhea, chlamydia, syphilis, herpes); and d) hypertension.

Possible effects of opioid use and its resultant lifestyle on the course of the pregnancy include toxemia, miscarriage, premature rupture of membranes, and infections. Possible short- and long-term effects on the baby include low birth weight, prematurity, stillbirth, neonatal abstinence syndrome, and sudden infant death syndrome (426, 479, 480). Approximately one-half of the infants born to women with opioid dependence are physiologically dependent on opioids and may experience a moderate to severe withdrawal syndrome requiring pharmacologic intervention. However, when socioeconomic factors (e.g., family disruption, poverty) are controlled for, mild to moderate neonatal withdrawal does not appear to affect psychomotor or intellectual development (480).

The goals of treatment for the pregnant opioid-using patient include ensuring physiologic stabilization and avoidance of opioid withdrawal; preventing further abuse of illicit drugs or alcohol; improving maternal nutrition; encouraging participation in prenatal care and rehabilitation; reducing the risk of obstetrical complications, including low birth weight and neonatal withdrawal, which can be lethal if untreated; and arranging for appropriate postnatal care when necessary.

Pregnant patients who lack the motivation or psychosocial supports to remain drug free should be considered for methadone maintenance regardless of their previous history of treatment. Withdrawal from methadone is not recommended, except in cases where methadone treatment is logistically not possible. In cases where medical withdrawal is necessary, there are no data to suggest that withdrawal in one trimester is worse than in any other. On the other hand, a narcotic antagonist should never be given to a pregnant substance-using patient because of the risk of spontaneous abortion, premature labor, or stillbirth. Data on the safety of clonidine for pregnant patients are not available.

In a randomized comparison of enhanced and standard methadone maintenance for pregnant opioid-dependent women, Carroll et al. (481) found that enhanced treatment—consisting of standard treatment (daily methadone medication, weekly group counseling, and thrice-weekly urine screening) plus weekly prenatal care by a nurse-midwife, weekly relapse-prevention groups, positive contingency awards for abstinence, and provision of therapeutic child care during treatment visits—resulted in improved neonatal outcomes (longer gestations and higher birth weights) but did not affect maternal drug use.

6. Age: children and adolescents

Some psychiatrists prefer to avoid methadone maintenance as a first-line treatment for opioid dependence in adolescents since it may become a lifelong therapy. Although therapeutic communities are sometimes recommended, most adolescents have difficulty tolerating prolonged confinement in such programs unless the programs are specifically tailored to meet the clinical needs of this age group.

VII.   Research Directions

The treatment of patients with substance use disorders would be improved by research focusing on the following broad areas:

A.   The factors that alter the development, clinical course, and prognosis of these disorders, including genetic, developmental, biological, cognitive, and sociocultural factors, as well as comorbidity and the impact of early experience with abusable substances.

B.   The effects of treatment modalities in current use, as well as those being developed, on short-, intermediate-, and long-term outcomes in specific patient populations.

C.   The differential efficacy of treatment programs, with specific attention to the site of treatment and the mix of specific treatment modalities used.

D.   The intensity and staging of treatment (i.e., using different treatments in different settings at different phases of the disorder) and the interactive (i.e., additive, synergistic, or antagonistic) effects of various treatment modalities when applied concurrently or in sequence.

E.   The impact of sociodemographic, psychiatric, and general medical characteristics, as well as patient treatment preferences, on treatment, participation, compliance, and outcome.

F.   Improved methods for the diagnosis and treatment of comorbid psychiatric and/or substance use disorders, including approaches for defining the precise temporal and etiologic relationships between substance use and other forms of psychopathology.

G.   The biological, cognitive, and behavioral factors contributing to development of the prolonged abstinence syndrome in patients previously dependent on alcohol, cocaine, or opioids.

H.   The acute and chronic effects of abused substances on the morphology, biochemistry, and physiology of the brain, as revealed through brain imaging or other assessment techniques, and the time course of recovery from these effects once patients are drug free.

I.   New pharmacotherapies that reduce craving in both active and abstinent substance users.

J.   New pharmacotherapies that may reverse the physiologic effects of chronic substance use on the functioning of the brain and other affected organs.

K.   Identification of both risk and protective factors that influence vulnerability to development of substance use disorders.

L.   Organizational and managerial factors in the cost-effectiveness of treatment programs.

M.   Programmatic approaches aimed at prevention and early intervention for these disorders.

Selected examples of *specific* types of research that are needed are the following:

A.   Studies to guide the identification of patient populations who will benefit from naltrexone for treatment of alcohol use disorders.

B.   The development of more-effective pharmacotherapies for the treatment of cocaine dependence, including agents that reduce short- and long-term craving for cocaine.

C.   The further development of pharmacotherapies with mixed agonist/antagonist properties that block the effects of opioids and reduce opioid craving. In addition, the development of nonopioid medications for opioid withdrawal with better risk-benefit ratios than those of currently available agents.

D.   Studies of the pathogenesis of substance-induced fetal abnormalities following in utero exposure to alcohol or cocaine.

E.   The development of new pharmacotherapies for pregnant substance-abusing women that do not affect the fetus.

F.   Studies of the efficacy of behavioral, psychosocial, and family-based interventions in the treatment of children and adolescents at risk for substance use disorders.

G.   Studies to identify the gene or genes that influence the heritability of alcoholism and the development of techniques to alter the genetic makeup of individuals carrying this gene or genes.

VIII.   Development Process

This practice guideline was developed under the auspices of the Steering Committee on Practice Guidelines. The process is detailed in a document available from the APA Office of Research, "APA Practice Guideline Development Process." Key features of the process included the following:

❖   initial drafting by a work group that included psychiatrists with clinical and research expertise in substance use disorders;

❖   a comprehensive literature review (see the following outline);

❖   the production of multiple drafts with widespread review by over 145 individuals and 36 organizations (see section IX);

❖   approval by the APA Assembly and Board of Trustees; and

❖   planned revisions at 3- to 5-year intervals.

Computerized searches of relevant literature were carried out for the period January 1980 to February 1993, and these were subsequently updated through March 1994. Databases accessed included MEDLINE and PsycLIT. In addition, specialized bibliographies were obtained from Ovid Technologies, from the Alcohol and Alcohol Problems Science Database of the National Institute on Alcohol Abuse and Alcoholism (NIAAA), and from the Office for Treatment Improvement of the Substance Abuse and Mental Health Services Administration (SAMHSA). The specific searches included the following:

A.   MEDLINE (*Index Medicus*) searches were conducted for the following periods:

1.   January 1980 to February 1993, with the following key words:

a.   "Substance abuse—treatment outcome," yielding 4,543 references.

2. January 1988 to February 1992, with the following key words:

   a. "Substance use disorders and substance dependence," yielding 2,427 references.
   b. "Alcoholism and substance abuse," yielding 8,515 references.

3. January 1992 to March 1994, with the following key words:

   a. "Substance abuse treatment outcome," yielding 83 references.

B. A PsycLIT search on CD-ROM (*Psychological Abstracts*) was conducted for the period January 1983 to December 1990, with the following key words:

1. "Drug abuse, substance abuse, alcoholism, aggressive behavior, violence," yielding 98 references.
2. "Alcohol abuse, alcoholism, aggressive behavior, violence," yielding 69 references.

C. A PsycLIT (Silver Platter 3.1) search was conducted for the following periods:

1. January 1987 to September 1992, with the following key words:

   a. "Alcohol and drug treatment outcome," yielding 14 references.
   b. "Drug abuse, relapse prevention, rehabilitation," yielding 25 references.

2. January 1980 to October 1993, with the following key words:

   "Drug abuse outcome," yielding 31 references.

D. Current Information Service (NIAAA) bibliographies from the Alcohol and Alcohol Problems Science Database (ETOH) for the period January 1992 to May 1993 were obtained for the following areas:

1. Evolution of DSM-III and DSM-IV, yielding 23 references.
2. Therapies for alcohol dependence, yielding 39 references.

E. An Ovid Technologies search was conducted in May 1990 for the period January 1983 to April 1990, with the following key words:

1. "Treatment of alcoholism," yielding 50 references.
2. "Clinical pharmacology of alcoholism," yielding 89 references.
3. "Dual diagnosis," yielding 62 references.

F. An Office for Treatment Improvement search was conducted for the period January 1987 to September 1990, with the following key words:

1. "Coexisting substance abuse and mental disorders," yielding 83 references.

Papers selected from the aforementioned databases for further review were those published in English-language, peer-reviewed journals. Preference was given to papers based on randomized, controlled clinical trials, or nonrandomized case-control studies, or cohort studies that used broadly accepted statistical techniques for analyzing data. Clinical reports involving descriptions of patients or groups of patients were also reviewed if the sample size was felt to be adequate for drawing conclusions about the efficacy of a given treatment or if an individual case report was thought to illustrate a particularly important clinical point. Epidemiologic studies and studies involving meta-analysis were also reviewed if the population sample or the number of studies was sufficiently large to constitute a representative sample of patients with substance use disorders or a specific patient subgroup.

Review articles and book chapters were also reviewed. Criteria for inclusion were publication in a well-regarded peer-reviewed psychiatric, substance abuse, or general medical journal or in a major psychiatric text published in the decade between 1983 and 1993.

IX. Individuals and Organizations That Submitted Comments

Allan J. Adler, M.D., F.R.C.P.(C)
John Ambre, M.D., Ph.D.
Lee H. Beecher, M.D.
Myron L. Belfer, M.D.
Thomas Beresford, M.D.
Mel Ira Blaustein, M.D.
Sheila B. Blume, M.D.
Peter A. Boxer, M.D., M.P.H.
Steve J. Brasington, M.D.
Peter Bridge, M.D.
William H. Bristow, Jr., M.D.
David W. Brook, M.D.
Mary D. Bublis, M.D.
Robert Byck, M.D.
Robert Paul Cabaj, M.D.
Jean Lud Cadet, M.D.
Kenneth Carter, M.D.
Domenic A. Ciraulo, M.D.
Wilson M. Compton, M.D.
Gerard J. Connors, Ph.D.
James R. Cooper, M.D.
Linda Cottler, Ph.D.
Francine Cournos, M.D.
Lino Covi, M.D.

Dorynne Czechowicz, M.D.
Amin N. Daghestani, M.D.
William C. Dalsey, M.D.
Dave M. Davis, M.D.
Prakash N. Desai, M.D.
O'Neil S. Dillon, M.D.
Stephen Dilts, M.D.
Edward F. Domino, M.D.
Mina K. Dulcan, M.D.
Robert L. DuPont, M.D.
Richard S. Epstein, M.D.
Juan B. Espinosa, M.D.
Cesar Fabiani, M.D.
Loretta Finnegan, M.D.
Phillip J. Flores, Ph.D.
Saul Forman, M.D.
Marshall Forstein, M.D.
Richard J. Frances, M.D.
Linda Fuller, D.O.
Marc Galanter, M.D.
Frank Henry Gawin, M.D.
William Goldman, M.D.
James Goodman, M.D.
Enoch Gordis, M.D.

David Gorelick, M.D.
Sheila Hafter Gray, M.D.
Michael K. Greenberg, M.D.
Shelly F. Greenfield, M.D., M.P.A.
Harry E. Gwirtsman, M.D.
Deborah Hasin, Ph.D.
Stephen T. Higgins, Ph.D.
Ken Hoffman, M.D., M.P.H.
Steven K. Hoge, M.D.
Kate Hudgins, Ph.D.
John R. Hughes, M.D.
Steven E. Hyman, M.D.
Christine L. Kasser, M.D.
Edward Kaufman, M.D.
Edward J. Khantzian, M.D.
Howard D. Kibel, M.D.
Lucy Jane King, M.D.
Donald F. Klein, M.D.
Thomas R. Kosten, M.D.
Mary Jeanne Kreek, M.D.
Barry J. Landau, M.D.
David C. Lanier, M.D.
Hyung Kon Lee, M.D.
Alan Leshner, Ph.D.
William L. Licamele, M.D.
Joyce H. Lowinson, M.D.
James F. Maddux, M.D.
Velandy Manohar, M.D.
Eric R. Marcus, M.D.
Sara Marriott, M.B.B.S., M.R.C.Psych.
Ronald L. Martin, M.D.
James R. McCartney, M.D.
James R. McKay, Ph.D.
Laura McNicholas, M.D.
Jack H. Mendelson, M.D.
Roger E. Meyer, M.D.
Norman S. Miller, M.D.
William R. Miller, Ph.D.
Kenneth Minkoff, M.D.
Peter M. Monti, Ph.D.
Jerome A. Motto, M.D.
Edgar P. Nace, M.D.
J.C. Negrete, M.D., F.R.C.P.(C)

Melvyn M. Nizny, M.D.
Edward V. Nunes, M.D.
Charles O'Brien, M.D., Ph.D.
Lisa Simon Onken, Ph.D.
John Peake, M.D.
Glen N. Peterson, M.D.
Herbert S. Peyser, M.D.
Ghulam Qadir, M.D.
Edward Reilly, M.D.
John A. Renner, Jr., M.D.
Vaughn I. Rickert, Psy.D.
E.B. Ritson, M.D.
Nicholas L. Rock, M.D.
Barbara R. Rosenfeld, M.D.
Richard Rothman, M.D.
A. John Rush, M.D.
Jane E. Sasaki, M.D.
Bernard Savariego, M.D.
Marc A. Schuckit, M.D.
Carlotta Schuster, M.D.
Edward J. Schwab, Ph.D.
Paul M. Schyve, M.D.
James H. Scully, M.D.
Linda Semlitz, M.D.
Edward C. Senay, M.D.
Cynthia M. Shappell, M.D.
Steven S. Sharfstein, M.D.
Dale Simpson, M.D.
Leslie Smith, M.D.
Mark B. Sobell, Ph.D.
Wesley E. Sowers, M.D.
Anderson Spickard, M.D.
Robert G. Stephens, M.D.
Robert S. Stephens, Ph.D.
Verner Stillner, M.D.
Richard T. Suchinsky, M.D.
William Tatomer, M.D.
Gene Tenelli, M.D.
Forest Tennant, M.D., Ph.D.
Jerome Tilles, M.D.
William G. Troyer, Jr., M.D.
Jalie A. Tucker, Ph.D.
George E. Vaillant, M.D.

Marsha L. Vannicelli, Ph.D.   H.G. Wittington, M.D.
John J. Verdon, Jr., M.D.   C. Roy Woodruff, Ph.D.
John G. Wagnitz, M.D., M.S.   George E. Woody, M.D.
Naimah Weinberg, M.D.   Henry H. Work, M.D.
Sidney Weissman, M.D.   Leon Wurmser, M.D.
Joseph J. Westermeyer, M.D., Ph.D.

Agency for Health Care Policy and Research
American Academy of Child and Adolescent Psychiatry
American Academy of Neurology
American Academy of Pediatrics
American Academy of Psychiatrists in Alcoholism and Addiction
American Association of Chairmen of Departments of Psychiatry
American Association of Community Psychiatrists
American Association of Pastoral Counselors
American Association of Psychiatric Administrators
American Association of Psychiatrists from India
American Association of Suicidology
American Board of Adolescent Psychiatry
American College of Emergency Physicians
American College of Neuropsychopharmacology
American Group Psychotherapy Association
American Medical Association
American Psychiatric Electrophysiology Association
American Psychoanalytic Association
American Psychological Association
American Psychosomatic Society
American Society of Group Psychotherapy and Psychodrama
Association for Academic Psychiatry
Association for Medical Education and Research in Substance Abuse
Association for the Advancement of Behavior Therapy
Baltimore-Washington Society for Psychoanalysis
Committee on Problems of Drug Dependence
Joint Commission on Accreditation of Healthcare Organizations
National Association of Psychiatric Health Systems
National Association of Veterans Affairs Chiefs of Psychiatry
National Institute of Mental Health
National Institute on Alcohol Abuse and Alcoholism
National Institute on Drug Abuse
Pakistan Psychiatric Society of North America
Royal College of Psychiatrists
Society for Adolescent Medicine
Society of Biological Psychiatry

X. References

The following coding system is used to indicate the nature of the supporting evidence in the summary recommendations and references:

[A] *Randomized clinical trial.*   A study of an intervention in which subjects are prospectively followed over time; there are treatment and control groups; subjects are randomly assigned to the two groups; both the subjects and the investigators are blind to the assignments.

[B] *Clinical trial.*   A prospective study in which an intervention is made and the results of that intervention are tracked longitudinally; study does not meet standards for a randomized clinical trial.

[C] *Cohort or longitudinal study.*   A study in which subjects are prospectively followed over time without any specific intervention.

[D] *Case-control study.*   A study in which a group of patients is identified in the present and information about them is pursued retrospectively or backward in time.

[E] *Review with secondary data analysis.*   A structured analytic review of existing data, e.g., a meta-analysis or a decision analysis.

[F] *Review.*   A qualitative review and discussion of previously published literature without a quantitative synthesis of the data.

[G] *Other.*   Textbooks, expert opinion, case reports, and other reports not included above.

1. Institute of Medicine: A study of the evolution, effectiveness and financing of public and private drug treatment systems, in Treating Drug Problems, vol 1. Edited by Gerstein DR, Harwood HJ. Washington, DC, National Academy Press, 1990 [G]

2. American Psychiatric Association: Diagnostic and Statistical Manual of Mental Disorders, 4th ed. Washington, DC, APA, 1994 [G]

3. Elliot DS, Huizinga D, Menard S: Multiple Problem Youth: Delinquency, Substance Use and Mental Health. New York, Springer-Verlag, 1989 [F]

4. Milan R, Halikas JA, Meller JE, Morse C: Psychopathology among substance abusing juvenile offenders. J Am Acad Child Adolesc Psychiatry 1991; 30:569–574 [D]

5. Christie-Burke K, Burke JD, Regier JD, Rae DS: Age at onset of selected mental disorders in five community populations. Arch Gen Psychiatry 1990; 47:511–518 [D]

6. Bukstein OG, Brent DA, Kaminer Y: Comorbidity of substance abuse and other psychiatric disorders in adolescents. Am J Psychiatry 1989; 146:1131–1141 [F]

7. Mirin SM, Weiss RD, Michael J: Psychopathology in substance abusers: diagnosis and treatment. Am J Drug Alcohol Abuse 1988; 14:139–157 [D]

8. Deykin EY, Levy JC, Wells V: Adolescent depression, alcohol and drug abuse. Am J Public Health 1987; 7:178–182 [D]

9. Treffert DA: Marijuana use in schizophrenia: a clear hazard. Am J Psychiatry 1978; 135:1213–1215 [D]

10. Alterman AI, Erdlen DL, Laporte DJ, Erdlen FR: Effects of illicit drug use in an inpatient psychiatric population. Addict Behav 1982; 7:231–242 [D]

11. Inman DJ, Bascue LO, Skoloda T: Identification of borderline personality disorders among substance abuse inpatients. J Subst Abuse Treat 1985; 2:229–232 [D]

12. Hesselbrock MN, Meyer RE, Keener JJ: Psychopathology in hospitalized alcoholics. Arch Gen Psychiatry 1985; 42:1050–1055 [D]

13. Lesieur HR, Blume SB: Pathological gambling, eating disorders, and the psychoactive substance use disorders. J Addict Dis 1993; 12:89–102 [F]

14. Batki SL, Sorensen JL, Faltz B, Madover S: Psychiatric aspects of treatment of i.v. drug abusers with AIDS. Hosp Community Psychiatry 1988; 39:439–441 [G]

15. Trocki KT, Leigh BD: Alcohol consumption and unsafe sex: a comparison of heterosexuals and homosexual men. J Acquir Immune Defic Syndr 1991; 4:981–986 [D]

16. Ausubel DP: Methadone maintenance treatment: the other side of the coin. Int J Addict 1983; 18:851–862 [F]

17. Donovan JE, Jessor R: Structure of problem behavior in adolescence and young adulthood. J Consult Clin Psychol 1985; 53: 890–904 [C]

18. Dupont RL: Getting Tough on Gateway Drugs: A Guide for the Family. Washington, DC, American Psychiatric Press, 1984 [G]

19. Brook DW, Brook JS: The etiology and consequences of adolescent drug use, in Prevention and Treatment of Drug and Alcohol Abuse. Edited by Watson RR. Clifton, NJ, Humana Press, 1990 [G]

20. National Household Survey on Drug Abuse: Main Findings, 1992. Washington, DC, US Department of Health and Human Services, 1992 [D]

21. Allen CA, Cooke DJ: Stressful life events and alcohol misuse in women: a critical review. J Stud Alcohol 1985; 46:147–152 [F]

22. Cloninger CR, Bohman M, Sigvardsson S: Inheritance of alcohol abuse: cross-fostering analysis of adopted men. Arch Gen Psychiatry 1981; 38:861–868 [D]

23. Cloninger CR: Neurogenetic adaptive mechanisms in alcoholism. Science 1987; 236:410–416 [G]

24. Bohman M, Sigvardsson S, Cloninger CR: Maternal inheritance of alcohol abuse: cross-fostering analysis of adopted women. Arch Gen Psychiatry 1981; 38:965–969 [D]

25. Kendler KS, Heath AC, Neale MC, Kessler RC, Eaves LJ: Alcoholism and major depression in women: a twin study of the causes of comorbidity. Arch Gen Psychiatry 1993; 50:690–698 [D]

26. Khantzian EJ: The self-medication hypothesis of addictive disorders: focus on heroin and cocaine dependence. Am J Psychiatry 1985; 142:1259–1264 [F]

27. Nurco DN, Stephenson PE, Hanlon TE: Aftercare/relapse prevention and the self-help movement. Int J Addict 1991; 25: 1179–1200 [F]

28. Vaillant GE, Milofsky MS: Natural history of male alcoholism, IV: paths to recovery. Arch Gen Psychiatry 1982; 39:127–133 [E]

29. Vaillant GE: The Natural History of Alcoholism: Causes, Patterns, and Paths to Recovery. Cambridge, MA, Harvard University Press, 1983 [E]

30. Vaillant GE: What can long-term follow-up teach us about relapse and prevention of relapse in addiction? Br J Addict 1988; 83:1147–1157 [C]

31. McLellan AT, Luborsky L, Woody GE, Druley KA, O'Brien CP: Predicting response to alcohol and drug abuse treatments: role of psychiatric severity. Arch Gen Psychiatry 1983; 40:620–625 [C]

32. Vaillant GE: A 20-year follow-up of New York addicts. Arch Gen Psychiatry 1973; 29:237–241 [C]

33. Brecht ML, Anglin MD, Woodward JA, Bonett DG: Conditional factors of maturing out: personal resources and preaddiction sociopathy. Int J Addict 1987; 22:55–69 [B]

34. Schuckit MA: Prediction of outcome among alcoholics. Drug Abuse and Alcoholism Newsletter 1988; 27(4) [F]

35. Institute of Medicine: Broadening the Base of Treatment for Alcohol Problems. Washington, DC, National Academy Press, 1990 [G]

36. Williams GD, Grant BF, Harford TC, Noble J: Population projections using DSM-III criteria: alcohol abuse and dependence, 1990–2000. Alcohol Health Res World 1989; 13:366–370 [D]

37. Annual Medical Examiner Data 1990: Data from the Drug Abuse Warning Network (DAWN) Statistical Series: Series 1, number 10-B, DHHS Publication (ADM) 91-1840. Rockville, MD, US Department of Health and Human Services, National Institute on Drug Abuse, 1991 [G]

38. US Centers for Disease Control: Alcohol-related mortality and years of potential life lost—United States, 1987. MMWR Morb Mortal Wkly Rep 1990; 39(11):173–177 [D]

39. US National Center for Health Statistics: Prevention Profile. Washington, DC, US Government Printing Office, 1992 [D]

40. Institute for Health Policy, Brandeis University: Substance Abuse: The Nation's Number One Health Problem: Key Indicators for Policy. Princeton, NJ, Robert Wood Johnson Foundation, October 1993 [G]

41. US Centers for Disease Control: Current trends: statewide prevalence of illegal drug use by pregnant women—Rhode Island. MMWR Morb Mortal Wkly Rep 1990; 39:225–227 [D]

42. Chasnoff IJ, Landress HJ, Barrett ME: The prevalence of illegal drug use or alcohol use during pregnancy and discrepancies in mandatory reporting in Pinellas County, Florida. N Engl J Med 1990; 322:1202–1206 [D]

43. Kessler RC, McGonagle KA, Zhao S, Nelson CB, Hughes M, Eshleman S, Wittchen H, Kendler KS: Lifetime and 12-month prevalence of DSM-III-R psychiatric disorders in the United States: results from the National Comorbidity Study. Arch Gen Psychiatry 1994; 51:8–19 [D]

44. Ross HE, Glaser FB, Germanson T: The prevalence of psychiatric disorders in patients with alcohol and other drug problems. Arch Gen Psychiatry 1988; 45:1023–1031 [D]

45. Mirin SM, Weiss RD: Substance abuse and mental illness, in Clinical Textbook of Addictive Disorders. Edited by Frances RJ, Miller SI. New York, Guilford Press, 1991 [G]

46. Mirin SM, Weiss RD: Psychiatric comorbidity in drug and alcohol addiction, in Comprehensive Handbook of Drug and Alcohol Addiction. Edited by Miller NS. New York, Guilford Press, 1991 [G]

47. Mirin SM, Weiss RD, Griffin ML, Michael JL: Psychopathology in drug abusers and their families. Compr Psychiatry 1991; 32: 36–51 [G]

48. Mirin SM, Weiss RD, Greenfield S: Psychoactive substance use disorders, in The Practitioner's Guide to Psychoactive Drugs, 3rd ed. Edited by Gelenberg A, Bassuk E, Schoonover S. New York, Plenum, 1991 [F]

49. Weiss RD, Mirin SM, Griffin ML, Michael JL: Psychopathology in cocaine abusers: changing trends. J Nerv Ment Dis 1988; 176:719–725 [C]

50. Weiss RD, Mirin SM, Griffin ML: Diagnosing major depression in cocaine abusers: the use of depression rating scales. Psychiatry Res 1989; 28:335–343 [E]

51. Crowley TJ, Chesluk D, Dilts S, Hart R: Drug and alcohol abuse among psychiatric admissions. Arch Gen Psychiatry 1974; 30: 13–20 [D]

52. Eisen SV, Grob MC, Dill DL: Substance Abuse in an Inpatient Population: A Comparison of Patients on Appleton and Generic Units: McLean Hospital Evaluative Service Unit Report 745. Belmont, MA, McLean Hospital, 1988 [C]

53. Marlatt GA, Larimer ME, Baer JS, Quigley LA: Harm reduction for alcohol problems: moving beyond the controlled drinking controversy. Behav Ther 1993; 24:461–504 [F]

54. Rawson RA, Obert JL, McCann MJ, Mann AJ: Cocaine treatment outcome: cocaine use following inpatient, outpatient and no treatment. NIDA Res Monogr 1986; 67:271–277 [C]

55. Rounsaville BJ, Anton SF, Carroll K, Budde D, Prusoff BA, Gawin F: Psychiatric diagnoses of treatment-seeking cocaine abusers. Arch Gen Psychiatry 1991; 48:43–51 [C]

56. Marlatt GA, Gordon JR (eds): Relapse Prevention: Maintenance Strategies in the Treatment of Addictive Behaviors. New York, Guilford Press, 1985 [F]

57. Wikler A, Pescor FT: Classical conditioning of a morphine abstinence phenomenon, reinforcement of opioid-drinking behavior and "relapse" in morphine addicted rats. Psychopharmacologia 1967; 10:255–284 [A]

58. Childress AR, Ehrman R, Rohsenow DJ, Robbins SJ, O'Brien CP: Classically conditioned actors in drug dependence, in Substance Abuse: A Comprehensive Textbook. Edited by Lowinson JH, Ruiz P, Millman RB. Baltimore, Williams & Wilkins, 1992 [F]

59. Wise RA: The neurobiology of craving: implications for the understanding and treatment of addiction. J Abnorm Psychol 1988; 97:118–132 [F]

60. McLellan AT, Alterman AI, Cacciola J, Metzger D, O'Brien CP: A quantitative measure of substance abuse treatment programs: the Treatment Services Review. J Nerv Ment Dis 1992; 180: 101–110 [G]

61. Khantzian EJ, Treece C: DSM-III psychiatric diagnosis of narcotic addicts: recent findings. Arch Gen Psychiatry 1985; 42: 1067–1071 [D]

62. Fleisch B: Approaches in the Treatment of Adolescents With Emotional and Substance Abuse Problems. Rockville, MD, US Department of Health and Human Services, 1991 [G]

63. Friedman AS, Beschner GM: Treatment Services for Adolescent Substance Abusers: DHHS Publication ADM 85-1342. Rockville, MD, National Institute on Drug Abuse, 1985 [G]

64. Horvath AO, Luborsky L: The role of the therapeutic alliance in psychotherapy. J Consult Clin Psychol 1993; 61:561–573 [F]

65. Luborsky L, McLellan AT, Woody GE, O'Brien CP, Auerbach A: Therapist success and its determinants. Arch Gen Psychiatry 1985; 42:602–611 [A]

66. Miller WR, Rollnick S: Motivational Interviewing: Preparing People to Change Addictive Behavior. New York, Guilford Press, 1991 [G]

67. Khantzian EJ: The primary care therapist and patient needs in substance abuse treatment. Am J Drug Alcohol Abuse 1988; 14:159–167 [F]

68. Galanter M: Network therapy for addiction: a model for office practice. Am J Psychiatry 1993; 150:28–36 [F]

69. Daley DC, Marlatt GA: Relapse prevention: cognitive and behavioral interventions, in Substance Abuse: A Comprehensive Textbook. Edited by Lowinson JH, Ruiz P, Millman RB. Baltimore, Williams & Wilkins, 1992 [F]

70. Miller WR, Hester RK: The effectiveness of alcoholism treatment: what research reveals, in Treating Addictive Behaviors: Processes of Change. Edited by Miller WR, Heather NH. New York, Plenum, 1986 [F]

71. Jaffe JH: Drug addiction and drug abuse, in Goodman and Gilman's The Pharmacological Basis of Therapeutics, 7th ed. Edited by Gilman AG, Gilman LS, Rall TW, Murad F. New York, Macmillan, 1985 [F]

72. Liskow BI, Goodwin D: Pharmacological treatment of alcohol intoxication withdrawal and dependence: a critical review. J Stud Alcohol 1987; 48:356–370 [F]

73. Jaffe JH, Ciraulo DA: Drugs used in the treatment of alcoholism, in Diagnosis and Treatment of Alcoholism. Edited by Mendelson JH, Mello NK. New York, McGraw-Hill, 1985 [G]

74. Kleber HD: Opioids: detoxification, in Textbook of Substance Abuse Treatment. Edited by Galanter M, Kleber HD. Washington, DC, American Psychiatric Press, 1994 [G]

75. Meyer RE, Mirin SM, Zackon F: Community outcome on narcotic antagonists, in The Heroin Stimulus: Implications for a Theory of Addiction. Edited by Meyer RE, Mirin SM. New York, Plenum, 1979 [B]

76. Meyer RE, Mirin SM: A psychology of craving: implications of behavioral research, in Substance Abuse: Clinical Problems and Perspectives. Edited by Lowinson JH, Ruiz P. Baltimore, Williams & Wilkins, 1991 [F]

77. Wikler A: Dynamics of drug dependence: implications of a conditioning theory for research and treatment. Arch Gen Psychiatry 1973; 28:611–616 [F]

78. Gragg DM: Drugs to decrease alcohol consumption (letter). N Engl J Med 1982; 306:747 [G]

79. Banys P: The clinical use of disulfiram (Antabuse): a review. J Psychoactive Drugs 1988; 20:243–261 [F]

80. Fuller RK, Branchey L, Brightwell DR, Derman RM, Emrick CD, Iber FL, James KE, Lacoursiere RB, Lee KK, Lowenstam I, Maaney I, Neiderheiser D, Nocks JJ, Shaw S: Disulfiram treatment of alcoholism: a Veterans Administration cooperative study. JAMA 1986; 256:1449–1455 [A]

81. Howard MO, Elkins RL, Rimmele C, Smith JW: Chemical aversion treatment of alcohol dependence. Drug Alcohol Depend 1991; 29:107–143 [F]

82. Frawley PJ, Smith JW: Chemical aversion therapy in the treatment of cocaine dependence as part of a multimodal treatment program: treatment outcome. J Subst Abuse Treat 1990; 7:21–29 [C]

83. Carroll KM, Rounsaville BJ, Nich C, Gordon LT, Wirtz PW, Gawin FH: One year follow-up of psychotherapy and pharmacotherapy for cocaine dependence: delayed emergence of psychotherapy effects. Arch Gen Psychiatry 1994; 51:989–998 [C]

84. Beck AT, Emery GE, Greenberg RL: Anxiety Disorders and Phobias: A Cognitive Perspective. New York, Basic Books, 1985 [F]

85. Wright FD, Beck AT, Newman CF, Liese BS: Cognitive therapy of substance abuse: theoretical rationale. NIDA Res Monogr 1993; 137:123–146 [F]

86. Annis HM, Davis CS: Relapse prevention, in Handbook of Alcoholism Treatment Approaches. Edited by Hester RK, Miller WR. New York, Pergamon Press, 1989 [F]

87. Annis HM: A relapse prevention model for treatment of alcoholics, in Treating Addictive Behaviors: Process of Change. Edited by Miller WR, Heather NH. New York, Plenum, 1986 [F]

88. Annis HM, Davis CS: Self-efficacy and the prevention of alcoholic relapse: initial findings from a treatment trial, in Assessment and Treatment of Addictive Disorders. Edited by Baker TB, Cannon DS. New York, Praeger, 1988 [B]

89. Carroll KM, Rounsaville B, Gawin F: A comparative trial of psychotherapies for ambulatory cocaine abusers: relapse prevention and interpersonal psychotherapy. Am J Drug Alcohol Abuse 1991; 17:229–247 [B]

90. Cooney NL, Kadden RM, Litt MD, Getter H: Matching alcoholics to coping skills or interactional therapies: two-year follow-up results. J Consult Clin Psychol 1991; 59:598–601 [B]

91. Kadden RM, Cooney NL, Getter H, Litt MD: Matching alcoholics to coping skills or interactional therapies: posttreatment results. J Consult Clin Psychol 1989; 57:698–704 [B]

92. Miller W: Motivational interviewing with problem drinkers. Behav Psychother 1983; 11:147–172 [G]

93. Miller WR: Motivation for treatment: a review. Psychol Bull 1985; 98:84–107 [F]

94. Miller WR, Benefield RG, Tonigan JS: Enhancing motivation for change in problem drinking: a controlled study of two therapist styles. J Consult Clin Psychol 1993; 61:455–461 [B]

95. Higgins ST, Delaney DD, Budney AJ, Bickel WK, Hughes JR, Foerg F, Fenwick JW: A behavioral approach to achieving initial cocaine abstinence. Am J Psychiatry 1991; 148:1218–1224 [C]

96. Higgins ST, Budney AJ, Bickel WK, Hughes JR, Foerg F, Badger G: Achieving cocaine abstinence with a behavioral approach. Am J Psychiatry 1993; 150:763–769 [A]

97. Higgins ST, Budney AJ, Bickel WK, Foerg FE, Donham R, Badger GJ: Incentives improve outcome in outpatient behavioral treatment of cocaine dependence. Arch Gen Psychiatry 1994; 51:568–576 [B]

98. Azrin NH: Improvements in the community-reinforcement approach to alcoholism. Behav Res Ther 1976; 14:339–348 [B]

99. Crowley TJ: Contingency contracting treatment of drug-abusing physicians, nurses, and dentists. NIDA Res Monogr 1984; 46:68–83 [F]

100. Niaura RS, Rohsenow DJ, Binkoff JA, Monti PM, Pedraza M, Abrams DB: Relevance of cue reactivity to understanding alcohol and smoking relapse. J Abnorm Psychol 1988; 97:133–152 [F]

101. Klajner F, Hartman LM, Sobell MB: Treatment of substance abuse by relaxation training: a review of its rationale, efficacy and mechanisms. Addict Behav 1984; 9:41–55 [F]

102. Childress A, Ehrman R, McLellan A, O'Brien C: Update on behavioral treatments for substance abuse. NIDA Res Monogr 1988; 90:183–192 [F]

103. Monti PM, Rohsenow DJ, Rubonis AV, Niaura RS, Sirota AD, Colby SM, Goddard P, Abrams DB: Cue exposure with coping skills treatment for male alcoholics: a preliminary investigation. J Consult Clin Psychol 1993; 61:1011–1019 [B]

104. O'Brien CP, Childress AR, McLellan T, Ehrman R: Integrating systemic cue exposure with standard treatment in recovering drug dependent patients. Addict Behav 1990; 15:355–365 [C]

105. Cannon DS, Baker TB, Wehl CK: Emetic and electric shock alcohol aversion therapy: six and twelve month follow-up. J Consult Clinical Psychol 1981; 49:360–368 [A]

106. Holder HD, Longabaugh R, Miller WR, Rubonis AV: The cost effectiveness of treatment for alcoholism: a first approximation. J Stud Alcohol 1991; 52:517–540 [E]

107. Woody GE, Luborsky L, McLellan AT, O'Brien CP, Beck AT, Blaine J, Herman I, Hole A: Psychotherapy for opiate addicts: does it help? Arch Gen Psychiatry 1983; 40:639–645 [B]

108. Woody GE, McLellan AT, Luborsky L, O'Brien C: Psychotherapy for substance abusers. Psychiatr Clin North Am 1986; 9: 547–562 [F]

109. Woody GE, McLellan AT, Luborsky L, O'Brien CP: Sociopathy and psychotherapy outcome. Arch Gen Psychiatry 1985; 42: 1081–1086 [B]

110. Luborsky L: Principles of Psychoanalytic Psychotherapy: A Manual for Supportive-Expressive Therapy. New York, Basic Books, 1984 [F]

111. Ohehagen A, Berglund M, Appel CP, Andersson K, Nilsson B, Skjaerris A, Wedlin-Toftenow AM: A randomized study of long-term out-patient treatment in alcoholics. Alcohol Alcohol 1992; 27:649–658 [A]

112. Klerman G, Weissman M, Rounsaville B, Chevron E: Interpersonal Psychotherapy of Depression. New York, Basic Books, 1984 [F]

113. Rounsaville BJ, Glazer W, Wilber CH, Weissman MM, Kleber HD: Short-term interpersonal psychotherapy in methadone-maintained opiate addicts. Arch Gen Psychiatry 1983; 40:629–636 [B]

114. Zinberg S, Wallace J, Blume SB: Practical Approaches to Alcoholism Psychotherapy. New York, Plenum, 1978 [G]

115. Brandsma J, Pattison EM: The outcome of group psychotherapy in alcoholics: an empirical review. Am J Drug Alcohol Abuse 1985; 11:151–162 [F]

116. Khantzian EJ, Halliday KS, McAuliffe WE: Addiction and the Vulnerable Self: Modified Dynamic Group Therapy for Substance Abusers. New York, Guilford Press, 1990 [F]

117. Yalom ID, Bloch S, Bond G, Zimmerman E, Qualls B: Alcoholics in interactional group therapy: an outcome study. Arch Gen Psychiatry 1978; 35:419–425 [B]

118. Vannicelli M: Removing Roadblocks: Group Psychotherapy With Substance Abusers and Family Members. New York, Guilford Press, 1992 [G]

119. McKay JR, Longabaugh R, Beattie MC, Maisto SA: The relationship of pretreatment family functioning to drinking behavior during follow-up by alcoholic patients. Am J Drug Alcohol Abuse 1992; 18:445–460 [C]

120. Steinglass P, Bennett L, Wolin S, Reiss D: The Alcoholic Family. New York, Basic Books, 1987 [F]

121. Stanton MD: Family treatment approaches to drug abuse problems: a review. Fam Process 1979; 18:251–280 [F]

122. Heath A, Atkinson B: Systematic treatment of substance abuse: a graduate course. J Marital Family Therapy 1988; 14:411–418 [G]

123. Stanton MD: Course-work and self-study in the family treatment of alcohol and drug abuse: expanding health and Atkinson's curriculum. J Marital Family Therapy 1988; 14:419–427 [B]

124. Stanton MD, Thomas TC: Family Therapy of Drug Abuse and Addiction. New York, Guilford Press, 1982 [G]

125. Kaufman E, Kaufman P: Family Therapy of Drug and Alcohol Abuse. New York, Gardner Press, 1979, pp 147–186 [G]

126. Heath AW, Stanton MD: Family therapy, in Clinical Textbook of Addictive Disorders. Edited by Frances RJ, Miller SI. New York, Guilford Press, 1991 [F]

127. Getter H, Litt MD, Kadden RM, Cooney NL: Measuring treatment process in coping skills and interactional group therapies for alcoholism. Int J Group Psychother 1992; 42:419–430 [B]

128. Roehrich L, Goldman MS: Experience-dependent neuropsychological recovery and the treatment of alcoholism. J Consult Clin Psychol 1993; 61:812–821 [B]

129. Rohsenow DJ, Monti PM, Binkoff JA, Liepman MR, Nirenberg TD, Abrams DB: Patient-treatment matching for alcoholic men in communication skills vs cognitive-behavioral mood management training. Addict Behav 1991; 16:63–69 [B]

130. Annis HM, Chan D: The differential treatment model: empirical evidence from a personality typology of adult offenders. Criminal Justice and Behavior 1983; 10:159–173 [D]

131. Miller WR: Client/treatment matching in addictive behaviors. Behavior Therapist 1992; 15:7–8 [G]

132. McKay JR, Longabaugh R, Beattie MC, Maisto SA, Noel N: Changes in family functioning during treatment and drinking outcomes for high and low autonomy alcoholics. Addict Behav 1993; 18:355–363 [A]

133. McKay JR, Longabaugh R, Beattie MC, Maisto SA, Noel N: Does adding conjoint therapy to individually focused alcoholism treatment lead to better family functioning? J Subst Abuse 1993; 5:45–59 [B]

134. McKay JR, Maisto SA, O'Farrell TJ: End-of-treatment self-efficacy, aftercare, and drinking outcomes of alcoholic men. Alcohol Clin Exp Res 1993; 17:1078–1083 [A]

135. McKay JR, Maisto SA: An overview and critique of advances in the treatment of alcohol use disorders. Drugs and Society 1993; 8:1–29 [F]

136. Longabaugh R, Beattie MC, Noel N, Stout R, Malloy P: The effect of social investment on treatment outcome. J Stud Alcohol 1993; 54:465–478 [B]

137. McLellan AT, Woody GE, Luborsky L, O'Brien CP, Druley KA: Increased effectiveness of substance abuse treatment: a prospective study of patient-treatment matching. J Nerv Ment Dis 1983; 171:597–605 [C]

138. Miller WR, Hester RK: Inpatient treatment for alcoholism: who benefits? Am Psychol 1986; 41:794–805 [F]

139. Miller WR, Hester R: Matching problem drinkers with optimal treatments, in Treating Addictive Behaviors: Processes of Change. Edited by Miller WR, Heather NH. New York, Plenum, 1986 [F]

140. Nace EP, Davis CW, Gaspari JP: Axis II comorbidity in substance abusers. Am J Psychiatry 1991; 148:118–120 [D]

141. Hoffmann N, Halikas J, Mee-Lee D: The Cleveland Admission, Discharge, and Transfer Criteria: Model for Chemical Dependency Treatment Programs. Cleveland, Northern Ohio Chemical Dependency Treatment Directors Association, 1987 [G]

142. Hoffmann NG, Mee-Lee D: Patient Placement Criteria for the Treatment of Psychoactive Substance Use Disorders. Washington, DC, American Society of Addiction Medicine, 1991 [G]

143. McKay JR, McLellan AT, Alterman AI: An evaluation of the Cleveland criteria for inpatient treatment of substance abuse. Am J Psychiatry 1992; 149:1212–1218 [C]

144. Prochaska JO, DiClemente CC, Norcross JC: In search of how people change: applications to addictive behaviors. Am Psychol 1992; 47:1102–1114 [F]

145. Project MATCH (Matching Alcoholism Treatment to Client Heterogeneity): rationale and methods for a multisite clinical trial matching patients to alcoholism treatment. Alcohol Clin Exp Res 1993; 17:1130–1145 [A]

146. Ball J, Ross A: The Effectiveness of Methadone Maintenance Treatment. New York, Springer-Verlag, 1991 [C]

147. Joe GW, Simpson DD, Hubbard RL: Treatment predictors of tenure in methadone maintenance. J Subst Abuse 1991; 3:73–84 [C]

148. McLellan AT, Arndt IO, Metzger DS, Woody GE, O'Brien CP: The effects of psychological services in substance abuse treatment. JAMA 1993; 269:1953–1959 [B]

149. McLellan AT, Grissom GR, Brill P, Durell J, Metzger DS, O'Brien CP: Private substance abuse treatments: are some programs more effective than others? J Subst Abuse Treat 1993; 10:243–254 [C]

150. McLellan AT, Alterman AI, Metzger DS, Grissom GR, Woody GE, Luborsky L, O'Brien CP: Similarity of outcome predictors across opiate, cocaine, and alcohol treatments: role of treatment services. J Consult Clin Psychol 1994; 62:1141–1158 [D]

151. Apsler R, Harding WM: Cost-effectiveness analysis of drug abuse treatment: current status and recommendations for future research, in Background Papers on Drug Abuse Financing and Services Approach: Drug Abuse Services Research Series, number 1, DHHS Publication (ADM) 91-17777. Rockville, MD, National Institute on Drug Abuse, 1991 [E]

152. Dackis CA, Gold MS: Psychiatric hospitals for treatment of dual diagnosis, in Substance Abuse: A Comprehensive Textbook. Edited by Lowinson JH, Ruiz P, Millman RB. Baltimore, Williams & Wilkins, 1992 [F]

153. Hayashida M, Alterman AI, McLellan AT, O'Brien CP, Purtell JJ, Volpicelli JR, Raphaelson AH, Hall CP: Comparative effectiveness and costs of inpatient and outpatient detoxification of patients with mild-to-moderate alcohol withdrawal syndromes. N Engl J Med 1989; 320:358–365 [B]

154. Friedman AS, Glickman NW: Residential program characteristics for completion of treatment by adolescent drug abusers. J Nerv Ment Dis 1987; 165:418–424 [D]

155. McLellan AT: The psychiatrically severe drug abuse patients: methadone maintenance or therapeutic community? Am J Drug Alcohol Abuse 1984; 10:77–95 [A]

156. De Leon G, Rosenthal MS: Treatment in residential therapeutic communities, in Treatments of Psychiatric Disorders: A Task Force Report of the American Psychiatric Association, vol 2. Washington, DC, APA, 1989 [G]

157. Simpson DD, Sells SB (eds): Opioid Addiction and Treatment: A 12 Year Follow-Up. Melbourne, FL, Robert E Krieger, 1990 [E]

158. De Leon GD, Wexler HK, Jainchill N: The therapeutic community: success and improvement rates 5 years after treatment. Int J Addict 1982; 17:703–747 [C]

159. De Leon G: The Therapeutic Community: Study of Effectiveness. NIDA Treatment Research Monograph Series, DHHS Publication (ADM) 85-1286. Rockville, MD, National Institute on Drug Abuse, 1984 [C]

160. Longabaugh R: Longitudinal outcome studies, in Alcoholism: Origins and Outcome. Edited by Rose RM, Barrett J. New York, Raven Press, 1988 [F]

161. Kleber HD, Slobetz F: Outpatient drug-free treatment, in Handbook on Drug Abuse. Edited by DuPont RL, Goldstein A, O'Donnell J. Rockville, MD, National Institute on Drug Abuse, 1979 [G]

162. McLellan AT, O'Brien CP, Metzger DS, Alterman AI, Cornish J, Urschel H: Is substance abuse treatment effective: compared to what? in Addictive States. Edited by O'Brien CP, Jaffe J. New York, Raven Press, 1992 [F]

163. Crumley FE: Substance abuse and adolescent suicidal behavior. JAMA 1990; 163:3051–3056 [F]

164. Schuckit MA: Primary male alcoholics with histories of suicide attempts. J Stud Alcohol 1986; 47:78–81 [D]

165. Rich CL, Young D, Fowler RC: San Diego suicide study, I: young vs old subjects. Arch Gen Psychiatry 1986; 43:577–582 [D]

166. Hawton K: Assessment of suicide risk. Br J Psychiatry 1987; 150:145–153 [F]

167. Murphy GE: Suicide and substance abuse. Arch Gen Psychiatry 1988; 45:593–594 [G]

168. Norstrom T: Alcohol and suicide in Scandinavia. Br J Addict 1988; 83:553–559 [E]

169. Dorpat TL: Drug automatism, barbiturate poisoning and suicide behavior. Arch Gen Psychiatry 1974; 31:216–220 [G]

170. Budde RD: Cocaine abuse and violent death. Am J Drug Alcohol Abuse 1989; 15:375–382 [D]

171. Langevin R, Paitich D, Orchard B, Handy L, Russon A: The role of alcohol, drugs, suicide attempts and situational strains in homicide committed by offenders seen for psychiatric assessment: a controlled study. Acta Psychiatr Scand 1982; 66:229–242 [D]

172. Luisada PV: The phencyclidine psychosis: phenomenology and treatment. NIDA Res Monogr 1978; 21:241–253 [C]

173. Brecher M, Wang BW, Wong H, Morgan JP: Phencyclidine and violence: clinical and legal issues. J Clin Psychopharmacol 1988; 8:398–401 [D]

174. Melges FT, Tinklenberg JR, Hollister LE, Gillespie HK: Temporal disintegration and depersonalization during marijuana intoxication. Arch Gen Psychiatry 1970; 23:204–210 [B]

175. Bowers MB Jr: Acute psychosis induced by psychotomimetic drug abuse, 1: clinical findings. Arch Gen Psychiatry 1972; 27: 437–439 [C]

176. Bowers MB Jr: Acute psychosis induced by psychotomimetic drug abuse, 2: neurochemical findings. Arch Gen Psychiatry 1972; 27:440–442 [C]

177. McLellan AT, Luborsky L, O'Brien CP: Alcohol and drug abuse treatment in three different populations: is there improvement and is it predictable? Am J Drug Alcohol Abuse 1986; 12:101–120 [C]

178. McLellan AT: "Psychiatric severity" as a predictor of outcome from substance abuse treatments, in Psychopathology and Addictive Disorders. Edited by Meyer RE. New York, Guilford Press, 1986 [G]

179. Penick EC, Powell BJ, Liskow BI, Jackson JO, Nickel EJ: The stability of coexisting psychiatric syndromes in alcoholic men after one year. J Stud Alcohol 1988; 49:395–405 [C]

180. Rounsaville BJ, Weissman MM, Wilber CH, Kleber HD: Pathways to opiate addiction: an evaluation of differing antecedents. Br J Psychiatry 1982; 141:437–446 [D]

181. Rounsaville BJ, Weissman MM, Kleber H, Wilber C: Heterogeneity of psychiatric diagnosis in treated opiate addicts. Arch Gen Psychiatry 1982; 39:161–166 [D]

182. Rounsaville BJ, Kosten TR, Weissman MM, Kleber HD: Prognostic significance of psychopathology in treated opioid addicts: a 2.5-year follow-up study. Arch Gen Psychiatry 1986; 43:739–745 [D]

183. Stone MH: The Fate of Borderline Patients: Successful Outcome and Psychiatric Practice. New York, Guilford Press, 1990 [G]

184. Tarter RE: Evaluation and treatment of adolescent substance abuse: a decision tree method. Am J Drug Alcohol Abuse 1990; 16:1–46 [G]

185. Rounsaville BJ, Dolinsky ZS, Babor TF, Meyer RE: Psychopathology as a predictor of treatment outcome in alcoholics. Arch Gen Psychiatry 1987; 44:505–513 [C]

186. Jaffe JH, Ciraulo DA: Alcoholism and depression, in Psychopathology and Addictive Disorders. Edited by Meyer RE. New York, Guilford Press, 1986 [F]

187. Hunt W, Barnet L, Branch L: Relapse rates in addiction programs. J Clin Psychol 1971; 27:455–456 [G]

188. Goodwin DW: Alcohol: clinical aspects, in Substance Abuse: A Comprehensive Textbook, 2nd ed. Edited by Lowinson JH, Ruiz P, Millman RB, Langrod JG. Baltimore, Williams & Wilkins, 1992 [G]

189. Bridge TP, Mirsky AF, Goodwin FK (eds): Psychological, Neuropsychiatric, and Substance Abuse Aspects of AIDS: Advances in Biochemical Psychopharmacology, vol 44. New York, Raven Press, 1988 [G]

190. Sorensen JL, Costantini MF, London JA: Coping with AIDS: strategies for patients and staff in drug abuse treatment programs. J Psychoactive Drugs 1989; 21:435–440 [F]

191. Ball JC, Lange WR, Myers CP, Friedman SR: Reducing the risk of AIDS through methadone maintenance treatment. J Health Soc Behav 1988; 29:214–226 [C]

192. Novick DM: The medically ill substance abuser, in Substance Abuse: A Comprehensive Textbook, 2nd ed. Edited by Lowinson JH, Ruiz P, Millman RB, Langrod JG. Baltimore, Williams & Wilkins, 1992 [G]

193. Tuberculosis and human immunodeficiency virus infection: recommendations of the Advisory Committee for the Elimination of Tuberculosis (ACET). MMWR Morb Mortal Wkly Rep 1989; 38:236–238, 243–250 [G]

194. Woods JR, Plessinger MA, Clark KA: Effect of cocaine on uterine blood flow and fetal oxygenation. JAMA 1987; 257:957–961 [G]

195. Szeto HH: Maternal-fetal pharmacokinetics and fetal dose-response relationships. Ann NY Acad Sci 1989; 562:42–55 [F]

196. Dattel BJ: Substance abuse in pregnancy. Semin Perinatol 1990; 14:179–187 [F]

197. Fulroth RF, Durand DJ, Nicherson BG, Espinoza AM: Prenatal cocaine exposure is not associated with a large increase in the incidence of SIDS (abstract). Pediatr Res 1989; 25:215A [C]

198. Fried PA: Postnatal consequences of maternal marijuana use. NIDA Res Monogr 1985; 59:61–72 [C]

199. Little RE, Asker RL, Sampson PD, Renwick JH: Fetal growth and moderate drinking in early pregnancy. Am J Epidemiol 1986; 123:270–278 [C]

200. Meeker JE, Reynolds PC: Fetal and newborn death associated with maternal cocaine use. J Anal Toxicol 1990; 14:378–382 [D]

201. Handler A, Kistin N, Davis F, Ferre C: Cocaine use during pregnancy: perinatal outcomes. Am J Epidemiol 1991; 133:818–824 [D]

202. Tabor BL, Smith-Wallace T, Yonekura ML: Perinatal outcome associated with PCP versus cocaine use. Am J Alcohol Abuse 1990; 16:337–348 [D]

203. Vinci R, Parker S, Bauchner H, Zuckerman B, Cabral H: Maternal cocaine use and impaired fetal oxygenation (abstract). Pediatr Res 1989; 25:231A [C]

204. Ciraulo DA, Shader RI: Clinical Manual of Chemical Dependence. Washington, DC, American Psychiatric Press, 1991 [F]

205. Finnegan LP, Kendall SR: Maternal and neonatal effects of alcohol and drugs, in Substance Abuse: A Comprehensive Textbook, 2nd ed. Baltimore, Williams & Wilkins, 1992 [G]

206. Blume SB: Is social drinking during pregnancy harmless? there is reason to think not. Adv Alcohol Subst Abuse 1985; 5:209–219 [F]

207. Griffin ML, Weiss RD, Mirin SM, Lange U: A comparison of male and female cocaine abusers. Arch Gen Psychiatry 1989; 46:122–126 [D]

208. Winfield I, George LK, Swartz M, Blazer DG: Sexual assault and psychiatric disorders among a community sample of women. Am J Psychiatry 1990; 147:335–341 [D]

209. Ladwig GB, Andersen MD: Substance abuse in women: relationship between chemical dependency of women and past reports of physical and/or sexual abuse. Int J Addict 1989; 24:739–754 [D]

210. Stevens S, Arbiter N, Glider P: Women residents: expanding their role to increase treatment effectiveness in substance abuse programs. Int J Addict 1989; 24:425–434 [G]

211. Reilly D: Family factors in the etiology and treatment of youthful drug abuse. Family Therapy 1976; 2:149–171 [G]

212. Stanton MD, Landau-Stanton J: Therapy with families of adolescent substance abusers, in Treatment Choices for Alcohol and Drug Abuse. Edited by Milkman HB, Sederer LI. Lexington, MA, Lexington Books, 1990 [G]

213. Catalano RF, Hawkins JD, Wells EA, Miller J, Brewer D: Evaluation of the effectiveness of adolescent drug abuse treatment, assessment of risks for relapse, and promising approaches for relapse prevention. Int J Addict 1991; 25:1085–1140 [F]

214. Barnes GM: Alcohol use among older persons: findings from a western New York State general population survey. J Am Geriatr Soc 1979; 27:244–250 [D]

215. McCourt WF, Williams AF, Schneider L: Incidence of alcoholism in a state mental hospital population. Q J Stud Alcohol 1971; 32:1085–1088 [D]

216. Atkinson JH, Schuckit MA: Geriatric alcohol and drug misuse and abuse. Advances in Substance Abuse 1983; 3:195–237 [G]

217. Atkinson RM (ed): Alcohol and Drug Abuse in Old Age. Washington, DC, American Psychiatric Press, 1984 [G]

218. Abrams RC, Alexopoulos G: Geriatric addictions, in Clinical Textbook of Addictive Disorders. Edited by Frances RJ, Miller SI. New York, Guilford Press, 1991 [G]

219. National Institute on Alcohol Abuse and Alcoholism: Alcohol and minorities. Alcohol Alert, issue 23 (PH 347), January 1994, pp 1–4 [G]

220. Institute of Medicine: The treatment of special populations: overview and definitions, in Broadening the Base of Treatment for Alcohol Problems. Washington, DC, National Academy Press, 1990 [G]

221. Dolan MP, Roberts WR, Penk WE, Robinowitz R, Atkins HG: Personality differences among black, white and Hispanic-American male heroin addicts on MMPI content scales. J Clin Psychol 1983; 39:807–813 [D]

222. Cabaj RP: Substance abuse in the gay and lesbian community, in Substance Abuse: A Comprehensive Textbook, 2nd ed. Edited by Lowinson JH, Ruiz P, Millman RB. Baltimore, Williams & Wilkins, 1992 [G]

223. Liles RE, Childs D: Similarities in family dynamics of incest and alcohol abuse. Alcohol Health and Res World 1986; Fall:66–69 [G]

224. Kosten TR, Rounsaville BJ, Kleber HD: Parental alcoholism in opioid addicts. J Nerv Ment Dis 1985; 173:461–469 [D]

225. O'Farrell T: Marital and family therapy in alcoholism treatment. J Subst Abuse Treat 1989; 6:23–29 [F]

226. Leukefeld CG, Tims FM: Compulsory treatment for drug abuse. Int J Addict 1990; 25:621–640 [F]

227. Beane EA, Beck JC: Court based civil commitment of alcoholics and substance abusers. Bull Am Acad Psychiatry Law 1991; 19:359–366 [D]

228. Anker AL, Crowley TJ: Use of contingency contracts in specialty clinics for cocaine abuse. NIDA Res Monogr 1981; 41:452–459 [B]

229. Conditions for the use of narcotic drugs, Code of Federal Regulations (CFR), 21 CFR Part 291.505, April 1994 [G]

230. Helzer JE, Burnam A, McEvoy LT: Alcohol abuse and dependence, in Psychiatric Disorders in America. Edited by Robins LN, Regier DA. New York, Free Press, 1991 [E]

231. Hasin DS, Grant B, Endicott J: The natural history of alcohol abuse: implications for definitions of alcohol use disorders. Am J Psychiatry 1990; 147:1537–1541 [C]

232. Rosenberg H: Prediction of controlled drinking by alcoholics and problem drinkers. Psychol Bull 1993; 113:129–139 [F]

233. Baer JS, Marlatt GA, Kivlahan DR, Fromme K, Larimer ME, Williams E: An experimental test of three methods of alcohol risk reduction with young adults. J Consult Clin Psychol 1992; 60:974–979 [A]

234. Kivlahan DR, Marlatt GA, Fromme K, Coppel DB, Williams E: Secondary prevention with college drinkers: evaluation of an alcohol skills training program. J Consult Clin Psychol 1990; 58:805–810 [A]

235. Apsler R: Evaluating the cost-effectiveness of drug abuse treatment services. NIDA Res Monogr 1991; 113:57–66 [E]

236. McLellan AT: Patient-Treatment Matching and Outcome Improvement in Alcohol Rehabilitation: Institute of Medicine Report on Future Directions in Research and Treatment of Alcohol Dependence. Washington, DC, National Academy of Sciences, 1989 [G]

237. McKay JR, Murphy R, Longabaugh R: The effectiveness of alcoholism treatment: evidence from outcome studies, in Psychiatric Treatment: Advances in Outcome Research. Edited by Mirin ST, Gossett J, Grob MC. Washington, DC, American Psychiatric Press, 1991 [F]

238. Moos RH, Finney JW, Cronkite RC: Alcoholism Treatment: Context, Process, and Outcome. New York, Oxford University Press, 1990 [F]

239. McCrady BS, Noel NE, Abrams DB, Stout RL, Nelson HF, Hay WM: Effectiveness of three types of spouse-involved behavioral alcoholism treatment. J Stud Alcohol 1986; 47:459–467 [A]

240. O'Farrell TJ, Cutter HS, Floyd FJ: Evaluating behavioral marital therapy for male alcoholics: effects on marital adjustment and communication from before to after treatment. Behav Ther 1985; 16:147–167 [A]

241. Bunn JY, Booth BM, Loveland Cook CA, Blow FC, Fortney JC: The relationship between mortality and intensity of inpatient alcoholism treatment. Am J Public Health 1984; 84:211–214 [C]

242. Walsh DC, Hingson RW, Merrigan DM, Morelock Levenson S, Cupples A, Heeren T, Coffman GA, Becker CA, Barker TA, Hamilton SK, McGuire TG, Kelly CA: A randomized trial of treatment options for alcohol-abusing workers. N Engl J Med 1991; 325:775–782 [A]

243. Annis HM: Is inpatient rehabilitation of the alcoholic cost-effective? in Controversies in Alcoholism and Substance Abuse. New York, Haworth Press, 1986 [F]

244. McCrady B, Longabaugh R, Fink E, Stout R, Beattie M, Ruggieri-Authelet A: Cost-effectiveness of alcoholism treatment in partial hospital versus inpatient settings after brief inpatient treatments: 12-month outcomes. J Consult Clin Psychol 1986; 54:708–713 [B]

245. Fink EB, Longabaugh R, McCrady BM, Stout RL, Beattie M, Ruggieri-Authelet A, McNiel D: Effectiveness of alcoholism treatment in partial versus inpatient settings: twenty-four-month outcomes. Addict Behav 1985; 10:235–248 [C]

246. McLachlan JFC, Stein RI: Evaluation of a day clinic for alcoholics. J Stud Alcohol 1982; 43:261–272 [G]

247. McKay JR, Alterman AI, McLellan AT, Snider EC: Treatment goals, continuity of care, and outcome in a day hospital substance abuse rehabilitation program. Am J Psychiatry 1994; 151: 254–259 [C]

248. Volpicelli JR, Alterman AI, Hagashida M, O'Brien CP: Naltrexone in the treatment of alcohol dependence. Arch Gen Psychiatry 1992; 49:876–880 [A]

249. O'Malley SS, Jaffe A, Chang G, Schottenfeld MD, Meyer RE, Rounsaville BJ: Naltrexone and coping skills therapy for alcohol dependence: a controlled study. Arch Gen Psychiatry 1992; 49:881–887 [A]

250. Eskelson CD, Hameroff SR, Kanel JS: Ethanol increases serum β-endorphin levels in rats. Anesth Analg 1980; 59(7) [G]

251. Wilkinson CW, Crabbe JC, Keith LD, Kendall JW, Dorsa DM: Influence of ethanol dependence on regional brain content of β-endorphin in the mouse. Brain Res 1986; 378:107–114 [G]

252. Stine SM, Freeman M, Burns B, Charney DS, Kosten TR: Effects of methadone dose on cocaine abuse in a methadone program. Am J Addictions 1992; 1:294–303 [B]

253. Marchner J: The pharmacology of alcohol-sensitizing drugs, in Pharmacological Treatments for Alcoholism. Edited by Edwards G, Littleton J. New York, Methuen, 1984 [F]

254. Peachey JE: A review of the clinical use of disulfiram and calcium carbamide in alcoholism treatment. Clin Psychopharmacol 1981; 1:368–375 [F]

255. Fox R: Disulfiram—alcohol side effects. JAMA 1968; 204:271–272 [B]

256. Fuller RF, Roth HP: Disulfiram for the treatment of alcoholism: an evaluation in 128 men. Ann Intern Med 1979; 90:901–904 [A]

257. Arana GW, Hyman SE: Handbook of Psychiatric Drug Therapy, 2nd ed. Boston, Little, Brown, 1991 [G]

258. Peachey JE, Brien JF, Loomis CW: A study of the calcium carbamide-ethanol interaction in man: symptom response. Alcohol Clin Exp Res 1980; 4:322–329 [A]

259. Peachey JE: Clinical uses of the alcohol-sensitizing drugs, in Pharmacological Treatments for Alcoholism. Edited by Little EG. New York, Croom Helm, 1984 [G]

260. Lister RG, Nutt DJ: Alcohol antagonists—the continuing quest. Alcohol Clin Exp Res 1988; 12:566–569 [G]

261. Keso L, Salaspuro M: Inpatient treatment of employed alcoholics: a randomized clinical trial of Hazelden-type and traditional treatment. Alcohol Clin Exp Res 1990; 14:584–589 [A]

262. Gerrein JR, Rosenberg CM, Manohar V: Disulfiram maintenance in outpatient treatment of alcoholism. Arch Gen Psychiatry 1973; 28:798–802 [A]

263. Ciraulo DA, Barnhill J, Boxenbaum H: Pharmacokinetic interaction of disulfiram and antidepressants. Am J Psychiatry 1985; 142:1373–1374 [B]

264. Fawcett J, Clark DC, Aagesen CA, Pisani VD, Tilkin JM, Sellers D, McGuire M, Gibbons RD: A double-blind, placebo-controlled trial of lithium carbonate therapy for alcoholism. Arch Gen Psychiatry 1987; 44:248–256 [A]

265. Dorus W, Ostrow D, Anton R, Cushman P, Collins JF, Schaefer M, Charles HL, Desai P, Hayashida M, Malkerneker U, Willengring M, Fiscella R, Sather MR: Lithium treatment of depressed and nondepressed alcoholics. JAMA 1989; 262:1646–1652 [A]

266. Mason BT, Kocsis JH: Desipramine treatment of alcoholism. Psychopharmacol Bull 1991; 27:155–161 [A]

267. Nunes EV, McGrath PJ, Quitkin FM, Stewart JP, Harrison W, Tricamo E, Ocepek-Welikson K: Imipramine treatment of alcoholism with comorbid depression. Am J Psychiatry 1993; 150: 963–965 [A]

268. Naranjo CA, Kadlec KE, Sanheuza P, Woodley-Remus D, Sellars EM: Fluoxetine differentially alters alcohol intake and other consummatory behavior in problem drinkers. Clin Pharmacol Ther 1990; 47:490–498 [B]

269. Lawrin MO, Naranjo CA, Sellars EM: Identification and testing of new drugs for modulating alcohol consumption. Psychopharmacol Bull 1986; 22:1020–1025 [G]

270. Cornelius JR, Salloum IM, Cornelius MD, Ehler JB, Perel JM: Fluoxetine vs placebo in depressed alcoholics. Presented at New Clinical Drug Evaluation Unit (NCDEU) Meeting, Marco Island, FL, June 1994 [A]

271. Silber A: Rationales for the technique of psychotherapy with alcoholics. Int J Psychoanal Psychother 1974; 2:328–347 [G]

272. Chaney EF: Social skills training, in Handbook of Alcoholism Treatment Approaches. Edited by Hester RK, Miller WR. New York, Pergamon Press, 1989 [F]

273. Monti PM, Abrams DB, Binkoff JA, Zwick WR, Liepman MR, Nirenberg TD, Rohsenow DJ: Communication skills training, communication skills training with family and cognitive behavioral mood management training for alcoholics. J Stud Alcohol 1990; 51:263–270 [A]

274. Longabaugh R, Rubin A, Malloy P, Beattie M, Clifford PR, Noel N: Drinking outcomes of alcohol abusers diagnosed as antisocial personality disorder. Alcohol Clin Exp Res 1994; 18:778–785 [B]

275. Miller WR, Munoz RF: How to Control Your Drinking, revised ed. Albuquerque, University of New Mexico Press, 1982 [F]

276. Sanchez-Craig M: Therapist's Manual for Secondary Prevention of Alcohol Problems: Procedures for Teaching Moderate Drinking and Abstinence. Toronto, Addiction Research Foundation, 1984 [F]

277. Bandura A: Self-efficacy: toward a unifying theory of behavioral change. Psychol Rev 1977; 84:191–215 [F]

278. Burling TA, Reilly PM, Moltzen JO, Ziff DC: Self-efficacy and relapse among inpatient drug and alcohol abusers: a predictor of outcome. J Stud Alcohol 1989; 50:354–360 [C]

279. Edwards G, Brown D, Duckitt A, Oppenheimer E, Sheehan M, Taylor C: Outcome of alcoholism: the structure of patient attributions as to what causes change. Br J Addict 1987; 82:533–545 [C]

280. Hunt GM, Azrin NH: A community reinforcement approach to alcoholism. Behav Res Ther 1973; 11:91–104 [A]

281. Chick J, Ritson B, Connaughton J, Stewart A, Chick J: Advice vs extended treatment for alcoholism: a controlled study. Br J Addict 1988; 83:159–170 [A]

282. Babor TF: Avoiding the Horrible and Beastly Sin of Drunkenness: Does Dissuasion Make a Difference? Storrs, University of Connecticut School of Medicine, 1992 [G]

283. Bien TH, Miller WR, Tonigan JS: Brief interventions for alcohol problems: a review. Addiction 1993; 88:315–336 [F]

284. Anderson P, Scott E: The effect of general practitioners' advice to heavy drinking men. Br J Addict 1992; 87:891–900 [A]

285. Moos RH, Moos B: The process of recovery from alcoholism, III: comparing functioning in families of alcoholics and matched control families. J Stud Alcohol 1984; 45:111–118 [F]

286. McCrady BS, Stout R, Noel N, Abrams D, Nelson HF: Effectiveness of three types of spouse-involved behavioral alcoholism treatment. Br J Addict 1991; 86:1415–1424 [F]

287. Bowers T, Al-Redha MR: A comparison of outcome with group/marital and standard/individual therapies with alcoholics. J Stud Alcohol 1990; 51:301–309 [A]

288. Noel NE, McCrady BS, Stout RL, Fisher-Nelson H: Predictors of attrition from an outpatient alcoholism treatment program for couples. J Stud Alcohol 1987; 48:229–235 [B]

289. Litt MD, Babor TF, DelBoca FK, Kadden RM, Cooney NL: Types of alcoholics, II: application of an empirically derived typology to treatment matching. Arch Gen Psychiatry 1992; 49: 609–614 [A]

290. Maisto SA, O'Farrell TJ, McKay JR, Connors GJ, Pelcovits M: Factors in maintaining sobriety following alcohol treatment. Alcohol Treatment Q 1989; 6:143–150 [C]

291. Walker RD, Donovan DM, Kivlahan DR, O'Leary MR: Length of stay, neuropsychological performance and aftercare: influences on alcoholism treatment outcome. J Clin Consult Psychol 1983; 51:900–911 [B]

292. McLatchie BH, Lomp KG: An experimental investigation of the influence of aftercare on alcohol relapse. Br J Addict 1988; 83: 1045–1054 [B]

293. Gilbert FS: The effect of type of aftercare follow-up on treatment outcome among alcoholics. J Stud Alcohol 1988; 49:149–159 [A]

294. Ito J, Donovan D: Aftercare in alcoholism treatment: a review, in Treating Addictive Behaviors: Processes of Change. Edited by Miller WR, Heather NH. New York, Plenum, 1986 [F]

295. O'Farrell TJ, Choquette KA, Cutter HS, Brown ED, McCourt WF: Behavioral marital therapy with and without additional couples relapse prevention sessions for alcoholics and their wives. J Stud Alcohol 1993; 54:652–666 [B]

296. Alcoholics Anonymous: The Big Book. New York, Alcoholics Anonymous World Services, 1973 [G]

297. Nowinski J, Baker S, Carroll K: 12 Step Facilitation Therapy Manual: DHHS Publication (ADM) 92–1893. Rockville, MD, US Department of Health and Human Services, 1992 [G]

298. Cross GM, Morgan CW, Mooney AJ, Martin CA, Rafter JA: Alcoholism treatment: a ten year follow-up study. Alcohol Clin Exp Res 1990; 14:169–173 [C]

299. Gilbert FS: Development of a "steps questionnaire." J Stud Alcohol 1991; 52:353–360 [C]

300. Emrick C: Alcoholics Anonymous: affiliation processes and effectiveness as treatment. Alcohol Clin Exp Res 1987; 11:416–423 [G]

301. McCrady BS, Irvine S: Self-help groups, in Handbook of Alcoholism Treatment Approaches. Edited by Hester RK, Miller WR. Elmsford, NY, Pergamon Press, 1989 [G]

302. Tallaksen CM, Bohmer T, Bell H: Blood and serum thiamin and thiamin phosphate esters concentrations in patients with alcohol dependence syndrome before and after thiamin treatment. Alcohol Clin Exp Res 1992; 16:320–325 [B]

303. Bond NW, Homewook J: Wernicke's encephalopathy and Korsakoff's psychosis: to fortify or not to fortify? Neurotoxicology 1991; 13:353–355 [F]

304. Blass JP, Gibson GE: Abnormality of a thiamine-requiring enzyme in patients with Wernicke-Korsakoff syndrome. N Engl J Med 1977; 297:1367–1370 [G]

305. Shaw JM, Kolesar GS, Sellers EM, Kaplan HL, Sandor P: Development of optimal treatment tactics for alcohol withdrawal. J Clin Psychopharmacol 1981; 1:382–389 [B]

306. Naranjo CA, Sellers EM, Chater K, Iversen P, Roach C, Sykora K: Nonpharmacologic intervention in acute alcohol withdrawal. Clin Pharmacol Ther 1983; 34:214–219 [A]

307. Whitfield CL, Thompson G, Lamb A, Spencer V, Pfeifer M, Browning-Ferrando M: Detoxification of 1,024 alcoholic patients without psychoactive drugs. JAMA 1978; 239:1409–1410 [B]

308. Femino J, Lewis DC: Clinical Pharmacology and Therapeutics of the Alcohol Withdrawal Syndrome: Monograph 272. Rockville, MD, National Institute on Alcohol Abuse and Alcoholism, 1982 [F]

309. Rosenbloom A: Emerging treatment options in the alcohol withdrawal syndrome. J Clin Psychiatry 1988; 49(Dec suppl):28–32 [G]

310. Victor M: Treatment of alcohol intoxication and the withdrawal syndrome: a critical analysis of the use of drugs and other forms of therapy. Psychosom Med 1966; 28:636–650 [G]

311. Saitz R, Mayo-Smith MF, Roberts MS, Redmond HA, Bernard DR, Calkins DR: Individualized treatment for alcohol withdrawal. JAMA 1994; 272:519–523 [A]

312. Bradley KA: Management of alcoholism in the primary care setting. West J Med 1992; 156:273–277 [F]

313. Woo E, Greenblatt DJ: Massive benzodiazepine requirements during acute alcohol withdrawal. Am J Psychiatry 1979; 136:821–823 [G]

314. Sellers EM, Naranjo CA: New strategies for the treatment of alcohol withdrawal. Psychopharmacol Bull 1983; 22:88–91 [F]

315. Seppala T, Aranko K, Mattila MJ, Shrotriay RC: Effects of alcohol on buspirone and lorazepam actions. Clin Pharmacol Ther 1982; 32:201–207 [A]

316. Gessner PK: Treatment of the alcohol withdrawal syndrome. Substance Abuse 1979; 1:2–5 [G]

317. Gessner PK: Drug withdrawal therapy of the alcohol withdrawal syndrome, in Biochemistry and Pharmacology of Ethanol, vol 2. Edited by Majchowicz E, Moble E. New York, Plenum, 1979 [G]

318. Gross GA: The use of propranolol as a method to manage acute alcohol detoxification. J Am Osteopathic Assoc 1982; 82:206–207 [B]

319. Zilm DH, Sellers EM, MacLeod SM: Propranolol effect on tremor in alcohol withdrawal. Ann Intern Med 1975; 83:234–236 [G]

320. Sellers EM, Zilm DH, Macleod SM: Chlordiazepoxide and propranolol treatment of alcoholic withdrawal (abstract). Clin Res 1975; 23:610A [A]

321. Kraus MI, Gottlieb LD, Horwitz RI, Anscher M: Randomized clinical trial of atenolol in patients with alcohol withdrawal. N Engl J Med 1985; 313:905–909 [A]

322. Wilkins AJ, Jenkins WJ, Steiner JA: Efficacy of clonidine in treatment of alcohol withdrawal state. Psychopharmacology (Berl) 1983; 81:78–80 [A]

323. Robinson BJ, Robinson GM, Maling TJ, Johnson RH: Is clonidine useful in the treatment of alcohol withdrawal? Alcohol Clin Exp Res 1989; 13:95–98 [A]

324. Smith DE: Use of psychotropic drugs in alcoholism treatment: a summary. Addictions Alert 1989; 2:47–48 [F]

325. Gorelick DA, Wilkins JN: Special aspects of human alcohol withdrawal. Rec Dev Alcohol 1986; 4:283–305 [G]

326. Greenblatt DJ, Shader RI: Treatment of the alcohol withdrawal syndrome, in Manual of Psychiatric Therapeutics. Edited by Shader RI. Boston, Little, Brown, 1975 [G]

327. Sandor P, Sellers EM, Dumbrell M, Khouw V: Effect of short- and long-term alcohol use on phenytoin kinetics in chronic alcoholics. Clin Pharmacol Ther 1981; 30:390–397 [G]

328. Shaw GK: Alcohol dependence and withdrawal. Br Med Bull 1982; 38:99–102 [F]

329. Rothstein E: Prevention of alcohol withdrawal seizure: the roles of diphenylhydantoin and chlordiazepoxide. Am J Psychiatry 1973; 130:1381–1382 [B]

330. Sampliner R, Iber FL: Diphenylhydantoin control of alcohol withdrawal seizures: results of a controlled study. JAMA 1974; 230:1430–1432 [A]

331. Wilbur R, Kulik FA: Anticonvulsant drugs in alcohol withdrawal: use of phenytoin, primidone, carbamazepine, valproic acid and the sedative anticonvulsants. Am J Hosp Pharm 1981; 38:1138–1148 [F]

332. Poutanen P: Experience with carbamazepine in the treatment of withdrawal symptoms in alcohol abusers. Br J Addict 1979; 74:201–204 [B]

333. Malcolm R, Ballenger JC, Sturgis ET, Anton R: Double-blind controlled trial comparing carbamazepine to oxazepam treatment of alcohol withdrawal. Am J Psychiatry 1989; 146:617–621 [A]

334. Chu NS: Carbamazepine: prevention of alcohol withdrawal seizures. Neurology 1979; 29:1397–1401 [G]

335. Post RM, Ballenger JC, Putnam F, Bunney WE: Carbamazepine in alcohol withdrawal syndromes: relationship to the kindling model (letter). J Clin Psychopharmacol 1983; 3:204 [G]

336. Wilson A, Vulcano B: A double-blind, placebo-controlled trial of magnesium sulfate in the ethanol withdrawal syndrome. Alcohol Clin Exp Res 1984; 8:542–545 [A]

337. Robins E: The Final Months: A Study of the Lives of 134 Persons Who Committed Suicide. New York, Oxford University Press, 1981 [D]

338. Berglund M: Suicide in alcoholism: a prospective study of 88 suicides, I: the multidimensional diagnosis at first admission. Arch Gen Psychiatry 1984; 41:888–891 [C]

339. Linnoila MI: Anxiety and alcoholism. J Clin Psychiatry 1989; 50:26–29 [G]

340. Nunes EV, Quitkin FM, Brady R, Stewart JW: Imipramine treatment of methadone maintenance patients with affective disorder and illicit drug use. Am J Psychiatry 1991; 148:667–669 [B]

341. Ciraulo DA, Jaffe JH: Tricyclic antidepressants in the treatment of depression associated with alcoholism. J Clin Psychopharmacol 1981; 1:146–150 [F]

342. Ciraulo DA, Barnhill JG, Jaffe JH: Clinical pharmacokinetics of imipramine and desipramine in alcoholics and normal volunteers. Clin Pharmacol Ther 1988; 43:509–518 [B]

343. Cornelius JR, Salloum IM, Cornelius MD, Perel JM, Thase ME, Ehler JG, Mann JJ: Fluoxetine trial in suicidal depressed alcoholics. Psychopharmacol Bull 1993; 29:195–199 [B]

344. Bruno F: Buspirone in the treatment of alcoholic patients. Psychopathology 1989; 22(suppl 1):49–59 [A]

345. Kranzler HR, Burleson JA, Del Boca FK, Babor TF, Korner P, Brown J, Bohn MJ: Buspirone treatment of anxious alcoholics: a placebo-controlled trial. Arch Gen Psychiatry 1994; 51:720–731 [A]

346. Schottenfeld RS, O'Malley SS, Smith L, Rounsaville BJ, Jaffe JH: Limitation and potential hazards of MAOI's for the treatment of depressive symptoms in abstinent alcoholics. Am J Drug Alcohol Abuse 1989; 15:339–344 [G]

347. Galamos JT: Alcoholic liver disease: fatty liver, hepatitis, and cirrhosis, in Gastroenterology. Edited by Berk JE. Philadelphia, WB Saunders, 1985 [G]

348. Lieber CS: Pathogenesis of alcoholic liver disease: an overview, in Alcohol and the Liver. Edited by Fisher MM, Rankin JG. New York, Plenum, 1977 [G]

349. Lieber CS, Leo MA: Alcohol and the liver, in Medical Disorders of Alcoholism: Pathogenesis and Treatment. Edited by Lieber CS. Philadelphia, WB Saunders, 1982 [G]

350. Mendelson JH, Babor TF, Mello NK, Pratt H: Alcoholism and prevalence of medical and psychiatric disorders. J Stud Alcohol 1986; 47:361–366 [D]

351. Van Thiel DH, Gavaler JS: Endocrine effects of chronic alcohol abuse: hypothalamic-pituitary-gonadal axis, in Alcohol and the Brain: Chronic Effects. Edited by Tarter RE, Van Thiel DH. New York, Plenum, 1985 [B]

352. Korsten MA, Lieber CS: Medical complications of alcoholism, in The Diagnosis and Treatment of Alcoholism. Edited by Mendelson JH, Mello NK. New York, McGraw-Hill, 1985 [G]

353. Gorenstein EE: Cognitive-perceptual deficit in an alcoholism spectrum disorder. J Stud Alcohol 1987; 48:310–318 [D]

354. Bowden SC: Separating cognitive impairment in neurologically asymptomatic alcoholism from Wernicke-Korsakoff syndrome: is the neuropsychological distinction justified? Psychol Bull 1990; 107:355–366 [F]

355. Rindi G: Alcohol and thiamine of the brain. Alcohol 1989; 24:493–495 [G]

356. Turner S, Daniels L, Greer S: Wernicke's encephalopathy in an 18-year-old woman. Br J Psychiatry 1989; 154:261–262 [G]

357. Naidoo DP, Bramdev A, Cooper K: Wernicke's encephalopathy and alcohol-related disease. Postgrad Med J 1991; 67:978–981 [C]

358. McNamara ME, Campbell JJ, Recupero PR: Wernicke-Korsakoff syndrome (letter). J Neuropsychiatry Clin Neurosci 1991; 3:232 [G]

359. Martin PR, Eckardt MJ, Linnoila M: Treatment of chronic organic mental disorders associated with alcoholism. Recent Dev Alcohol 1989; 7:329–350 [G]

360. Saravay S, Pardes H: Auditory elementary hallucinations in alcohol withdrawal psychosis. Arch Gen Psychiatry 1967; 16: 652–658 [D]

361. Williams CM, Skiller AE: The cognitive effects of alcohol abuse: a controlled study. Br J Addict 1990; 85:911–917 [B]

362. Lemoine P, Harroussea H, Borteyru JP: Les enfants de parents alcooliques: anomalies observées à propos de 127 cas. Ouest Medical 1968; 25:477–482 [C]

363. Clarren SK, Smith DW: The fetal alcohol syndrome. N Engl J Med 1978; 298:1063–1067 [G]

364. Liskow BI, Rinck C, Campbell J: Alcohol withdrawal in the elderly. J Stud Alcohol 1989; 50:414–421 [D]

365. Kofoed LL, Tolson RL, Atkinson RM, Toth RL, Turner JA: Treatment compliance of older alcoholics: an elder-specific approach is superior to "mainstreaming." J Stud Alcohol 1987; 48:47–51 [B]

366. Gorelick DA: Progression of dependence in male cocaine addicts. Am J Drug Alcohol Abuse 1992; 18:13–19 [C]

367. Alterman AI, O'Brien CP, August DS, Snider EC, Droba M, Cornish JW, McLellan AT, Hall CP, Raphaelson AH, Schrade FX: Effectiveness and costs of inpatient versus day hospital cocaine rehabilitation. J Nerv Ment Dis 1994; 182:157–163 [A]

368. Budde D, Rounsaville B, Bryant K: Inpatient and outpatient cocaine abusers: clinical comparisons at intake and one-year follow-up. J Subst Abuse Treat 1992; 9:337–342 [C]

369. Kosten TR: Pharmacotherapeutic interventions for cocaine abuse: matching patients to treatments. J Nerv Ment Dis 1989; 177:379–389 [F]

370. Gorelick DA: Overview of pharmacologic treatment approaches for alcohol and other drug addiction. Psychiatr Clin North Am 1993; 16:141–156 [F]

371. Kosten TR, McCance-Katz E: New pharmacotherapies, in American Psychiatric Press Review of Psychiatry, vol 14. Edited by Oldham J, Riba MB. Washington, DC, American Psychiatric Press, 1995 [G]

372. Gawin FH, Kleber HD: Abstinence symptomatology and psychiatric diagnosis in chronic cocaine abusers. Arch Gen Psychiatry 1986; 43:107–113 [B]

373. Weddington WW, Brown BS, Haertzen CA, Cone EJ, Dax EM, Herning RI, Michaelson BS: Changes in mood, craving and sleep during short-term abstinence reported by male cocaine addicts. Arch Gen Psychiatry 1990; 47:861–868 [C]

374. Gawin FH, Kleber HD, Byck R, Rounsaville BJ, Kosten TR, Jatlow PI, Morgan C: Desipramine facilitation of initial cocaine abstinence. Arch Gen Psychiatry 1989; 46:117–121 [A]

375. Arndt I, Dorozynsky L, Woody G, McLellan AT, O'Brien CP: Desipramine treatment of cocaine abuse in methadone maintenance patients. NIDA Res Monogr 1989; 95:322–323 [A]

376. Weddington WW Jr, Brown BS, Haertzen CA, Hess JM, Mahaffey JR, Kolar AF, Jaffee JH: Comparison of amantadine and desipramine combined with psychotherapy for treatment of cocaine dependence. Am J Drug Alcohol Abuse 1991; 17:137–152 [A]

377. Kosten TP, Morgan CM, Falcione J, Schottenfeld RS: Pharmacotherapy for cocaine-abusing methadone-maintained patients using amantadine or desipramine. Arch Gen Psychiatry 1992; 49:894–898 [A]

378. Halikas JA, Crosby RD, Carlson GA, Crea F, Graves NM, Bowers LD: Cocaine reduction in unmotivated crack users using carbamazepine versus placebo in a short-term, double-blind crossover design. Clin Pharmacol Ther 1991; 50:81–95 [A]

379. Cornish JW, Alterman AA, Maany I, Droba M, O'Brien CP: Amantadine and carbamazepine treatment for cocaine abuse, in CME Syllabus and Scientific Proceedings in Summary Form, 145th Annual Meeting of the American Psychiatric Association. Washington, DC, APA, 1992 [G]

380. Montoya ID, Levin FR, Fudala P, Gorelick DA: A double-blind comparison of carbamazepine and placebo treatment of cocaine dependence. NIDA Res Monogr 1994; 141:435 [A]

381. Malcolm R, Hutto BR, Phillips JD, Ballenger JC: Pergolide mesylate treatment of cocaine withdrawal. J Clin Psychiatry 1991; 52:39–40 [C]

382. Wolfsohn R, Angrist B: A pilot trial of levodopa/carbidopa in early cocaine abstinence (letter). J Clin Psychopharmacol 1990; 10:440–442 [C]

383. Pollack MH, Rosenbaum JF: Fluoxetine treatment of cocaine abuse in heroin addicts. J Clin Psychiatry 1991; 52:31–33 [E]

384. Batki SL, Manfredi LB, Jacob P III, Jones RT: Fluoxetine for cocaine dependence in methadone maintenance: quantitative plasma and urine cocaine/benzoylecgonine concentrations. J Clin Psychopharmacol 1993; 13:243–250 [B]

385. Gawin FH, Allen D, Humblestone B: Outpatient treatment of "crack" cocaine smoking with flupenthixol decanoate: a preliminary report. Arch Gen Psychiatry 1989; 46:322–325 [B]

386. Margolin A, Kosten T, Petrakis I, Avants SK, Kosten T: An open pilot study of bupropion and psychotherapy for the treatment of cocaine abuse in methadone-maintained patients. NIDA Res Monogr 1991; 105:367–368 [B]

387. Kosten TR, Morgan CH, Schottenfeld RS: Amantadine and desipramine in the treatment of cocaine abusing methadone maintained patients. NIDA Res Monogr 1991; 105:510–511 [A]

388. Brotman AW, Witkie SM, Gelenberg AJ, Falk WE, Wojcik J, Leahy L: An open trial of maprotiline for the treatment of cocaine abuse: a pilot study. J Clin Psychopharmacol 1988; 8:125–127 [C]

389. Golwyn DH: Cocaine abuse treated with phenelzine. Int J Addict 1988; 23:897–905 [B]

390. Kosten TR, Kleber HD, Morgan C: Treatment of cocaine abuse with buprenorphine. Biol Psychiatry 1989; 26:170–172 [C]

391. Gastfriend DR, Mendelson JH, Mello NK, Teoh SK: Preliminary results of an open trial of buprenorphine in the outpatient treatment of combined heroin and cocaine dependence. NIDA Res Monogr (in press) [B]

392. Johnson RE, Jaffe JH, Fudala PJ: A controlled trial of buprenorphine treatment for opioid dependence. JAMA 1992; 267: 2750–2755 [A]

393. Schottenfeld RS, Pakes J, Ziedonis D, Kosten TR: Buprenorphine: dose-related effects on cocaine and opioid use on cocaine-abusing opioid-dependent humans. Biol Psychiatry 1993; 34: 66–74 [B]

394. Rosecan JS: The treatment of cocaine addiction with imipramine, L-tyrosine, and L-tryptophan. Presented at the VII World Congress of Psychiatry, Vienna, July 11–16, 1983 [G]

395. Dackis CA, Gold MS: Bromocriptine as treatment of cocaine abuse. Lancet 1985; 1:1151–1152 [E]

396. Gutierrez-Esteinou R, Baldessarini RJ, Cremens MC, Campbell A, Teicher MH: Interactions of bromocriptine with cocaine (letter). Am J Psychiatry 1988; 145:1173 [E]

397. Gawin FH: Neuroleptic reduction of cocaine-induced paranoia but not euphoria? Psychopharmacology (Berl) 1986; 90:142–143 [G]

398. Margolin A, Azants SK, Kosten TR, Nichou C: A double-blind study of mazindol for the treatment of cocaine abuse in newly abstinent cocaine abusing methadone-maintained patients: a preliminary report. NIDA Res Monogr 1994; 141:446 [A]

399. Washton AM: Treatment of cocaine abuse. NIDA Res Monogr 1986; 67:263–270 [B]

400. Kang S-Y, Kleinman PH, Woody GE, Millman RB, Todd TC, Kemp J, Lipton DS: Outcomes for cocaine abusers after once-a-week psychosocial therapy. Am J Psychiatry 1991; 148:630–635 [A]

401. Schiffer F: Psychotherapy of nine successfully treated cocaine abusers: techniques and dynamics. J Subst Abuse Treat 1988; 5:131–137 [E]

402. Spitz HI: Cocaine abuse: therapeutic group approaches, in Cocaine Abuse: New Directions in Treatment and Research. Edited by Spitz HI, Rosecan JS. New York, Brunner/Mazel, 1987 [G]

403. Carroll KM, Rounsaville BJ, Gordon LT, Nich C, Jatlow P, Bisighini RM, Gawin FH: Psychotherapy and pharmacotherapy for ambulatory cocaine abusers. Arch Gen Psychiatry 1994; 51: 177–187 [B]

404. Carroll KM, Rounsaville BJ: Psychosocial treatments, in American Psychiatric Press Review of Psychiatry, vol 14. Edited by Oldham JM, Riba MB. Washington, DC, American Psychiatric Press, 1995 [G]

405. Wesson DR, Smith DE: Cocaine: treatment perspectives. NIDA Res Monogr 1985; 61:193–203 [F]

406. Washton AM: Cocaine Addiction. New York, WW Norton, 1989 [F]

407. Galanter M, Egelko S, DeLeon G, Rohrs C: A general hospital day program combining peer-led and professional treatment of cocaine abusers. Hosp Community Psychiatry 1993; 44:644–649 [C]

408. Satel SL, Price LH, Palumbo JM, McDougle CJ, Krystal JH, Gawin F, Charney DS, Heninger GR, Kleber HD: Clinical phenomenology and neurobiology of cocaine dependence: a prospective inpatient study. Am J Psychiatry 1991; 148:1712–1716 [C]

409. Goldfrank LR, Hoffman RS: The cardiovascular effects of cocaine. Ann Emerg Med 1991; 20:165–175 [F]

410. Satel SL, Southwick SM, Gawin FH: Clinical features of cocaine-induced paranoia. Am J Psychiatry 1991; 148:495–498 [C]

411. Handelsman L, Chordia PL, Escovar IL, Marion IJ, Lowinson JH: Amantadine for treatment of cocaine dependence in methadone-maintained patients (letter). Am J Psychiatry 1988; 145: 533 [C]

412. Tennant FS, Sagherian AA: Double-blind comparison of amantadine hydrochloride and bromocriptine mesylate for ambulatory withdrawal from cocaine dependence. Arch Intern Med 1987; 147:109–112 [A]

413. Giannini AJ: Bromocriptine therapy in cocaine withdrawal. J Clin Pharmacol 1987; 27:267–270 [A]

414. Teller DW, Devenyi P: Bromocriptine in cocaine withdrawal—does it work? Int J Addict 1988; 23:1197–1205 [C]

415. Moscovitz H, Brookoff D, Nelson L: A randomized trial of bromocriptine for cocaine users presenting to the emergency department. J Gen Intern Med 1993; 8:1–4 [A]

416. Nunes EV, McGrath PJ, Wager S, Quitkin FM: Lithium treatment for cocaine abusers with bipolar spectrum disorders. Am J Psychiatry 1990; 147:655–657 [B]

417. Cocores JA, Patel MD, Gold MS, Pottash AC: Cocaine abuse, attention deficit disorder, and bipolar disorder. J Nerv Ment Dis 1987; 175:431–432 [G]

418. Gawin FH, Kleber HD: Cocaine abuse treatment: open trial with desipramine and lithium carbonate. Arch Gen Psychiatry 1984; 41:903–909 [B]

419. Weiss RD, Pope HG Jr, Mirin SM: Treatment of chronic cocaine abuse and attention deficit disorder, residual type, with magnesium pemoline. Drug Alcohol Depend 1985; 15:69–72 [E]

420. Khantzian EJ: An extreme case of cocaine dependence and marked improvement with methylphenidate treatment. Am J Psychiatry 1983; 140:784–785 [G]

421. Giannini AJ, Malone DA, Giannini MC, Price WA, Loiselle RH: Treatment of depression in chronic cocaine and phencyclidine abuse with desipramine. J Clin Pharmacol 1986; 26:211–214 [C]

422. Arndt IO, McLellan AT, Dorozynsky L, Woody G, O'Brien CP: Desipramine treatment for cocaine dependence: role of antisocial personality disorder. J Nerv Ment Dis 1994; 182:151–156 [A]

423. Ziedonis DM, Kosten TR: Depression as a prognostic factor for pharmacological treatment of cocaine dependence. Psychopharmacol Bull 1991; 27:337–343 [A]

424. Urogenital anomalies in the offspring of women using cocaine during early pregnancy—Atlanta, 1968–1980. MMWR Morb Mortal Wkly Rep 1989; 38:536, 541–542 [D]

425. Chasnoff IJ, Burns WJ, Schnoll SH: Cocaine use in pregnancy. N Engl J Med 1985; 313:666–669 [F]

426. Ward SLD, Bautista DB, Derry MK, Mills KSC, Durfee M, Lisbin A, Keens TG: Incidence of SIDS in infants of substance abusing mothers (abstract). Pediatr Res 1989; 25:106A [D]

427. Fulroth RF, Phillips B, Durand DJ: Perinatal outcome of infants exposed to cocaine and/or heroin in utero. Am J Dis Child 1989; 143:905–910 [C]

428. Schneider JW, Chasnoff IJ: Cocaine abuse during pregnancy: its effects on infant motor development—a clinical perspective. Topics in Acute Care and Trauma Rehabilitation 1987; 2:59–69 [F]

429. Neuspiel DR, Hamel SC, Hochberg E, Greene J, Campbell D: Maternal cocaine use and infant behavior. Neurotoxicol Teratol 1991; 13:229–233 [C]

430. Delaney-Black V, Roumell N, Shankaran S, Bedard M: Maternal cocaine use and infant outcomes (abstract). Pediatr Res 1990; 25:242A [G]

431. Robins LN, Regier DA (eds): Psychiatric Disorders in America. New York, Free Press, 1991 [G]

432. Metzger DS, Woody GE, McLellan AT, O'Brien CP, Druley P, Navaline H, DePhillippis D, Stolley P, Abrutyn E: Human immunodeficiency virus seroconversion among intravenous drug users in- and out-of-treatment: an 18-month prospective follow-up. J Acquir Immune Defic Syndr 1993; 6:1049–1056 [C]

433. Schottenfeld RS, Kleber HD: Methadone maintenance, in Comprehensive Textbook of Psychiatry, 6th ed. Edited by Kaplan HI, Sadock BJ. Baltimore, Williams & Wilkins, 1995 [F]

434. Hubbard RL, Marsden ME, Rachal JV: Drug Abuse Treatment: A National Study of Effectiveness. Chapel Hill, University of North Carolina Press, 1989 [C]

435. General Accounting Office: Methadone Maintenance: Some Treatment Programs Are Not Effective; Greater Federal Oversight Needed: Publication GAO/HRD90-104. Washington, DC, US Government Printing Office, 1990 [G]

436. Tennant FS Jr, Rawson RA, Pumphrey E, Seecof R: Clinical experiences with 959 opioid-dependent patients treated with levo-alpha-acetylmethadol (LAAM). J Subst Abuse Treat 1986; 3:195–202 [B]

437. Ling W, Klett CJ, Gillis RD: A cooperative clinical study of methadyl acetate. Arch Gen Psychiatry 1978; 35:345–353 [B]

438. Zangwell BC, McGahan P, Dorozynsky L, McLellan AT: How effective is LAAM treatment? clinical comparison with methadone. NIDA Res Monogr 1986; 67:249–255 [B]

439. Des Jarlais DC, Joseph H, Dole VP: Long-term outcomes after termination from methadone maintenance treatment. Ann NY Acad Sci 1981; 362:231–238 [C]

440. McGlothlin WH, Anglin DM: Shutting off methadone: costs and benefits. Arch Gen Psychiatry 1981; 38:885–892 [B]

441. Gonzalez JP, Brogden RD: Naltrexone: a review of its pharmacodynamic and pharmacokinetic properties and therapeutic efficacy in the management of opioid dependence. Drugs 1988; 35:192–213 [F]

442. Brewer C, Rezae H, Bailey C: Opioid withdrawal and naltrexone induction in 48–72 hours with minimal drop-out, using a modification of the naltrexone-clonidine technique. Br J Psychiatry 1988; 153:340–343 [B]

443. Anton RF, Hogan I, Jalali B, Riordan CE, Kleber HD: Multiple family therapy and naltrexone in the treatment of opiate dependence. Drug Alcohol Depend 1981: 8:157–168 [A]

444. Kleber HD: Treatment of drug dependence: what works. Int Rev Psychiatry 1989; 1:81–100 [F]

445. Washton AM, Pottash AC, Gold MS: Naltrexone in addicted business executives and physicians. J Clin Psychiatry 1984; 45: 39–41 [B]

446. Woody GE, McLellan AT, O'Brien CP: Treatment of behavioral and psychiatric problems associated with opiate dependence. NIDA Res Monogr 1984; 46:23–35 [G]

447. Woody GE, McLellan AT, Luborsky L, O'Brien CP: Twelve-month follow-up of psychotherapy for opiate dependence. Am J Psychiatry 1987; 144:590–596; correction, 1989; 146:1651 [B]

448. Woody GE, McLellan AT, Luborsky L, O'Brien CP: Psychotherapy in community methadone programs: a validation study. Am J Psychiatry 1995; 152:1302–1308 [B]

449. Stitzer ML, Iguchi MY, Felch LJ: Contingent take-home incentive: effects on drug use of methadone maintenance patients. J Consult Clin Psychol 1992; 60:927–934 [B]

450. Brahen LS, Henderson RK, Capone T, Kordal N: Naltrexone treatment in a jail work-release program. J Clin Psychiatry 1984; 45:49–52 [A]

451. McAuliffe WE: A randomized controlled trial of recovery training and self-help for opioid addicts in New England and Hong Kong. J Psychoactive Drugs 1990; 22:197–209 [B]

452. Kleber HD: Detoxification from narcotics, in Substance Abuse: Clinical Problems and Perspectives. Edited by Lowinson J, Ruiz P. Baltimore, Williams & Wilkins, 1981 [F]

453. Jasinski DR, Johnson RE, Kuchel TR: Clonidine in morphine withdrawal: differential effects on signs and symptoms. Arch Gen Psychiatry 1985; 42:1063–1076 [B]

454. Kleber HD, Topazian M, Gaspari J, Riordan CE, Kosten T: Clonidine and naltrexone in the outpatient treatment of heroin withdrawal. Am J Drug Alcohol Abuse 1987; 13:1–17 [B]

455. Gold MS, Pottash AC, Sweeny DR, Kleber HD: Opiate withdrawal using clonidine. JAMA 1980; 243:343–346 [B]

456. Vining E, Kosten TR, Kleber HD: Clinical utility of rapid clonidine-naltrexone detoxification or opioid abuse. Br J Addict 1988; 83:567–575 [B]

457. Charney DS, Heninger GR, Kleber HD: The combined use of clonidine and naltrexone as a rapid, safe, and effective treatment of abrupt withdrawal from methadone. Am J Psychiatry 1986; 143:831–837 [B]

458. O'Connor PG, Waugh ME, Schottenfeld RS, Diakogiannis IA, Rounsaville BJ: Ambulatory opiate detoxification and primary care: a role for the primary care physician. J Gen Intern Med 1992; 7:532–534 [B]

459. Mello NK, Mendelson JH: Buprenorphine suppresses heroin use by heroin addicts. Science 1980; 207:657–659 [A]

460. Ellison F, Ellison W, Daulouede JP, Daubech JF, Pautrizel B, Bourgeois M, Tignol J: Opiate withdrawal and electro-stimulation: double-blind experiments. Encephale 1987; 13:225–229 [A]

461. Alling A, Johnson BD, Elmoghazy E: Cranial electro stimulation (CES) use in the detoxification of opiate dependent patients. J Subst Abuse Treat 1990; 7:173–180 [F]

462. Ter Riet G, Kleijnen J, Knipschild P: A meta-analysis of studies into the effect of acupuncture on addiction. Br J Gen Pract 1990; 40:379–382 [E]

463. National Council Against Health Fraud: Acupuncture: the position paper of the National Council Against Health Fraud. Am J Acupuncture 1991; 19:273–279 [F]

464. Brewington V, Smith M, Lipton D: Acupuncture as a detoxification treatment: an analysis of controlled research. J Subst Abuse Treat 1994; 11:289–307 [G]

465. Ulett GA: Beyond Yin and Yang: How Acupuncture Really Works. St Louis, Warren H Green, 1992, pp 1–170 [G]

466. Wen HL, Cheung SYC: Treatment of drug addiction by acupuncture and electrical stimulation. Am J Acupuncture 1973; 1:71–75 [B]

467. Whitehead PC: Acupuncture in the treatment of addiction: a review and analysis. Int J Addict 1978; 13:1–16 [F]

468. Kleber HD, Weissman MM, Rounsaville BJ: Imipramine as treatment for depression in addicts. Arch Gen Psychiatry 1983; 40:649–653 [A]

469. Sellers EM, Ciraulo DA, DuPont RL, Griffiths RR, Kosten TR, Romach MK, Woody GE: Alprazolam and benzodiazepine dependence. J Clin Psychiatry 1993; 54(suppl 10):64–75 [F]

470. Griffiths RR, McLeod DR, Bigelow GE, Liebson IA, Roache JD, Nowowieski P: Comparison of diazepam and oxazepam: preference, liking and extent of abuse. J Pharmacol Exp Ther 1984; 229:501–508 [A]

471. Kosten TR, Schumann B, Wright D, Carney MK, Gawin FH: A preliminary study of desipramine in the treatment of cocaine abuse in methadone maintenance patients. J Clin Psychiatry 1987; 48:442–444 [B]

472. Kosten TR, Gawin FH, Rounsaville BJ, Kleber HD: Cocaine abuse among opioid addicts: demographic and diagnostic factors in treatment. Am J Drug Alcohol Abuse 1986; 12:1–16 [C]

473. Kosten TR, Rounsaville BJ, Kleber HD: A 2.5-year follow-up of cocaine use among treated opioid addicts: have our treatments helped? Arch Gen Psychiatry 1987; 44:281–284 [C]

474. Condelli WS, Fairbank JA, Dennis ML, Rachal JV: Cocaine use by clients in methadone programs: significance, scope and behavioral interventions. J Subst Abuse Treat 1991; 8:203–212 [F]

475. Anglin MD, Almog IJ, Fisher DG, Peters KR: Alcohol use by heroin addicts: evidence for an inverse relationship: a study of methadone maintenance and drug-free treatment samples. Am J Drug Alcohol Abuse 1989; 15:191–207 [D]

476. Stimmel B, Cohen M, Sturiano V, Hanbury R, Korts D, Jackson G: Is treatment for alcoholism effective in persons on methadone maintenance? Am J Psychiatry 1983; 140:862–866 [B]

477. American Thoracic Society: Diagnostic standards and classification of tuberculosis. Am Rev Respir Dis 1990; 142:725–735; correction, 1990; 142:1470 [G]

478. Dooley SW Jr, Castro KG, Hutton MD, Mullan RJ, Polder JA, Snider DE Jr: Guidelines for preventing the transmission of tuberculosis in health-care settings, with special focus on HIV-related issues. MMWR Morb Mortal Wkly Rep 1990; 39:1–29 [G]

479. Kaltenbach KK, Nathanson L, Finnegan LP: Temperament characteristics of infants born to drug dependent women (abstract). Pediatr Res 1989; 25:15A [D]

480. Suffet F, Brotman R: A comprehensive care program for pregnant addicts: obstetrical, neonatal and child development outcomes. Int J Addict 1984; 19:199–219 [C]

481. Carroll KM, Chang G, Behr H, Clinton B, Kosten TR: Improving treatment outcome in pregnant, methadone-maintained women. Am J Addiction 1995; 4:56–59 [B]

APPENDIX

American Psychiatric Association Practice Guideline Development Process

---

I. Background and Definition

In 1991, the American Psychiatric Association (APA), through its Assembly and Board of Trustees, embarked on the process of developing practice guidelines. Since its inception, the APA has generated, under many different formats, guidelines for psychiatric practice. *Practice guidelines* as defined by this project, however, are systematically developed documents appearing in a standardized format presenting patient care strategies to assist psychiatrists in clinical decision making. Importantly, although guidelines may be used for a variety of purposes, their primary purpose is to assist psychiatrists in their care of patients.

Both the American Medical Association (AMA) and the Institute of Medicine (IOM) have sought to define the key features necessary to ensure that practice guidelines are of high quality. The AMA's attributes apply to the development process, stating that practice guidelines should 1) be developed by or in conjunction with physician organizations, 2) use reliable methodologies that integrate relevant research findings and clinical expertise, 3) be as comprehensive and specific as possible, 4) be based on current information, and 5) be widely disseminated. The IOM's attributes are criteria for evaluating the finished product: validity, based on the strength of the evidence, expert judgment, and estimates of health and cost outcomes compared with alternative practices; reliability/reproducibility; clinical applicability and flexibility; clarity; attention to multidisciplinary concerns; timely updates; and documentation. Taken together, these prescriptives have essentially set national standards for guideline efforts.

II. Topic Selection

The APA Steering Committee on Practice Guidelines oversees the development of APA practice guidelines. The Steering Committee selects topics for practice guidelines according to the following criteria:

1. Degree of public importance (prevalence and seriousness)
2. Relevance to psychiatric practice
3. Availability of information and relevant data

4.   Availability of work already done that would be useful in the development of a practice guideline

5.   The area is one in which increased psychiatric attention and involvement would be helpful for the field

III.   Contributors

APA practice guidelines are developed by a work group of psychiatrists in active clinical practice, including academicians or researchers who spend a significant percentage of their time in the clinical care of patients. Work group members are selected on the basis of their knowledge and experience in the topic area, their commitment to the integrity of the guideline development process as outlined by the AMA and IOM, and their representativeness of the diversity of American psychiatry.

Work group members are asked to decline participation if they feel there are possible conflicts of interest or biases that could impact their ability to maintain scientific objectivity.

IV.   Evidence Base

The evidence base for practice guidelines is derived from two sources—research studies and clinical consensus. Where gaps exist in the research data, evidence is derived from clinical consensus, obtained through extensive review of multiple drafts of each guideline (see section VI). Both research data and clinical consensus vary in their validity and reliability for different clinical situations; guidelines state explicitly the nature of the supporting evidence for specific recommendations so that readers can make their own judgments regarding the utility of the recommendation.

The literature review process is explicitly described in the guideline. The literature review includes other guidelines addressing the same topic, when available. Whenever possible, evidence tables are constructed to illustrate the data regarding risks and benefits for each treatment. In many cases, however, evidence tables are used only to assist in writing the text and do not appear in the guideline.

V.   Format

Each practice guideline is presented in a standardized format, with variations as appropriate (e.g., a guideline about psychiatric evaluation or a procedure may vary from that about a specific illness).

The standard outline is as follows:

I. Executive Summary of Recommendations
II. Disease Definition, Epidemiology, Natural History
III. Review of Available Treatments: Goals, Efficacy, Side Effects, Implementation
IV. Development of a Treatment Plan for the Individual Patient
V. Clinical Features Influencing Treatment
VI. Research Directions
VII. Reviewers and Consultants
VIII. Organizations Submitting Comments

Section I provides an overview of the organization and scope of recommendations contained in subsequent sections, with each recommendation identified as falling into one of three categories of endorsement:

[I]   Recommended with substantial clinical confidence
[II] Recommended with moderate clinical confidence
[III] Options that may be recommended on the basis of individual circumstances

Section II presents the characteristics of the illness using current DSM criteria. Differential diagnosis, appropriate diagnostic procedures, aspects of the epidemiology and natural history with important treatment implications, and issues concerning special patient characteristics are outlined in this section.

Section III presents a review of the available data on all potential treatments, organized according to three broad categories: 1) psychiatric management, 2) psychosocial interventions, and 3) somatic interventions. For each treatment, this information is presented in a standard format:

a)   Goals of treatment
b)   Efficacy data
c)   Side effects and safety
d)   Implementation issues (e.g., patient selection, laboratory testing, dosing, frequency, duration)

Section IV presents a synthesis of the information in section III, directed at providing a framework for clinical decision making for the individual patient.

Section V addresses psychiatric, general medical, and demographic factors influencing treatment, including comorbidities. Relevant ethnic, cross-cultural, social, or extrinsic factors (e.g., cultural mores, family, support system, living situation, health care beliefs, etc.) that could potentially preclude or modify the practical application of guidelines and may play a role in health care decisions are emphasized.

Section VI identifies directions for further research.

Section VII lists all persons submitting substantive comments on guideline drafts.

Section VIII lists all organizations submitting a response on guideline drafts.

VI.   Review, Dissemination, and Updates

Each practice guideline is extensively reviewed at multiple draft stages. Draft 1 is reviewed by the Steering Committee. Draft 2 is reviewed by approximately 50 reviewers with expertise in the topic. Draft 3 is reviewed by members of the APA Assembly, the District Branches, Joint Reference Committee, Board of Trustees, Council on Research, other components related to the subject area, any APA member by request, the *American Journal of Psychiatry,* and representatives of approximately 100 related organizations. Draft 4 is approved by the Assembly, the Board of Trustees, and the *American Journal of Psychiatry* prior to publication.

After publication, each practice guideline is disseminated through a variety of mechanisms, including publication in the *American Journal of Psychiatry,* publication in a variety of formats through American Psychiatric Press, Inc., and use in specially designed training programs. Each practice guideline is revised at 3- to 5-year intervals to reflect new knowledge in the field.

INDEX

Bipolar disorder. *See also* Depression, Mania
  acute phase treatment, 150–151, 156–157, 159, 166–167, 172
  children and adolescents, 184–185
  clinical features influencing treatment, 182–188
  cocaine use disorders and, 277
  comorbid medical conditions, 184
  comorbid psychiatric disorders, 183
  cultural issues, 187
  depressive episodes, 170–171, 177–179, 190–191
  diagnosis, 143–144
  differential diagnosis, 144
  DSM-IV criteria, 143
  eating disorders and, 47
  elderly persons, 185–186
  electroconvulsive therapy, 166–168
  epidemiology, 145
  family history, 144, 145, 184
  gender issues, 186–187
  history and course, 144–145
  maintenance treatment, 151–152, 157, 160, 180–181, 180–182, 191–192
  major depressive disorder and, 108, 117
  manic episodes, 171, 176–177, 190
  mixed episodes and ultrarapid cycling, 179–180, 191
  pharmacological treatments, 149–166
  pregnancy and, 186–187
  psychiatric management, 146–149, 189
  psychotherapeutic treatments, 168–172
  with psychotic or catatonic features, 182
  puerperal psychosis and, 113
  recommendations, 188–192
  research issues, 192–193
  sleep patterns and, 148, 169, 181, 192
  substance use disorders and, 183, 225
  suicide or violence risk, 173, 182–183
  support groups, 172
  treatment compliance, 147–148
  treatment plan, 172–182, 189
  treatment principles, 146
  treatment setting, 188–189
  use of life charts, 149, 181, 188
Birth control pills. *See* Oral contraceptives

Birth defects
  mood stabilizers and, 186
Borderline personality disorder
  eating disorders and, 47
  major depressive disorder and, 113
  substance use disorders and, 250
Breastfeeding
  antidepressants and, 113, 187
Brief interventions
  alcohol use disorders, 219, 263–264
  major depressive disorder, 93
Bromocriptine
  cocaine use disorders treatment, 273
  cocaine use disorders with comorbid ADHD treatment, 277
  cocaine withdrawal treatment, 221, 276–277
Bulimia nervosa
  assessment principles, 58–60
  DSM-III-R criteria, 45
  epidemiology and characteristics, 46–47
  goals of treatment, 48–49
  pharmacologic treatments, 56–57, 64–65
  prognosis, 57
  psychosocial treatments, 55–57, 65
  recommendations, 64–66
  research issues, 66
  sexual abuse and, 47
  substance use disorders and, 65
  treatment setting, 54, 64
  twelve-step programs, 65–66
Buprenorphine
  cocaine use disorders treatment, 273
  opioid use disorders treatment, 222, 280
  opioid withdrawal treatment, 287
Bupropion
  anorexia nervosa treatment, contraindicated, 52–53
  bipolar disorder treatment, 164, 165
  cocaine use disorders treatment, 273
  depression in elderly persons treatment, 118
  depression with
    atypical features treatment, 110
    cardiac disease treatment, 114–115
    dementia treatment, 115
    glaucoma treatment, 115
    obstructive uropathy treatment, 116